Psychosomatic Medicine

Psychosomatic Medicine

Edited by

Kurt D. Ackerman, MD, PhD

Western Psychiatric Institute and Clinic of UPMC
University of Pittsburgh School of Medicine
Pittsburgh, PA

Andrea F. DiMartini, MD

Western Psychiatric Institute and Clinic of UPMC
Starzl Transplant Institute
University of Pittsburgh School of Medicine
Pittsburgh, PA

OXFORD
UNIVERSITY PRESS

OXFORD
UNIVERSITY PRESS

Oxford University Press is a department of the University of
Oxford. It furthers the University's objective of excellence in research,
scholarship, and education by publishing worldwide.

Oxford   New York
Auckland   Cape Town   Dar es Salaam   Hong Kong   Karachi
Kuala Lumpur   Madrid   Melbourne   Mexico City   Nairobi
New Delhi   Shanghai   Taipei   Toronto

With offices in
Argentina   Austria   Brazil   Chile   Czech Republic   France   Greece
Guatemala   Hungary   Italy   Japan   Poland   Portugal   Singapore
South Korea   Switzerland   Thailand   Turkey   Ukraine   Vietnam

Oxford is a registered trademark of Oxford University Press
in the UK and certain other countries.

Published in the United States of America by
Oxford University Press
198 Madison Avenue, New York, NY 10016

© Oxford University Press 2015

Library of Congress Cataloging-in-Publication Data
Psychosomatic medicine (Ackerman)
Psychosomatic medicine / edited by Kurt D. Ackerman, Andrea F. DiMartini.
p. ; cm.
Includes bibliographical references and index.
ISBN 978–0–19–932931–1 (alk. paper)
I. Ackerman, Kurt, editor.   II. DiMartini, Andrea F., editor.   III. Title.
[DNLM: 1. Psychophysiologic Disorders.   2. Mental Disorders—complications.
3. Psychosomatic Medicine—methods. WM 90]
RC454
616.89—dc23
2014041733

Series Introduction

We stand on the threshold of a new Golden Age of clinical and behavioral neuroscience with psychiatry at its fore. With the Pittsburgh Pocket Psychiatry series, we intend to encompass the breadth and depth of our current understanding of human behavior in health and disease. Using the structure of resident didactic teaching, we will be able to ensure that each subject area relevant to practicing psychiatrists is detailed and described. New innovations in diagnosis and treatment will be reviewed and discussed in the context of existing knowledge, and each book in the series will propose new directions for scientific inquiry and discovery. The aim of the series as a whole is to integrate findings from all areas of medicine and neuroscience previously segregated as "mind" or "body," "psychological" or "biological." Thus, each book from the Pittsburgh Pocket Psychiatry series will stand alone as a standard text for anyone wishing to learn about a specific subject area. The series will be the most coherent and flexible learning resource available.

David Kupfer, MD
Michael Travis, MD
Michelle Horner, DO

Preface

Psychosomatic medicine (PM) is a rapidly developing sub-specialty of psychiatry focusing on psychiatric care of patients with other medical disorders. PM specialists work to diagnose and manage psychiatric symptoms in a variety of medical settings, help optimize the medical care of their patients, and expand knowledge regarding the role of psychological factors in health and disease, applying this knowledge in the prevention and treatment of illness. PM practitioners may function as consultants in hospital-based wards, as primary providers in med-psych units, or as collaborative practitioners integrated with inpatient and outpatient medical teams. PM practitioners must strive to stay informed about the latest research and practice guidelines in a burgeoning field involving complex interactions and combinations of illnesses. To help address these challenges, this book provides practical instruction from PM clinicians, educators, and researchers, covering core clinical concepts routinely used in practice.

This book is intended to serve as an educational resource on salient psychosomatic medicine topics for trainees and colleagues in psychiatry and other medical specialties. A history of PM contextualizes the field, and an overview of the process of psychiatric consultation in the general medical setting emphasizes the specifics of psychosomatic interviewing, physical examination, and collaboration with primary services. The remaining chapters cover the diagnosis and management of conditions commonly encountered by the psychosomatic psychiatrist, including the assessment and treatment of psychiatric disorders in a medical setting; core areas of PM, such as assessment of decisional capacity; use of psychotropic medication in medically compromised patients; management of somatoform disorders, delirium, and cognitive disorders; psychiatric manifestations of neurologic and other general medical conditions; emergent complications of medication and illicit substance use; and special topics pertinent to PM. Finally, potential future directions in PM are explored.

Each chapter is organized in a standard format. Tables and diagrams are used to organize selected important information. At the end of each chapter, Key Points summarize important facts and ideas to remember, Suggested Readings include both text references and additional resources, and Exercises test the reader's comprehension of material covered. Unique abbreviations will be defined in the text as they occur. Common medical abbreviations such as EKGs are included in the glossary at the end of the book.

We hope readers will find *Psychosomatic Medicine—Pittsburgh Pocket Psychiatry* a useful clinical guide that will enhance their understanding and practice of psychosomatic medicine.

Kurt D. Ackerman, MD, PhD
Andrea F. DiMartini, MD

Contents

Acknowledgments

The authors would like to acknowledge the hard work and dedication of our residents and colleagues who helped shape the development this book, and who provided excellent editorial feedback. In particular, we are grateful for the invaluable assistance of Jane Ackerman, Nicole Bates, Amanda Brinson, Jack Cahalane, Matthew Conlon, Sarah Faeder, Karen Fielding, Shabana Khan, Erik Loraas, Wynne Lundblad, Darcy Moschenross, Barbara Nightingale, Mehak Sharma, Monique Simpson, Loren Sobel, Layla Soliman, Christie Urquhart, Sabina Vaichys, Robin Valpey, and Courtney Walker.

Contributors

Michael Gary Abesamis, MD

Department of Emergency
  Medicine/Medical Toxicology
University of Pittsburgh School of
  Medicine
Pittsburgh, PA

Kurt D. Ackerman, MD, PhD

Western Psychiatric Institute and
  Clinic of UPMC
Department of Psychiatry
University of Pittsburgh School of
  Medicine
Pittsburgh, PA

Pierre N. Azzam, MD

Western Psychiatric Institute and
  Clinic of UPMC
Department of Psychiatry
University of Pittsburgh School of
  Medicine
Pittsburgh, PA

Bradford Bobrin, MD

Western Psychiatric Institute and
  Clinic of UPMC
Department of Psychiatry
University of Pittsburgh School of
  Medicine
Pittsburgh, PA

Traci D'Almeida, MD

Western Psychiatric Institute and
  Clinic of UPMC
Department of Psychiatry
University of Pittsburgh School of
  Medicine
Pittsburgh, PA

Mary Amanda Dew, PhD

Western Psychiatric Institute and
  Clinic of UPMC
Departments of Psychiatry,
  Psychology and Epidemiology
University of Pittsburgh School of
  Medicine
Pittsburgh, PA

**Ann Louise DiBarry,
PMHCNS-BC**

Western Psychiatric Institute and
  Clinic of UPMC
Pittsburgh, PA

Andrea F. DiMartini, MD

Western Psychiatric Institute and
  Clinic of UPMC
Starzl Transplant Institute
Departments of Psychiatry and
  Surgery
University of Pittsburgh School of
  Medicine
Pittsburgh, PA

Christopher R. Dobbelstein, MD

Western Psychiatric Institute and
  Clinic of UPMC
Department of Psychiatry
University of Pittsburgh School of
  Medicine
Pittsburgh, PA

**Jacqueline Dunbar-Jacob,
RN, PhD**

School of Nursing
University of Pittsburgh
Pittsburgh, PA

Mary G. Fitzgerald, MSN,
PMHCNS-BC

Western Psychiatric Institute and
Clinic of UPMC
Pittsburgh, PA

Jody Glance, MD

Western Psychiatric Institute and
Clinic of UPMC
Department of Psychiatry
University of Pittsburgh School of
Medicine
Pittsburgh, PA

Ronald M. Glick, MD

Western Psychiatric Institute and
Clinic of UPMC
Center for Integrative Medicine at
UPMC Shadyside
Departments of Psychiatry
and Physical Medicine and
Rehabilitation
University of Pittsburgh School of
Medicine
Pittsburgh, PA

Priya Gopalan, MD

Western Psychiatric Institute and
Clinic of UPMC
Department of Psychiatry
University of Pittsburgh School of
Medicine
Pittsburgh, PA

Ghennady V. Gushchin,
MD, PhD

Western Psychiatric Institute and
Clinic of UPMC
Department of Psychiatry
University of Pittsburgh School of
Medicine
Pittsburgh, PA

Christopher R. Hope,
MD, MHA

Western Psychiatric Institute and
Clinic of UPMC
Pittsburgh, PA

Robert H. Howland, MD

Western Psychiatric
Institute and Clinic of
UPMC
Department of Psychiatry
University of Pittsburgh School of
Medicine
Pittsburgh, PA

Robert Hudak, MD

Western Psychiatric Institute and
Clinic of UPMC
Department of Psychiatry
University of Pittsburgh School of
Medicine
Pittsburgh, PA

Julie A. Hugo, MD

Western Psychiatric Institute and
Clinic of UPMC
Department of Psychiatry
University of Pittsburgh School of
Medicine
Pittsburgh, PA

Rolf G. Jacob, MD

Western Psychiatric Institute and
Clinic of UPMC
Department of Psychiatry
University of Pittsburgh School of
Medicine
Pittsburgh, PA

Abhishek Jain, MD

Western Psychiatric Institute and
Clinic of UPMC
Department of Psychiatry
University of Pittsburgh School of
Medicine
Pittsburgh, PA

Francis E. Lotrich, MD, PhD

Western Psychiatric Institute and
Clinic of UPMC
Department of Psychiatry
University of Pittsburgh School of
Medicine
Pittsburgh, PA

Kevin R. Patterson, MD

Western Psychiatric Institute and
    Clinic of UPMC
Department of Psychiatry
University of Pittsburgh School of
    Medicine
Pittsburgh, PA

Donna M. Posluszny, PhD

Biobehavioral Oncology
    Program
University of Pittsburgh
    Cancer Institute of
    UPMC
University of Pittsburgh School of
    Medicine
Pittsburgh, PA

Alin J. Severance, MD

Western Psychiatric Institute and
    Clinic of UPMC
Department of Psychiatry
University of Pittsburgh School of
    Medicine
Pittsburgh, PA

Ellen M. Whyte, MD

Western Psychiatric Institute and
    Clinic of UPMC
Department of Psychiatry and
    Department of Physical
    Medicine and Rehabilitation
University of Pittsburgh School of
    Medicine
Pittsburgh, PA

Part I

Introduction

History of Psychosomatic Medicine and Consultation-Liaison Psychiatry

Rolf G. Jacob, Julie A. Hugo, and Jacqueline Dunbar-Jacob

Early History

Psychosomatic medicine explores how psychological, behavioral, and social factors influence an individual's health and quality of life. The ancestral roots of psychosomatic medicine extend back to ancient Greece. The syllable "psych" in "psychosomatic" stems from the ancient Greek term *psyche*, usually translated as "soul." It was thought to be present in humans and animals, but not in plants. Located in the heart, its function included emotions and sense perception (Huffman, 2012). The ancient Greek root *soma*, or *sōmat*, refers to the "body." Another meaning of "psychosomatic" emphasizes the role of the "mind." The term for "mind" used in ancient Greece was *nous*. However, this term had broader connotations, ranging from "intellect" to "pantheistic" sentiments, including the "spiritual" or "divine." The conceptualization of some illnesses, such as epilepsy, included magical elements. The rejection of the magical is attributed to Hippocrates, who declared that epilepsy was not a sacred disease (Alexander & Selesnik, 1966).

Over the ensuing centuries, conceptualizations of psychological influences were slow to develop. In the Roman era, the power of the psychological or behavioral domain was explicitly recognized by Cicero, who emphasized personal responsibility for illness (Alexander & Selesnik, 1966). The Middle Ages saw a discussion of psychological influences in the writings of St. Augustine, with his pioneering use of introspection as a psychological tool. In the seventeenth century, Robert Burton's *The Anatomy of Melancholy* recognized psychological elements.

In ancient times, a distinction between mind and body was not yet clearly articulated. A deeper understanding of mechanisms underlying psychosomatic influences first required a better understanding of *organic* illness. However, "organic medicine" as practiced today did not begin to establish itself until the mid-1800s.

Credit for the original use of the word "psychosomatic" goes to Johann Christian August Heinroth, a German holistic psychiatrist, who, in 1818, published a textbook titled *Of Disturbances of Mental Life* in which he states, "Usually the causes for sleeplessness are *psycho-somatic*; however, each of these two spheres alone can contain its full cause" (Steinberg & Herman-Lingen, 2013). However, he never used the term in any subsequent writings.

In the relatively modern era, i.e. around the turn of the 20th century, further understanding developed of the "inner" workings of the mind, and as a result, methods were developed to study and influence behavior. For example, I. P. Pavlov studied classical conditioning; E. Thorndike formulated the law of effect that anticipated B. F. Skinner's operant conditioning; and Sigmund Freud developed psychoanalysis, using the technique of free association. By this time, organic medicine had developed to a point that physiological mechanisms of psychological influences on bodily function could be appreciated, and the field of psychophysiology was born. An early example is Cannon's fight-or-flight response mediated by the sympathetic nervous system. Later came Selye's endocrinologically mediated "General Adaptation Syndrome," and most recently an entire new field was established, psychoneuroimmunology, which examines the health impact of communication between the central nervous system and immune systems (see Chapter 22).

Psychodynamic Formulations for Psychosomatic Illnesses

In the United States, psychosomatic medicine as a programmatic science began in the 1930s, pursuing a hypothesis that certain illnesses were caused by the physiological effects of excessive, repeated, or chronic emotional activation. The psychoanalyst sought for the causative agent of such activation in the psychodynamic makeup of the person. That is, psychodynamic formulations look at an individual's symptoms and behaviors as a reflection of unconscious psychological processes, incorporating the patient's character pathology, personality strengths, and defense mechanisms, as well as processes of transference and resistance. Often the underlying problem is seen as a motivational conflict of which the patient is unaware, but which can be uncovered with the help of psychoanalysis. The diseases considered psychosomatic included those popularly referred to as the "Holy Seven": peptic ulcer, asthma, rheumatoid arthritis, neurodermatitis, essential hypertension, hyperthyroidism, and chronic inflammatory bowel disease. Psychoanalysts observed certain patterns in the psychodynamic histories of these patients, suggesting that specific illnesses were related to specific underlying dynamics, a phenomenon referred to as "organ specificity."

For example, Helen Flanders Dunbar, the founder of the American Psychosomatic Society, described the psychological profile of patients with hypertension as follows (with 13 additional variables not listed here; Flanders Dunbar, 1943):

Area of focal conflict: Aggression and passivity; rivalry and self-defeat
Neurotic traits: Perfectionism, rage outbursts
Characteristic behavior pattern: Urge to keep peace
Attitude toward father: Ambivalent
Attitude toward mother: Passive, fearful, or hostile.

This conceptualization recognized hostility among these causative factors. The impact of hostility was thought to be mediated by changes in sympathetic nervous system activity. Franz Alexander (Alexander, 1950), who had initiated this type of investigation at the Chicago Psychoanalytic Institute in 1932, developed the following model for hypertension:

Hostile and competitive impulses
→ Intimidation due to retaliation and failure
→ Increase in dependent longings
→ Inferiority feelings
→ Reactivation of hostile and competitive impulses
→ Anxiety and resulting inhibition of aggressive hostile impulses
⟹ *Hypertension*

Patients with peptic ulcer, on the other hand, were believed to have conflicts emanating from dependency needs that activated the parasympathetic nervous system, resulting in gastric hypersecretion:

Frustration in oral receptive longings
→ Oral aggressive response
→ Guilt
→ Anxiety
→ Overcompensation...by actual...accomplishments in responsible activities

→ Increased unconscious oral-dependent cravings as a reaction to excessive effort and concentration

→ Gastric hypersecretion

⟹ *Peptic ulcer*

Are such dynamics indeed specific for particular psychosomatic disorders? In a study, internists and psychoanalysts were asked to infer the underlying psychosomatic diagnosis by matching blinded transcripts of psychoanalytic interviews of a large number of patients to one of the seven psychosomatic disorders. The transcripts were blinded by editing out cues that directly would give the answer away, such as medical symptoms or diagnosis. The psychoanalysts classified about half (45%) of the interviews correctly, whereas the internists correctly classified only 25% (Pollock, 1959, cited in Alexander & Selesnik, 1966). The likelihood of agreement by random chance would have been 14% (1/7). Thus, just based on the dynamics, the psychoanalysts could diagnose the psychosomatic disorder better than chance, but half were still misclassified.

Taking a history for the diagnosis by inferred dynamics must have been quite demanding. For example, the profiles developed by Flanders Dunbar involved narrative specifications of about 18 independent variables (depending on how many subcategories are counted), including family history, personal data, health record, injuries, education, work record, income and vocational level, social relationships, sexual adjustment, attitude toward mother, attitude toward father, attitude toward current family, characteristic behavior pattern, neurotic traits, addictions, life situation immediately prior to onset, reaction to illness, and area of focal conflict and characteristic reaction (Flanders Dunbar, 1943).

Other obstacles to psychodynamic approaches existed as well. Therapy, even in shortened versions, aimed at providing a "corrective emotional experience" (Alexander et al., 1946), was time intensive, and was difficult to integrate with the busy demands of inpatient medical care (Bronheim, 2006). More time-efficient psychopharmacological treatment was becoming widespread. Furthermore, some individuals resented the implication that the origin of their disorder was "all in their head."

Also, as illustrated by the fate of the psychosomatic status of peptic ulcer disease, our understanding of the psychosomatic nature of diseases has evolved over time. Until the 1980s, many believed that peptic ulcer largely had psychosomatic origins. In 1947 it was written that "all aspects of the disease were intricately bound up with the character structure of the patient" (Zane, 1947). Through much of the twentieth century, the pathogenesis of the disease was believed to be due to stress and dietary factors, and the subsequent treatment prescribed was bed rest and the ingestion of special bland foods. It was not until the discovery of the spiral-shaped bacteria, later identified as *Helicobacter pylori*, that a bacterial etiology was seriously considered (Marshall & Warren, 1984). Today, while the eradication of this bacteria with antimicrobial agents is the mainstay of treatment, psychological stress is still recognized as a confounding and complicating factor in the etiology of peptic ulcers (Overmier & Murison, 2013).

Disciplines and Organizations That Practice Psychosomatic Medicine

The history of psychosomatic medicine described above forms a common background from which a number of subspecialties and scientific societies focusing on psychosomatic medicine developed; these are described below.

American Psychosomatic Society: Its mission focuses on how psychological, behavioral, and social factors influence health and disease (http://www.psychosomatic.org).

Society of Behavioral Medicine: This group explores the interaction of behavior, biology, and the environment, and its application to health (http://www.sbm.org/about).

The Academy of Psychosomatic Medicine (APM): The mission of this organization is to advance the treatment of those with comorbid psychiatric and medical illness (http://www.apm.org).

Consultation-Liaison Psychiatry

This field has been described as an "offspring of psychobiology, general hospital psychiatry, and psychosomatic medicine" (Lipowski, 1992). In their daily practice, consultation-liaison (C-L) psychiatrists often are asked to comment on psychological factors contributing to a general medical condition, such as cyclic vomiting syndrome. Such requests are grounded in the conceptual framework of psychodynamic psychosomatic medicine described earlier. In addition, C-L psychiatrists are skilled in interview techniques handed down from the psychoanalytic tradition. However, psychosomatic medicine is just one of several roots of C-L psychiatry. Another major root is "hospital psychiatry," or the development of psychiatric departments and psychiatric units within the medical hospital. Prior to this, individuals with serious mental illness were most often confined within asylums. Hospital psychiatry contributed knowledge in psychopharmacology and the deep understanding of pathophysiology for which physicians are uniquely trained.

Development of C-L Departments Within the Medical Hospital

The history of C-L psychiatry dates back to the turn of the twentieth century. It has been described in previous papers by Z. J. Lipowski in 1986 and John J. Schwab in 1989, with both authors separating the development of this subspecialty into four overlapping phases. Though we present a brief synopsis of these phases here, we direct the reader to the above papers for a more detailed historical account.

The first of these four phases (1900–1930) involved the development of hospital psychiatry as a field. World War I created an increased awareness of the field of psychiatry among the American public, as many young men were rejected or discharged from the military for psychiatric reasons, and large numbers of men returned from the war with "shell shock" (Schwab, 1989). Adolf Meyer, considered by many to be the "father of psychobiology," was one of the earliest professionals to identify the importance of psychiatry's involvement in medical care (Karl & Holland, 2013). In a 1929 paper, George Henry detailed his psychiatric work in an Albany, New York, hospital, describing initial indifference and sometimes even resistance to the idea of the inclusion of psychiatry within the general medical hospital. He noted that even some of the best medical schools at the time had no department of psychiatry, and in some schools instruction in psychiatry was provided by physicians in internal medicine. After considering his clinical observations of 300 psychiatric consultations, he concluded that every general hospital should have a psychopathic department and at least one attending psychiatrist, and the psychiatrist should participate in all staff conferences to allow for an exchange of ideas and discussion of cases that contain psychiatric components (Henry, 1929).

Following this phase of initial engagement within the medical hospital, the second of the four phases (1931–late 1950s) began with the Rockefeller Foundation's donation of $11 million for psychiatry, neurology, and related fields to general medical hospitals over a 10-year period (Schwab, 1989). The ultimate goal of these donations was to integrate the field of psychiatry, which until then had been relatively off on its own, into the standard practice and teaching of medicine. Beneficiaries included the University of Colorado, where in 1934 a Psychiatric Liaison Department, directed by Edward G. Billings, was developed. This department functioned as a team and provided all of the elements still considered important today in C-L psychiatry, including clinical service, teaching, and research (Lipowski, 1986).

World War II also served to enhance awareness of psychiatric applications to medical illness. While the period before World War II had led to the emigration of many psychoanalysts to America, there was also criticism that the field of psychosomatic medicine up through the end of the war had been too dominated by psychoanalysts (Hawkins, 1982). Within the field, there were competing opinions on how psychiatric consultation should function within the general medical hospital, how much emphasis should be placed on consultation activity versus liaison work, and how to balance clinical service with teaching needs (Lipowski, 1986). The economic ramifications of having a consultative service were also being explored by Edward Billings, as he believed that early recognition of psychiatric problems and subsequent treatment would be economically beneficial to both the hospital and the community (Thompson & Suddath, 1987). The American Psychosomatic Society was also founded during this time, and collaboration between psychiatrists and other physicians was becoming more common.

Following this phase, C-L psychiatry underwent a developmental period in the 1960s and 1970s. Different strategies of consultation were developed, with the target of the consultation varying from the patient to the consultee, the situation, and the subsequent interactions between the patient and the clinical team. C-L psychiatry experienced tremendous growth as a field during this time, and C-L psychiatrists were practicing as part of more medically specialized services. Research in the field also increased, and in 1974 the National Institute of Mental Health provided grant funding for fellowships in C-L work.

Up until this final period, Lipowski's and Schwab's descriptions of the history of C-L psychiatry had been rather harmonious with one another. In the last stage, beginning in 1975, Lipowski describes a period of rapid growth within the field extending to the publication of his review in 1986, whereas Schwab has alternatively described a period of consolidation and retrenchment in the field from 1980 to 1989. In the 1980s, training in psychiatric C-L was made a requirement for residencies in general psychiatry. By 1991, there were 55 C-L fellowships registered through the Academy of Psychosomatic Medicine. The APM initially applied to the American Board of Psychiatry and Neurology for subspecialty status in 1992; however, there was concern regarding the name of the subspecialty and the scope of practice. After much discussion, the official name of the subspecialty was adopted as psychosomatic medicine, and in 2003 it received approval as a subspecialty field of psychiatry.

Developments in Europe

As the field was continuing its evolution in the United States, by the 1980s practitioners of C-L psychiatry had yet to form any formal networks in Europe. In 1987 the European Consultation Liaison Workgroup (ECLW) for General Hospital Psychiatry and Psychosomatics was founded. With funding from the European community, the ECLW Collaborative Study was developed as a large multicenter epidemiological study with the purpose of examining psychiatric C-L service delivery in Europe. It examined the structure of C-L services, as well as the type of patients who required psychiatric consultation and the purpose of the consultations. The expectation was that more developed services would see more patients as well as a wider variety, with a larger goal of the study being to provide European data for future healthcare planning and research (Huyse et al., 1996; Huyse et al., 2001).

The study collected information on over 14,000 cases, and included 226 consultants and 56 psychiatric C-L services in 11 different countries (Huyse et al., 1996). For the most part, C-L service delivery in Europe appeared to function as "an emergency mental health service in a general hospital" (Huyse et al., 2001). Similar to its service functions in the United States, C-L psychiatry in Europe was found to serve a fairly complex population, with at least a large part of each service contributing to the care of the severely medically ill and the elderly, with the services acting as a link between primary, general medical, and psychiatric care.

The ECLW Collaborative Study provided an opportunity for collaboration within the field throughout Europe, and toward the end of this study, an international association within Europe was in its initial stages of development (Leentjens & Lobo, 2011). The association was named the European Association of Consultation-Liaison Psychiatry and Psychosomatics (EACLPP). Similar to the Academy of Psychosomatic Medicine in the United States, the EACLPP was created with the aim of promoting the treatment of individuals with concurrent psychiatric and medical illness, as well as advancing medical knowledge and practice within the field (Leentjens & Lobo, 2011). The EACLPP merged with the European Network of Psychosomatic Medicine (ENPM) in June 2012, forming a new society named the European Association of Psychosomatic Medicine (EAPM; Söllner & Schüssler, 2012).

History of Psychosomatic Terminology in the *DSM*: Somatic Symptom and Related Disorders

As mentioned earlier, a clinical role for the C-L psychiatrist is to help in the management of difficult patients in the medical setting, in particular those whose illness behaviors are appraised as excessive. Depending on the clinical specialty setting, such patients may receive diagnoses such as irritable bowel syndrome, cyclic vomiting syndrome, fibromyalgia, non-cardiac chest pain, chronic fatigue syndrome, multiple chemical sensitivities, temporomandibular joint dysfunction, chronic subjective dizziness, non-ulcer dyspepsia, and so on. Many of these are defined within the subspecialty by specific criteria based on the core symptoms.

As a group, these disorders have been given designations such as "functional somatic syndromes," "medically unexplained physical symptoms," "body distress syndromes," and "somatoform disorders," among others. There are several reasons for "lumping" the different functional somatic syndromes into superordinate categories. The core or defining symptoms of these syndromes show considerable overlap, and patients frequently exhibit comorbidity. Patients with somatic disorders frequently, but not always, have comorbid anxiety and depression. Also, these patients share other features, such as association with female gender (Wessely et al., 1999). Mechanisms proposed to underlie the development of these disorders include somatization, symptom amplification, and alexithymia. Somatization refers to "a tendency to experience and communicate somatic distress in response to psychosocial stress and to seek medical help for it" (Lipowski, 1988). Symptom amplification occurs when patients excessively and obsessively focus their attention on bodily sensations and reinterpret them as dangerous symptoms (Barsky, 1992). Alexithymia refers to a personality construct, the facets of which include (a) difficulty identifying feelings or distinguishing feelings from bodily sensations, and (b) difficulty describing one's feelings to others (Bagby et al., 1993). These features are thought to lead to chronic affect dysregulation and symptom formation (Taylor et al., 2010).

In psychiatry, the taxonomic systems of the previous editions of the *Diagnostic and Statistical Manual of Mental Disorders* (*DSM-III* and *DSM-IV*) referred to these conditions as "somatoform" disorders. The "form" in "somatoform" connotes a mental disorder masquerading as a medical illness. In the *DSM-III*, published in 1980, the specific mental disorders subsumed under this category included somatization disorder, conversion disorder (or hysterical neurosis, conversion type), psychogenic pain disorder, hypochondriasis (or hypochondriacal neurosis), and atypical somatoform disorder. In addition, psychological factors affecting physical condition constituted a category of its own, as did factitious disorder.

In the *DSM-III-R*, published in 1987, these disorders were retained, with minor changes in criteria. The "neurosis" labels were dropped for conversion disorder and hypochondriasis. Atypical somatoform disorder was subdivided into undifferentiated somatoform disorder and somatoform disorder not otherwise specified (NOS). In addition, the diagnosis of body dysmorphic disorder (dysmorphophobia) was included. The *DSM-IV* (1994) and *DSM-IV-TR* (2000) did not introduce any major changes, except for details in the symptom requirements for somatization disorder.

The 10th revision of the *International Classification of Diseases* (*ICD-10*), published in 1992, is of interest, as it is, within the foreseeable future, the system used for billing codes in the United States. Here, the main individual somatoform disorders include, similar to *DSM-III-R*, somatization disorder, undifferentiated somatization disorder, hypochondriacal disorder, and persistent somatoform pain disorder, as well as a new entity, somatoform autonomic dysfunction (e.g., irritable bowel syndrome). In addition, conversion disorder was put under "dissociative [conversion] disorders," and was split into dissociative motor disorders, dissociative convulsions, and dissociative anesthesia and sensory loss. Dysmorphophobia is not a separate disorder, but is included under hypochondriasis.

In the *DSM-IV* and *ICD-10*, diagnosis of a somatoform disorder required the symptoms to be medically unexplained. This requirement proved to be problematic for several reasons. First, the distinction presupposes a mind-body dualism that biases unknown etiologies to be assigned a "psychogenic" status (Jacob et al., 2001). Second, as already discussed, patients often resent the implication that their symptom is "mental" (i.e., "not real") rather than physical (i.e., "real"). Third, doctors may disagree on whether or not the symptom is unexplained: the reliability of the explained/unexplained distinction is poor. Fourth, distress from symptoms tends to be related to the total number of symptoms rather than just the unexplained ones.

For these reasons, in the current APA psychiatric diagnostic system (the fifth edition, or *DSM-5*), the "medically unexplained" requirement was abandoned, as was the syllable "form" in "somatoform." *DSM-5* introduced "somatic symptom and related disorders" to characterize the spectrum of psychiatric distress based on somatic symptoms. Similar to the older term "psychiatric overlay," the new definition focuses on the emotional and psychological reactions to somatic symptoms rather than on their etiology. The individual disorders are somatic symptom disorder, illness anxiety disorder, conversion disorder (functional neurological symptom disorder), psychological factors affecting other medical conditions, and factitious disorder (see Chapter 5 for details). Body dysmorphic disorder was moved to the category of obsessive-compulsive and related disorders. The "medically unexplained" concept survives only as a connotation of medical implausibility in conversion disorder and factitious disorder. It is anticipated that *ICD-11* will adopt a similar approach to understanding and categorizing somatic disorders.

Summary

Historically, the growth of psychosomatic medicine evolved from a holistic but rudimentary understanding of illness to more elaborate theorizing of psychodynamic processes, and finally to a broadly comprehensive "biopsychosocial" view, focused on integration of the psychological and behavioral with the pathophysiology of disease. Organizationally, the psychiatric subspecialty has developed from disparate practitioners to hospital C-L departments and formalized education as a subspecialty of psychiatry. While the American Board of Psychiatry and Neurology adopted the term "psychosomatic medicine" for C-L psychiatry as a subspecialty, this does not mean that psychosomatic medicine is the only foundation of C-L psychiatry, or, conversely, that C-L psychiatry is actually psychosomatic medicine. Future progress in C-L psychiatry might include subspecialization to service-specific medical subspecialties. This might include a greater emphasis on the "liaison" part, and further expansion into the general medicine outpatient environment.

Today, one of psychosomatic medicine's primary research objectives continues to be to explore how psychological, behavioral, and social factors influence the biological mechanisms of disease. With the advent of functional neuroimaging, coupled with greater gains in the fields of genetics and neuroscience, researchers in psychosomatic medicine are able to better explore the relationships between the mind, brain, and body, and how these dynamics affect and are influenced by the disease state. From investigations into the psychosocial influences on disease, to behavioral medicine's contributions to the understanding and treatment of pain, to the exciting developments in the study of psychoneuroimmunology—psychosomatic medicine as a whole, with its emphasis on interdisciplinary collaboration, is poised to have a profound impact on the future of medicine.

Key Points

- Psychophysiological terms in ancient Greece included *psyche* (soul), *sōma* (body), and *nous* (mind).
- Psychosomatic medicine was more clearly defined after the emergence of organic medicine, but risked becoming synonymous with "unexplained medical symptoms."
- The first use of the term "psychosomatic" is attributed to Johann Christian August Heinroth (1818).
- In the United States, psychosomatic medicine began in the 1930s as a psychodynamic understanding of conflicts affecting organic function mediated by the autonomic nervous system.
- The "Holy Seven" psychosomatic disorders include peptic ulcer, asthma, rheumatoid arthritis, neurodermatitis, essential hypertension, hyperthyroidism, and chronic inflammatory bowel disease. Today, most of these are no longer considered to be purely psychosomatic.
- Patients may resent psychosomatic attributions as being dismissive.
- Organizations or fields that today practice psychosomatic medicine include the American Psychosomatic Society, the Society of Behavioral Medicine, and the psychiatric subspecialty of consultation-liaison (C-L) psychiatry, the Academy of Psychosomatic Medicine.
- C-L psychiatry began when departments of psychiatry became accepted in medical schools.
- Early practitioners of C-L psychiatry included George Henry (Albany, New York, 1929) and Edward G. Billings (University of Colorado, 1934).
- After C-L psychiatry was renamed "psychosomatic medicine," it became recognized as a psychiatric subspecialty in 2003.
- In Europe, C-L psychiatry began in 1987 as the European Consultation Liaison Workgroup (ECLW) which, in 2011, founded the European Association of Consultation-Liaison Psychiatry and Psychosomatics (EACLPP); in 2012 this merged with the European Network of Psychosomatic Medicine (ENPM) to form the European Association of Psychosomatic Medicine (EAPM).

Disclosures

Dr. Jacob has no conflicts of interest.

Dr. Hugo has no conflicts of interest.

Dr. Dunbar-Jacob has no conflicts of interest.

Further Reading

Alexander F (1950). *Psychosomatic Medicine, Its Principles and Applications*. New York: W. W. Norton & Company.

Alexander F, French TM, Ewing T (1946). *Psychoanalytic Therapy: Principles and Application*. New York: Ronald Press Company.

Alexander FG, Selesnik ST (1966). *The History of Psychiatry*. New York: The New American Library.

American Psychiatric Association (2013). *Diagnostic and Statistical Manual of Mental Disorders*, 5th ed. Arlington, VA: American Psychiatric Publishing.

Bagby RM, Parker JA, Graeme JT (1994). The 20-item Toronto-alexithymia-scale. 1: Item selection and cross-validation of the factor structure. *J Psychosom Res.*, 38(1), 23–32.

Barsky AJ (1992). Amplification, somatization, and the somatoform disorders. *Psychosomatics*, 33(1), 28–34.

Bronheim H (2006). Psychotherapy. In Blumenfeld MS and Strain JJ (Eds.), *Psychosomatic Medicine*. Philadelphia: Lippincott Williams & Wilkins.

Flanders Dunbar H (1943). *Psychosomatic Diagnosis*. New York: Paul B. Hoeber.

Gitlin DF, Levenson JL, Lyketsos CG (2004). Psychosomatic medicine: A new psychiatric subspecialty. *Acad Psychiat.*, 28, 1–8.

Hawkins DR (1982). The role of psychoanalysis in consultation-liaison psychiatry. *Psychosomatics*, 23(11), 113–120.

Henry GW (1929). Some modern aspects of psychiatry in general hospital practice. *Am J Psychiat.*, 86(3), 481–499.

Huffman C. (Summer 2012 Edition). Philolaus. In Zalta EN (Ed.), *The Stanford Encyclopedia of Philosophy*. Retrieved from http://plato.stanford.edu/archives/sum2012/entries/philolaus/.

Huyse FJ, Herzog T, Lobo A, Malt UF, Opmeer BC, Stein B, et al. (2001). Consultation-liaison psychiatric service delivery: Results from a European study. *Gen Hosp Psychiat.*, 23, 124–132.

Huyse FJ, Herzog T, Malt UF, Lobo A, the ECLW. (1996). The European consultation-liaison workgroup (ECLW) Collaborative Study: General outline. *Gen Hosp Psychiat.*, 18, 44–55.

Karl SR, Holland JC (2013). Looking at the roots of psychosomatic medicine: Adolf Meyer. *Psychosomatics*, 54, 111–114.

Keefe FJ (2011). Behavioral medicine: A voyage to the future. *Ann Behav Med.*, 41, 141–151.

Kiecolt-Glaser JK, McGuire L, Robles TF, Glaser R (2002). Psychoneuroimmunology and psychosomatic medicine: Back to the future. *Psychosom Med.*, 64, 15–28.

Lane RD, Waldstein SR, Chesney MA, Jennings JR, Loyallo WR, Kozel PJ, et al. (2009). The rebirth of neuroscience in psychosomatic medicine, Part I: Historical context, methods, and relevant basic science. *Psychosom Med.*, 71, 117–134.

Lane RD, Waldstein SR, Critchley HD, Derbyshire SW, Drossman DA, Wager TD, et al. (2009). The rebirth of neuroscience in psychosomatic medicine, Part II: Clinical applications and implications for research. *Psychosom Med.*, 71, 135–151.

Leentjens AFG, Lobo A (2011). On the history of European Association of Consultation-Liaison Psychiatry and Psychosomatics. *J Psychosom Res.*, 70, 575–577.

Lipowski ZJ (1974). Consultation-liaison psychiatry: An overview. *Am J Psychiat.*, 131, 623–630.

Lipowski ZJ (1986). Consultation-liaison psychiatry: The first half century. *Gen Hosp Psychiat.*, 8, 305–315.

Lipowski ZJ (1992). Consultation-liaison psychiatry at century's end. *Psychosomatics*, 33(2), 128–133.

Lipsitt DR (2001). Consultation-liaison psychiatry and psychosomatic medicine: The company they keep. *Psychosom Med.*, 63, 896–909.

Marshall BJ, Warren JR (1984). Unidentified curved bacilli in the stomach of patients with gastritis and peptic ulceration. *Lancet*, 323(8390), 1311–1315.

Overmier JB, Murison R (2013). Restoring psychology's role in peptic ulcer. *Applied Psychol Health Well-Being*, 5, 5–27.

Schwab JJ (1985). Psychosomatic medicine: Its past and present. *Psychosom Med.*, 26(7), 583–593.

Schwab JJ (1989). Consultation-liaison psychiatry: A historical overview. *Psychosomatics*, 30(3), 245–254.

Söllner W, Schüssler G (2012). New 'European Association of Psychosomatic Medicine' founded. *J Psychosom Res.*, 73, 343–344.

Steinberg H, Herman-Lingen C (2013). Johann Christian August Heinroth: Psychosomatic medicine eighty years before Freud. *Psychiat Danub.*, *25*(1), 11–16.

The Rockefeller Archive Center. *100 Years: The Rockefeller Foundation.* Retrieved January 1, 2014, from http://rockefeller100.org/exhibits/show/health/psychiatry.

Taylor GJ, Bagby RM, Parker JD (2003). The 20-item Toronto Alexithymic Scale: IV. Reliability and factorial validity in different languages and cultures. *J Psychosom Res.*, *55*(3), 277–283.

Thompson TL, Suddath RL (1987). Edward G. Billings, MD: Pioneer of consultation-liaison psychiatry. *Psychosomatics*, *28*(3), 153–156.

Wessely S, Nimnuan C, Sharpe M (1999). Functional somatic syndromes: One or many? *Lancet*, *354*(9182), 936–939.

Zane MD (1947). Psychosomatic considerations in peptic ulcer. *Psychosom Med.*, *9*(6), 372–380.

Chapter 2

Psychiatric Consultation in the Inpatient General Medical Setting

Abhishek Jain, Ann Louise DiBarry, Priya Gopalan, Pierre N. Azzam, and Ellen M. Whyte

Introduction

The prevalence and impact of psychiatric symptoms on physical illness, quality of life, medical outcomes, and healthcare costs have led to increasing integration of psychiatric care in medical settings (Bronheim et al., 1998). In a 2011 study, Desan et al. found that a proactive psychiatric consultation service significantly reduced the hospital length of stay and resulted in a favorable cost-benefit ratio.

In addition to direct consultation for patient care, mental health professionals may take on various roles in the hospital setting, including staff education, participation in medicolegal and ethics teams, and hospital policy formulation. Some consultants may be embedded as members of a multidisciplinary treatment team and may routinely provide psychiatric screening and recommendations on all of the team's patients; other consultants may be available to a hospital system and provide psychiatric input and patient consultation only on an as-requested basis. Consultations also range from a brief "curbside" evaluation with focused recommendations to a comprehensive psychiatric assessment. An overall challenge and "art" of providing consultation involves understanding when a more focused approach versus a more comprehensive approach is needed.

Psychiatric consultation in each type of general clinical setting (e.g., outpatient, inpatient, skilled nursing facility), hospital environment (e.g., academic, community), or specialized hospital unit (e.g., intensive care unit, oncology unit) may present unique demands, challenges, and opportunities. The purpose of this chapter is to help optimize the (1) interview, (2) cognitive evaluation, (3) physical examination, (4) lethality assessment, (5) diagnosis, case formulation, and recommendations, and (6) documentation required for psychiatric consultation in an inpatient medical setting. These principles may need to be tailored to individual settings, patient types, and consultation questions, as described in specific chapters throughout this book.

Interview

Prior to the Interview

The consultation process usually begins when a primary medical service requests psychiatric input regarding a specific patient care issue. Common reasons for psychiatric consultation include altered mental status, anxiety, depression, substance use disorders, suicide risk, decision-making capacity, and psychological contribution to physical illness. Prior to beginning the patient interview, the following steps and considerations can prepare the consultant for an efficient and effective consultation.

1. *Contact the referring team and clarify the consultation request.* This can help streamline the consultation process and ensure that the referring team's questions are addressed. The consultant should try to understand relevant medical history, behavioral observations, whether the patient is aware of and agreeable to the consultation request, pending procedures or diagnostic tests, the anticipated length of hospital stay, and disposition plans.

2. *Establish the psychiatric service's role.* Institutional culture and specific clinical scenarios may determine whether the psychiatric consultant provides recommendations to the primary service or directly assists in patient care (e.g., placing orders for tests and medications). Establishing your role with the primary team is important for patient care, so that critical recommendations are not "lost."

3. *Review relevant records.* Review of the most salient medical and psychiatric records (e.g., reason for admission, current medical problems, home and current medications, labs, diagnostic tests, and prior psychiatric records) can typically be completed in 10–15 minutes and helps to frame the consultation question, facilitate communication with the primary medical service, and guide the psychiatric interview.

4. *Discuss with the patient's immediate care team.* Prior to entering the patient's room, the consultant may briefly obtain input from a team member currently working with the patient, such as a nurse or, if ordered, a safety sitter. This can help paint a picture of the patient's most recent presentation, highlight specific concerns, elucidate any safety or social issues, and assure staff that you are aware of the consultation request.

During the Interview

The patient assessment begins immediately after entering the patient's room. The consultant should take note of the patient's appearance, behavior, and environment, including visitors and supporting staff, food trays, personal belongings, acute medical care, and medical equipment (e.g., intravenous lines, infusions, catheters, oxygen supplementation, restraints, etc.).

At the beginning of the interview, the consultant typically explains his or her role and the purpose of the visit. To reduce distractions and improve patient engagement and attention, the consultant may ask the patient to mute or turn off the television, open the blinds, turn on lights, and close the hallway door. These should be posed as a request, as the patient should understand that he or she has control over the environment. Sitting in a chair next to the patient allows for improved communication. In one study, spine surgery patients perceived that providers who sat during the clinical interaction spent more time with them, leading to improved patient satisfaction and adherence (Swayden et al., 2012).

Depending on the clinical circumstance, visitors and other staff may be asked to leave during the interview to facilitate the patient's privacy, engagement, and openness with information. However, the patient may also reasonably request that a family member remain in the room for support or to provide relevant history. If the patient is sharing the room with another patient, acknowledge the limits of privacy and consider arrangements to optimize the patient's comfort (e.g., drawing a curtain or possibly taking the patient to a private meeting room).

Although fundamental skills for building rapport and engaging patients in an inpatient medical setting are similar to those used in other settings, psychiatric consultants must adapt to time constraints, interruptions from other care providers, and the patient's medical needs. The consultant's interaction style often needs to be flexible, such as moving from open-ended questions to more direct, close-ended questions as patients tire. For topics that may be potentially embarrassing or uncomfortable for the patient, the consultant should clarify which information will be included in the medical record. It is often possible to complete the consultation while limiting disclosure of personal history unrelated to safety, diagnoses, and consult recommendations.

Box 2.1 provides the general elements of an initial comprehensive consultation interview and assessment. Although each element may be helpful when providing psychiatric care, not all consultations are conducive to such detail, nor do they require it. Clinical judgment determines which areas must be covered.

Box 2.1 Outline for Initial Comprehensive Psychiatric Consultation Interview and Documentation

- **Patient demographics** (including age, gender/sex, marital status, birth date, admission date, reason for hospital admission)
- **Consultation information** (admitting service, hospital unit, requesting physician, date of consult, and reason for consult)
- **Patient's chief complaint**
- **History of present illness** (onset, frequency, duration, severity of symptoms)
- **Psychiatric review of symptoms** (pertinent symptoms related to depression, mania, anxiety disorders, psychosis, cognitive impairment, lethality, etc.)
- **Substance use history** (types, frequency, pattern, withdrawals, most recent use, treatment history [e.g., rehabilitation or counseling])
- **Psychiatric history** (diagnoses, hospitalizations, suicide attempts and self-injurious behavior, aggressive behavior, past and current mental health providers, past medications/treatments, duration and effectiveness of treatment)
- **Psychiatric medications immediately prior to admission** (adherence and prescribers, over-the-counter medications, supplements)
- **Medications during current admission** (scheduled and PRN medications [medical and psychiatric]; PRN psychiatric medications recently administered)
- **Allergies and non-allergic drug reactions**
- **Family psychiatric history**
- **Medical and surgical history**
- **Social history** (current living condition, household members, support system, marital status, employment, financial limitations, healthcare access, activities of daily living, driving)
- **Legal history** (past, ongoing, pending)
- **Relevant diagnostic and laboratory findings**
- **Medical review of systems**
- **Mental status and physical examinations** (see "Cognitive Evaluation" and "Physical Examination" sections)
- **Diagnostic impression**
- **Clinical assessment** (biopsychosocial formulation, lethality assessment)
- **Recommendations**
- **Follow-up and disposition plan** (including how often psychiatric follow-up will occur in the hospital and contact information for further questions).

Cognitive Evaluation

Cognitive evaluation tasks allow an objective assessment of the patient's orientation, attention, concentration, memory, executive functioning, language, fund of knowledge, abstract thinking, insight, and judgment. A cognitive function snapshot is useful and sometimes necessary for accurate diagnosis; for example, bedside cognitive testing may differentiate delirium, dementia, and pre-existing intellectual disability. Repeated bedside cognitive evaluations may even further clarify the diagnosis; for example, a patient's daily performance will likely fluctuate more with delirium than with dementia.

Clinicians may employ various testing methods when assessing cognition. A standardized instrument (e.g., Montreal Cognitive Assessment [MoCA]) can help assess a patient's overall cognitive status and provide more accurate test results. However, a patient may be too physically, psychiatrically, or cognitively impaired to participate in an extensive assessment (see "Standardized Cognitive Assessments" section for more details).

Attention and concentration should generally be assessed in all patients because impairment in these domains is suggestive of delirium, which is commonly present in inpatient medical settings. Furthermore, a patient with severe impairment in attention and concentration will likely perform poorly in all other cognitive domains, possibly rendering any further cognitive testing inaccurate.

The following are examples of questions and tests for each cognitive domain.

Orientation

Ask the patient:
Person: Patient's name and birthdate
Place: Building, floor, city, and state
Time: Day of the week, date, month, season, year
Situation: Reason for admission and treatment plan.

Attention

Read a list of about 20–30 random letters and ask the patient to tap a finger when he or she hears the letter "A." A patient with intact attention will typically have less than two errors (either failing to tap when hearing the letter "A" or incorrectly tapping when hearing another letter [adapted from the MoCA]).

An alternate test is "digit span," in which the patient is asked to repeat a sequence of random digits of increasing length (forward and backward). Normal range is repeating at least 5 digits forward and at least 3 digits backward.

Concentration

Ask the patient to state the months of the year or days of the week backward, spell "WORLD" backward, or serially subtract 7s from 100 ("100–93–86–79–72–65") or 3s from 20. A patient with intact concentration would typically have no more than one error with each test. Baseline impairment in knowledge, spelling, or calculation should be taken into account. Failure to perform the relatively easier tasks (e.g., days backward or serial 3s) suggests greater impairment than failure to perform the more difficult tasks (e.g., months backward or serial 7s).

Memory

Registration and immediate recall: Ask the patient to repeat three unrelated words (e.g., Chicago, table, and banana), and to remember these words for later recall.

Delayed recall: Three minutes after performing other tasks, ask the patient to repeat the previously registered three words. If the patient does not recall one or more words, provide categorical cues (e.g., "One of the words was the name of a city"). If the patient still does not recall the word, then provide multiple choices. Typically, a patient should be able to recall at least two out of three words without any cues or choices, and recall all words after being given cues and choices.

If patients have significant expressive language impairment, memory can be tested by showing them three unrelated objects, asking them to remember these three objects, and then after three minutes asking them identify the three objects from a selection of six objects.

Executive Functioning

One test of executive functioning is the Clock Drawing test, in which the patient is asked to draw a clock face with the hands showing a specific time, such as "10 past 11." Several methods exist for scoring this test. One method scores one point for each of the following: accurately drawing a circle, placing all numbers in sequence, placing all numbers in the proper spatial position, drawing two hands, and indicating the correct time - for a total of five points. A score of three or lower suggests impairment in executive functioning. While this is a useful test, its findings may be confounded if the patient has visuospatial impairment.

Another test of executive functioning is the Luria Maneuvers test, in which a patient is asked to mimic the clinician demonstrating three sequential maneuvers (e.g., tapping with the side of an open hand, then with a fist, then with an open palm) in a repeated pattern, then asked to perform this pattern without guidance. Failure to repeat three correct cycles without guidance is considered abnormal (Weiner et al., 2011).

Language

Repetition: Ask the patient to repeat a phrase.
Naming: Ask the patient to name two items (e.g., pen or watch).
Comprehension: Ask the patient to follow a verbal command (e.g., "Touch your nose").
Reading comprehension: Ask the patient to read and follow an instruction.
Writing: Ask the patient to write a complete sentence with a subject and verb.

Fund of Knowledge

Ask the patient to name the current and immediate past US presidents, discuss current events, or discuss a topic of the patient's interest (e.g., sports), which can also be integrated into the general interview to build rapport and to assess depression and anhedonia (loss of interest).

Abstract Thinking

Ask the patient to explain the meaning of a proverb (e.g., "Don't judge a book by its cover") or to explain similarities (e.g., "How are an apple and an orange similar?").

Insight

Ask the patient about his or her medical and psychiatric conditions and their relationship to the patient's current situation (e.g., insight into alcohol abuse and its possible connection with liver failure).

Judgment

Ask the patient how he or she would solve real-life problems (e.g., ask an elderly person what she would do if she were at home alone and smelled smoke).

Standardized Cognitive Assessments

We highlight two assessment tools: the Confusion Assessment Method (CAM), a test for delirium (Inouye et al., 1990), and the Montreal Cognitive Assessment (MoCA), a test of global cognition (Nasreddine et al., 2005). Both are widely used and have practical utility in an inpatient general medical setting.

The CAM is available online, is copyright protected, and should be acknowledged when used for clinical purposes. It has been translated into at least six languages and is designed for non-psychiatric medical providers. In a systematic literature review, the CAM was found to have a 94% sensitivity and an 89% specificity in identifying delirium (Wei et al., 2008).

The MoCA is available online free of charge (www.mocatest.org), has been translated into many languages, provides a version for patients with visual impairment, and has three English-language versions (allowing for retesting). In one study, a score of 25 or less (out of 30) demonstrated an 83% sensitivity and a 50% specificity in detecting at least mild cognitive impairment (Smith et al., 2007). Paying attention to the patient's performance in each subsection (visuospatial/executive, naming, memory, attention, language, abstraction, delayed recall, and orientation) can be clinically useful in determining the specific type of neurocognitive disorder that may be present.

Physical Examination

The Academy of Psychosomatic Medicine's *Practice Guidelines for Psychiatric Consultation in the General Medical Setting* recommends reviewing the results of previous physical examinations, supplementing with focused neurologic and physical assessments, and evaluating organ-specific complaints and medication side effects (Bronheim et al., 1998). Factors such as disruption of the psychiatrist-patient relationship may warrant exam completion by a non-psychiatric provider.

The physical examination begins by observing the patient's general appearance and behavior, and noting any obvious evidence of trauma, self-injury, abnormal physical movements, or drug abuse. Intoxication and withdrawal states can often be differentiated by their unique physical findings. For example, opioid intoxication is associated with respiratory depression and pupillary constriction, while opioid withdrawal is associated with pupillary dilation, piloerection, lacrimation, and rhinorrhea.

A focused physical examination is particularly useful when evaluating patients with altered mental status (e.g., toxidromes, intoxication), psychiatric symptoms secondary to organic conditions (e.g., hypothyroidism, Wilson's disease), neurologic conditions (e.g., strokes, seizures), and suspected psychosomatic disorders (e.g., conversion disorder, factitious disorder). Careful attention to physical findings may help distinguish psychiatric pathology (e.g., mood, anxiety, or psychotic disorder) from medical conditions (e.g., endocrine, metabolic, or rheumatologic abnormalities).

A neurologic examination (including cranial nerves, motor strength, coordination, gait, reflexes, frontal release signs, and ocular findings) may help identify syndromes such as catatonia, neurocognitive disorders, or specific toxidromes such as serotonin syndrome. For example, hyperreflexia, clonus (particularly ocular clonus), autonomic instability, and hyperactive bowel sounds suggest serotonin toxicity; lead-pipe rigidity, tremor, autonomic instability, and marked fever suggest neuroleptic malignant syndrome.

Specialized examinations may help differentiate psychosomatic disorders from physiological conditions. For example, Hoover's test for nonorganic weakness involves involuntary extension of the unimpaired leg when genuinely trying to flex the impaired leg. Waddell's signs for nonorganic back pain include superficial or non-anatomic *tenderness; simulation* of movement causing pain; *overreaction* based on subjective reaction to testing; *regional* symptoms that do not correspond to accepted neuroanatomy; and *distraction* tests in which symptoms, such as pain with straight leg raise, are not present when the patient is distracted.

Lethality Risk Assessment and Mitigation of Risk Factors

Suicide

In the United States, suicide is the 10th leading cause of death, and approximately 650,000 hospital visits yearly are due to self-harm. In one study (Luoma et al., 2002), about 45% of patients who completed suicide had seen a primary medical provider within the previous month. Risk of suicide is particularly elevated in medical diseases or trauma associated with a chronic course, intolerable pain, insomnia, disfigurement, or disability, such as with HIV/AIDS, cancer, multiple sclerosis, and spinal cord injuries.

Assessment of Suicide Risk

Primary medical teams often request psychiatric consultation to evaluate and manage patients who make suicidal statements or evidence risk for suicide. Furthermore, screening for suicide risk is a routine component of psychiatric evaluations even when consulting on unrelated issues. The psychiatric consultant may discover that a patient has a passive death wish, suicidal ideation, suicidal intent, or a previous attempt unknown to the medical team or family. Such a finding would trigger further assessment of the patient's suicide risk. A detailed risk assessment may include the following:

- Eliciting details (frequency, intensity, duration) about the patient's current suicidal thoughts, plans, intent, and behaviors;
- Evaluating the intentionality of any recent self-harm;
- Obtaining details about any specific plans, including timing, location, likelihood of discovery, access to methods, expectations of survival, rehearsal, and preparation for death (e.g., saying goodbye to loved ones);
- Understanding the patient's immediate risk factors, such as hopelessness, psychosocial stressors, recent losses or perceived losses, limited supports, social isolation, receptivity and access to mental healthcare, recent release from an inpatient psychiatric setting without established outpatient treatment, easy access to suicide methods (e.g., firearms);
- Compiling information on chronic risk factors, including demographics, past attempts, psychiatric history and current symptoms, medical history, family history of suicide, childhood trauma or neglect;
- Comparing any recent suicide attempts to past attempts to understand whether the attempts are becoming increasingly lethal;
- Assessing the patient's coping strategies, frustration tolerance, impulsivity, and threshold for self-harm;
- Considering protective factors such as problem-solving skills and conflict resolution, religious or moral prohibition, sense of responsibility toward others or pets, social supports, engagement in psychiatric and medical care, future planning, hopefulness, and willingness to communicate any future suicidal thoughts.

Two significant risk factors for suicide are prior suicide attempts and the presence of one or more psychiatric disorders. An estimated 10–20% of individuals who attempt suicide proceed to complete suicide, the risk of suicide is elevated in almost every major psychiatric disorder, and at least 90% of patients who complete suicide meet the criteria for a probable psychiatric diagnosis.

Access to lethal suicide methods has been associated with higher risk for suicide throughout scientific literature, such as commonly cited studies involving Golden Gate Bridge jumpers and United Kingdom suicides using coal gas. In general, minimizing access to lethal suicide methods may reduce the risk for suicide, especially in those who may be at risk for impulsive attempts. A hot-button political issue is firearm access and gun legislation regarding individuals with mental illness. Although laws continue to evolve and may be jurisdiction-specific, discussing access to and removal of firearms can be a useful clinical component of risk assessment and management. According to a recent meta-analysis of 16 studies, individuals with firearm access had more than a threefold risk of suicide and a doubled risk of homicide compared to individuals without firearm access (Anglemyer et al., 2014).

Management and Documentation of Suicide Risk

Due to the difficulty of predicting suicide, a realistic goal is not to "eliminate" suicide risk, but rather to weigh the acute and chronic risk and protective factors, and to develop a treatment plan to target immediate safety concerns, reduce future risk, and guide discharge planning. Identifying and addressing modifiable risk factors (e.g., inpatient alcohol rehabilitation for suicidal thoughts during alcohol use) are particularly useful.

Each risk and protective factor is individual and does not carry equal weight. If a patient only has one identifiable, yet serious, risk factor (e.g., a detailed suicide plan with clear intent) in the face of multiple protective factors, the clinician may still assess the patient to be at high risk and may recommend inpatient psychiatric admission. Obtaining consultation from a colleague can be helpful, especially in complex cases.

Though suicide is a rare event in medical hospitals, it is the second most commonly reported sentinel event, after wrong-site surgery. The most common method for suicide in the medical hospital is jumping, and the second most common is hanging. For patients identified as being at high risk for self-harm in a medical hospital, the psychiatric consultant may consider ordering elopement precautions, 1:1 safety sitters, and/or environmental modification (e.g., limiting access to sharp silverware).

Examples of documentation that synthesize the risk and protective factors to help outline a treatment plan include the following:

1. Although Mr. Smith denies any current suicidal ideation, has an established outpatient psychiatric provider, and is applying for financial assistance, based on his suicide attempt (overdose) two days ago, ongoing severely depressed mood, poor social supports, financial and housing instability, chronic pain, and alcohol and opioid abuse, he is at high risk for suicide and would require treatment in a locked inpatient psychiatric unit.

2. Ms. Johnson's suicide risk factors (past suicide attempt; history of schizophrenia; poor medication compliance; and unemployment) place her at a chronically elevated risk for suicide. However, based on her current protective factors (disavowing any current suicidal ideation, plan, or intent; strong family supports; sense of responsibility toward nieces and nephew; strong religious belief system with prohibition against suicide; stable housing; and close follow-up with Assertive Community Treatment), she is at relatively low risk for imminent self-harm, does not require inpatient psychiatric admission, and can continue following up with her outpatient providers upon discharge. The following treatment plan will further reduce her overall risk for self-harm by targeting her modifiable risk factors: (a) consideration for long-term injectable depot antipsychotic medication to decrease symptoms related to poor adherence; and (b) referral to occupational and vocational rehabilitation.

Violence

Psychiatric consultants may be asked to evaluate patients at risk for aggression toward others or at risk for being victims of violence. Although severe psychiatric illness, especially with comorbid substance use, has a modest association with violence, media bias and fictional portrayals may overinflate and overgeneralize the relationship between mental illness and violence. The majority of those with a history of mental illness are not violent, the majority of violence in the general population is not attributable to those with a history of mental illness, and individuals with a history of mental illness are more likely to be victims than perpetrators of violence (Choe et al., 2008). In one recent large study, mental illness alone did not predict violence; violence was more associated with other factors such as past violence, socioeconomics, and substance abuse (Elbogen, 2009).

Identifying the intentionality and potential cause of a patient's aggression helps further guide treatment, disposition, and safety planning (e.g., continued medical treatment for agitation in acute delirium, admission to a psychiatric hospital for aggression stemming from symptoms of schizophrenia, or possible criminal charges for violent antisocial behavior). A psychiatric consultant ought to pay particular attention to hospital safety and security policies, and be aware of local laws regarding duty to warn or protect third parties from violence, mandatory child or elder abuse reporting, and domestic violence considerations.

Overall, similar to a psychiatric consultant's role in assessing and managing suicide risk, a realistic goal is not to "eliminate" violence risk, but to weigh the risk and protective factors, and to outline a reasonable treatment plan to manage and mitigate risk. Although an exhaustive review of violence risk assessment is beyond the scope of this text, the general principles outlined earlier for suicide risk assessment, management, and documentation can also be applied to violence.

Diagnosis, Case Formulation, and Recommendations

The diagnostic impression, clinical assessment, recommendations, and follow-up plan are often the "bottom line" when primary teams seek consultation. Although the inpatient medical setting and acute medical problems may limit the precision of psychiatric diagnosis, psychiatric consultants should attempt to clarify the nature of psychiatric symptoms, outline any limitations with rendering a diagnosis, and identify a plan (such as reassessment or additional testing) to help reach accurate diagnoses. When summarizing the clinical assessment, using a biopsychosocial case formulation, with relevant predisposing, precipitating, perpetuating, and protective factors, can help succinctly capture a complex patient presentation. When possible, and with appropriate patient consent, obtaining collateral information from outpatient medical or mental health providers, family members, or others who know the patient can clarify the patient's baseline psychiatric and cognitive status and help focus diagnoses and recommendations.

As discussed above, psychiatric consultants may either provide recommendations to the primary service or directly assist in patient care (e.g., placing orders for tests and medications). Establishing the role of the consultant and clarifying who (i.e., the consultant or the primary team) will execute the treatment plan is important. It is also helpful to provide clear and specific recommendations, such as medication dosing and laboratory tests. The follow-up plan is often the most sought-after element of the treatment recommendation and should include whether and how often the psychiatric team will follow up, how to contact the psychiatric team for further questions, and any outpatient or disposition recommendations.

Documentation

With the almost universal use of electronic medical records, documentation is more readily accessed and relied upon as the primary mode of communication among medical providers. Medical documentation often serves multiple purposes, such as communicating with other medical disciplines, providing pertinent background information to fellow team members and other outpatient psychiatric providers, and summarizing treatment needs for third-party payers. Patients or their families are also increasingly requesting access to their medical records. Considering these various purposes and audiences, consultation records should aim to be organized, concise, accurate, objective, and relevant. Psychiatric jargon and unclear abbreviations should be avoided (e.g., "SCD" may be confusing and could refer to sleep continuity disturbance, sickle cell disease, sudden cardiac death, etc.).

Many electronic health record systems have an established consult template, and information such as demographics and medication lists can often be incorporated automatically into the note, while details of medical information can be referenced elsewhere in the medical record. The goal of the consultation note is to provide sufficient details to clarify diagnoses and treatment recommendations, while avoiding distracting, sensitive, or prejudicial patient information.

Overall, the consultation record should flow in a structured, logical, practical, and predictable pattern; it should follow the pattern of most other medical consultations, and it should include the relevant elements from Box 2.1.

Key Points

- Psychiatric consultation may range from a brief "curbside" phone conversation to a comprehensive psychiatric assessment. Understanding when to use a more focused or comprehensive approach is a common challenge and requires clinical judgment.
- Prior to the patient interview, contacting the referring team and clarifying the consultation request, establishing the psychiatric service's role, reviewing relevant records, and discussing the case with the patient's immediate care team can be useful.
- Patient assessment begins immediately upon entering the patient's room and observing the patient's appearance, behavior, and environment, and typically involves explaining the consultant's role, creating a reasonably conducive interview environment, and adapting psychiatric interview skills to the medical setting.
- Box 2.1 provides the general elements for a comprehensive initial consultation interview and assessment.
- Clinicians may reasonably employ various methods when assessing cognition.
- Conducting relevant physical and neurological examinations and reviewing the results of previous physical examinations can help clarify diagnoses.
- When assessing suicide or violence risk, a realistic goal is not to "eliminate" risk, but to outline a reasonable treatment plan to manage and mitigate risk.
- Documentation generally includes the elements of a typical psychiatric interview and evaluation, and often serves multiple purposes; particular attention should be paid when documenting challenging cases, such as those involving suicide or violence risk.

Disclosures

Dr. Jain has no conflicts of interest to disclose.

Ms. DiBarry has no conflicts of interest to disclose.

Dr. Gopalan has no conflicts of interest to disclose.

Dr. Azzam has no conflicts of interest to disclose.

Dr. Whyte has no conflicts of interest to disclose.

Further Reading

Anglemyer A, Horvath T, et al. (2014). The accessibility of firearms and risk for suicide and homicide victimization among household members: a systematic review and meta-analysis. *Ann Intern Med.*, *160*(2), 101–10.

Bronheim HE, Fulop G, et al. (1998). The Academy of Psychosomatic Medicine practice guidelines for psychiatric consultation in the general medical setting. *Psychosomatics*, *39*(4), S8–30.

Centers for Disease Control and Prevention. *National Suicide Statistics at a Glance*. Retreived from http://www.cdc.gov/violenceprevention/suicide/statistics/index.html.

Choe JY, Teplin LA, et al. (2008). Perpetration of violence, violent victimization, and severe mental illness: Balancing public health concerns. *Psychiatr Serv.*, *59*(2), 153–164.

Desan PH, Zimbrean PC, et al. (2011). Proactive psychiatric consultation services reduce length of stay for admissions to an inpatient medical team. *Psychosomatics*, *52*(6), 513–520.

Elbogen EB, Johnson SC (2009). The intricate link between violence and mental disorder: Results from the National Epidemiologic Survey on Alcohol and Related Conditions. *Arch Gen Psychiat.*, *66*(2), 152–161.

Luoma JB, Martin CE, et al. (2002). Contact with mental health and primary care providers before suicide: a review of the evidence. *Am J Psychiat.*, *159*(6), 909–916.

Nasreddine ZS, Phillips NA, et al. (2005). The Montreal Cognitive Assessment, MoCA: a Brief Screening Tool for Mild Cognitive Impairment. *J Am Geriatr Soc.*, *53*(4), 695–699.

Scott CL, Resnick PJ (2006). Violence risk assessment in persons with mental illness. *Aggress Violent Beh.*, *11*, 598–611.

Smith T, Gildeh N, et al. (2007). The Montreal Cognitive Assessment: Validity and utility in a memory clinic setting. *Can J Psychiat.*, *52*(5), 329–332.

Swayden KJ, Anderson KK, et al. (2012). Effect of sitting vs. standing on perception of provider time at bedside: A pilot study. *Patient Educ Couns.*, *86*(2), 166–171.

Weiner MF, Hynan LS, et al. (2011). Luria's three-step test: What is it and what does it tell us? *Int Psychogeriatr.*, *23*(10), 1602–1606.

Wei LA, Fearing MA, et al. (2008). The Confusion Assessment Method: A systematic review of current usage. *J Am Geriatr Soc.*, *56*(5), 823–830.

Exercises

1. Roughly what percentage of patients who completed suicide had seen a primary medical provider within the previous month?
   a. 5%
   b. 20%
   c. 45%
   d. 87%

2. Which cognitive domain is most helpful to evaluate when assessing delirium?
   a. Attention
   b. Memory
   c. Abstract thinking
   d. Executive functioning

3. Waddell's signs are physical examination findings suggestive of
   a. Non-organic weakness
   b. Non-organic seizures
   c. Non-organic amnesia
   d. Non-organic back pain

4. The psychiatric consultant in an inpatient general medical setting must adapt to
   a. Privacy limitations
   b. Interruptions from other care providers
   c. The patient's medical needs
   d. All of the above.

Answers: (1) c (2) a (3) d (4) d

Part II

Psychiatric Diagnosis and Management in the General Medical Setting

Mood Disorders and Insomnia in the General Medical Setting

Alin J. Severance and Christopher R. Hope

Epidemiology and Etiology

Mood disorders are very common in the general population, and they are generally two to three times more common among patients hospitalized for medical concerns. There is a high co-occurrence of depression and heart disease, diabetes, cancer, chronic obstructive pulmonary disease, stroke, and many other illnesses that may result in an inpatient admission (see Table 3.1, adapted from Berman & Pomili, 2005). Due to a variety of biological and psychosocial mechanisms, untreated mood disorders can increase morbidity and mortality in a number of chronic medical illnesses. Clinical outcomes may improve with proper psychiatric care.

Why are mood disorders more common in certain disease states? There are a number of possible mechanisms, including inflammation, altered levels of neurotransmitters, endocrine abnormalities, structural changes in the CNS, and genetic factors. Medical illness is also often associated with financial hardship, physical disability, caregiver burnout, social isolation, and the threat of pain and/or death. No single explanatory model applies to all cases of a mood disorder, and multiple etiological factors are often at play simultaneously (see Kendler et al., 2006).

For example, depression has been studied extensively in cardiovascular disease (see Chapter 13 for additional discussion), given the high level of comorbidity and a two- to fourfold increase of cardiovascular morbidity and mortality in the presence of major depression. As atherosclerosis progresses, neurohormonal, cytokine, and adrenergic systems act to compensate for a declining ability to supply the body with oxygenated blood. These signaling molecules may directly impact mood. In addition, after myocardial infarction (MI), patients must often adapt to decreased exercise tolerance, cognitive impairment, and sexual dysfunction. Post-hoc analyses of the Enhancing Recovery in Coronary Heart Disease Patients (ENRICHD) trial (Berkman et al., 2003) found that antidepressant treatment was associated with a lower rate of death and nonfatal myocardial infarction, in addition to reduced symptoms of depression.

Table 3.1 Point Prevalence of Major Depression

General population	8%
Rheumatoid arthritis	13%–20%
Stroke	22%
Coronary artery disease	15%–20%
End-stage renal disease	17%
Cancer (especially oropharyngeal, pancreatic, breast, and lung)	20%–25%
Chronic obstructive pulmonary disease	20%
Huntington's disease	50%
Parkinson's disease	25%–45%

Stress and depression are often interrelated; while stressful events increase an individual's risk for a depressive episode, depression may increase susceptibility to stressful life events. In the case of medical illness, depression can interfere with both seeking and adhering to effective medical treatment. People with depression often feel overwhelmed by their problems, and they may feel that they are beyond and/or unworthy of help. When faced with a new stressor, they are less able to identify a solution or to enlist assistance from supports in their life. Thought processes slow, concentration requires significant effort, and fond memories are increasingly difficult to recall. Sleep quality and energy decline, the digestive system is disrupted (with changes in appetite as well as bowel habits), pain experience is heightened, and libido is diminished. Problems begin to accumulate and fester, contributing to a sense of despair and diminishing the ability to take pleasure in normally enjoyable activities. Suffering may become all-consuming and may begin to make people around them miserable as well, especially when attempts to provide relief are unsuccessful. In social isolation, they are closed off to positive experiences and begin to question their own self-worth. In the extreme, they may conclude that suicide would be a kindness for themselves and others.

Differential Diagnosis of Mood Disorders in a Medical Setting

A review of the medical record prior to meeting the patient can help to both broaden the range of possible diagnoses and narrow the focus of clinical concern. What laboratory abnormalities were recorded, and what laboratory studies were omitted? Was a toxicology screen or blood alcohol level completed? Is their CNS imaging suggestive of cerebrovascular disease, neurodegenerative disease, or neoplasia? What do the social work and nursing notes say about family, housing, and/or recent stressors?

The primary aim of the consult may change after a thorough examination. When consulted for a "depressed patient" with weight loss and apathy, you might instead encounter a patient with vascular dementia, as evidenced by a Montreal Cognitive Assessment (MoCA) score of 12 and apraxia involving utensils. Likewise, a "difficult patient" with a recurrence of lung cancer who is refusing blood draws and medications might be so depressed that he has given up hope that he will ever recover.

A biopsychosocial formulation will both help answer the clinical question and identify additional areas of concern. Medical illness is often associated with loss of employment, financial ruin, family discord, and many other problems that may not come to light during a medical history. The elevated rates of depression in women with breast cancer may have as much to do with how our culture views breasts as with the misery related to chemotherapy treatment. Empowering a man with anhedonia and suicidal ideation to extricate himself from a physically abusive relationship may be just as important as choosing an appropriate antidepressant.

Mood symptoms tend to be broadly associated with medical conditions that are prolonged, incurable, painful, and/or disfiguring. Table 3.2 lists illnesses and substances that are commonly associated with depression or mania.

Please note that a normal grief/stress reaction, an adjustment disorder with disturbance of mood, and a primary mood disorder may each present with a spectrum of distress and impairment that vary over time and with intervention. Someone who is struggling in the face of significant medical illness may present with sadness, sleep disturbance, and even social withdrawal, though she likely will retain some confidence about her ability to cope in the future. Significant losses, such as the death of a spouse or child, may be accompanied by marked impairment that can be expected to improve with time. In contrast, a person with an adjustment disorder is viewed as having distress out of proportion to the stressor, but does not meet full criteria for a major depressive episode. Nevertheless, his impairment may interfere with his medical care and may even prolong his hospital stay. Depression is distinguished from an adjustment disorder and from normal grief not only by the number of symptoms but also by their severity and chronicity (as an adjustment disorder is expected to remit after the stressor is resolved). Whatever the diagnosis, we should first consider whether treatment is warranted and which treatment would be most effective. Treatment may differ for

Table 3.2 Illnesses and Substances Commonly Associated with Mood Symptoms. The majority can produce either manic, depressive, or mixed mood symptoms. Where manic (m) or depressive (d) symptoms predominate, it has been indicated.

Autoimmune conditions	Systemic lupus erythematosus, rheumatoid arthritis (d)
Organ failure	Myocardial infarction (d), renal failure (d), liver failure (d), chronic obstructive pulmonary disease (d)
Drugs of abuse and toxins	All drugs of abuse are associated with mood symptoms whether during intoxication, withdrawal, or during chronic use. Heavy metals, paint/gasoline inhalation, organophosphates, carbon monoxide, nerve gases are associated primarily with depression.
Endocrine conditions	Adrenal insufficiency, Addison's disease, Cushing's syndrome, diabetes mellitus, hypothyroidism, hyperthyroidism, hyperparathyroidism, hypoparathyroidism
Infectious diseases	Creutzfeldt-Jakob disease, HIV, Lyme disease, neurosyphilis, mononucleosis
Medications	Anabolic steroids, anticonvulsants, antidepressants (m), antihypertensives (d); clonidine, guanethidine, reserpine, methyldopa, beta blockers, antihistamines, benzodiazepines, bronchodilators (m), contraceptives (d) (especially if high estrogen content), chemotherapeutics (e.g., interferons, procarbazine, vincristine), corticosteroids, decongestants (m), dopamine agonists (m), efavirenz, GnRH agonists, H_2 blockers, isoretinoin, sulfonamides, triptans, tamoxifen, varenicline
Malignancy	Brain tumors, pancreatic cancer (d), oropharyngeal cancers (d), paraneoplastic syndromes
Neurologic	Delirium, dementia, epilepsy, Huntington's disease, multiple sclerosis, Parkinson's disease (d), stroke (especially left frontal and basal ganglia infarcts), anoxic brain injury, traumatic brain injury, Wilson's disease
Vitamin deficiencies	Vitamin B12 deficiency (d), folate deficiency (d), vitamin D deficiency (d)

grief, adjustment disorder, and depression, with more emphasis on social supports and pastoral care for grief and adjustment disorders and more emphasis on medications and psychotherapy for major depression or bipolar disorder. The level of impairment, rather than the presence of specific symptoms, should direct your decision-making process.

Additionally, there are a number of factors specific to the general medical setting that complicate appropriate diagnosis and treatment (see also Chapter 2):

1. Though hospitalized patients and their families occasionally request a psychiatric consultation, a psychiatric evaluation is generally requested by the medical provider. Unlike in the majority of behavioral health settings, the patient is not coming to you, and the patient may not even be aware that a psychiatric consultation was requested. You may be the first psychiatrist that the patient has ever met. Fear and hostility are common, especially if the patient's primary medical concerns are not being met and/or the psychiatric consult is experienced as a judgment against his or her sanity. In cases like these, it may take greater effort and creativity to develop an alliance. Letting a patient know that most consultations are for people with no psychiatric history, and normalizing the psychological distress associated with medical illness, may be fruitful strategies.

2. Even in patients with no psychiatric history, being hospitalized is frequently associated with some combination of sadness, anxiety, reduced interest, sleep deprivation, loss of appetite, fatigue, and poor concentration. Individuals with the best of prognoses still have to contend with the deconditioning, indignity, and temporary loss of agency that comes with being tethered to a hospital bed. Many patients are grappling with life-changing losses—loss of bodily functions, loss of financial independence or productivity, or even loss of loved ones. Thoughts of death, or even passive death wishes, are common in patients with terminal illnesses or chronic pain, and must be differentiated from actual suicidal ideation (see Chapters 20 and 21).

Diagnostic Approaches

In the fifth edition of the *Diagnostic and Statistical Manual of Mental Disorders* (DSM-5), the primary mood disorders (major depressive disorder, bipolar I disorder, and bipolar II disorder) have an exclusionary criterion for episodes that can be attributed to a substance or a medical condition. Furthermore, the description of major depression cautions that individual symptoms should not be included if they can be attributed to another medical condition. This serves to minimize over-diagnosis of primary mood disorders, especially in individuals with no history of mood symptoms who, for example, develop depression only during treatment with interferon, or who develop manic symptoms while being treated with high-dose glucocorticoids (cases in which a diagnosis of substance-induced mood disorder may be more appropriate). However, determination of etiology is rarely so straightforward, especially in a patient whom you have just met, and many hospital patients have medical conditions and medications that can be associated with mood symptoms. A more representative case might be someone with a history of major depression who reports a worsening of symptoms with prominent apathy following a left frontal stroke. How do you decide if her difficulty concentrating is due to the stroke or due to the depression?

Since the publication of the third edition (*DSM-III*) in 1980, the *Diagnostic and Statistical Manual of Mental Disorders* has prioritized diagnostic reliability through the use of simple, descriptive criteria for each diagnosis. There are at least three diagnostic approaches (reviewed in Table 3.3) to use in the context of comorbid medical illness: inclusive, exclusive, and substitutive approaches.

The inclusive approach counts all symptoms toward the diagnosis of depression or mania, even if there may be medical causes at play. Sleep disturbance is counted toward a psychiatric diagnosis, even if arguably due to postoperative pain and constant sounds from monitoring equipment in the ICU. While this approach has a high sensitivity, the risk of this strategy is poor specificity, leading to unnecessary treatment. Consider using an inclusive strategy when the depressive symptoms predate the medical illness, when the depressive symptoms are severe, or when a low threshold for treatment is desired.

The exclusive approach to psychiatric diagnosis omits symptom criteria that may be caused by medical illness or substances. For example, anorexia and fatigue, being common in patients with cancer, would not count toward a diagnosis of depression. Instead of requiring five of nine criteria for diagnosis of a major depressive episode, an individual with pancreatic cancer might have to meet five of only seven criteria. Likewise, irritability, insomnia, and poor concentration might be ignored for a diagnosis of mania in someone on intravenous steroids for severe postoperative pain. This approach reduces the number of false positives, but at the expense of reduced sensitivity, and some individuals with a potentially disabling mood episode may go without treatment. Consider using this strategy when a higher threshold for diagnosis is desired (e.g., if the patient is very reluctant to pursue treatment, if the mood symptoms are mild, or if the medical condition is acute and is likely to resolve).

Table 3.3 Diagnostic Approaches

Inclusive	All symptoms are counted (high sensitivity; low specificity)
Exclusive	Only symptoms that are independent of current medical illness are counted (low sensitivity; high specificity)
Substitutive	Somatic symptoms that overlap with medical illness are replaced with affective or cognitive symptoms (potentially maximizing both sensitivity and specificity) Potential substitutions: Sleep disturbance → social withdrawal and diminished speech Fatigue → guilt and pessimism Impaired concentration → reduced emotional reactivity Appetite disturbance → tearfulness

The substitutive approach attempts to replace somatic symptoms with criteria that are more specific to altered mood states, such as social withdrawal, tearfulness, and pessimism, with the goal of maximizing both sensitivity and specificity. This approach may be most useful with patients who have chronic and progressive illnesses with significant symptom overlap, such as end-stage renal disease, stroke, and metastatic cancer. Unfortunately, there is no expert consensus on which symptoms should replace the nonspecific criteria, and this approach is biased against those individuals who experience mood symptoms more in somatic terms than emotional. For example, an elderly man with no prior psychiatric history may express his distress more in terms of fatigue, diffuse pain, loss of appetite, and amotivation than in terms of sadness. In cultures where psychiatry is not widely practiced or accepted, or where emotional distress is largely a private experience, it may be especially important to pay attention to "nonspecific" physical symptoms without evident etiology. For example, despite significant symptom overlap, it is more common in China to diagnose someone with neurasthenia (*shenjing shuairuo*) than depression, perhaps due to its lack of social stigma (neurasthenia emphasizes headaches, insomnia, muscle weakness, and neuralgia; see Kleinman, 1991).

Experienced clinicians often use a combination of all approaches, depending on the severity and persistence of symptoms, the patient's age and cultural background, and collateral history. Consider a woman who reports tearfulness, insomnia, and worthlessness in the setting of inadequately managed pain, following a traumatic amputation that will likely prevent her dream of cycling across the country. Antidepressants might not be welcomed, or even effective, and she may continue to feel this way for weeks or even months as part of a normal grieving process. However, if the symptoms are interfering with physical therapy, or if a family member reports that the patient has been talking about being better off dead, then the risk of withholding treatment might outweigh the risks of over-diagnosing someone who is struggling with a life-changing event.

Treatment Approaches

Given the diagnostic challenges discussed above, it is often prudent for the choice of treatment to be guided by the symptoms of concern, especially when the etiology is ambiguous. Table 3.4 suggests different medications depending on which symptoms predominate. It is also worth noting that most efficacy studies for psychiatric medications exclude patients with comorbid medical conditions. While the treatment options are the same as in a behavioral health setting, you will need to pay much more attention to medication side effects, drug-drug interactions, altered metabolism, and absorption (Chapter 6 reviews this in detail). For example, you might consider starting sertraline at a reduced dose, or you might try another agent, in a patient with Crohn's disease, given that sertraline commonly causes nausea and diarrhea. With the advent of selective serotonin reuptake inhibitors (SSRIs), the risk/benefit analysis is often tilted toward treatment given their relative safety and favorable side-effect profile. On the other hand, they are often withheld in the perioperative period to minimize bleeding risk, and doses may need to be adjusted in the presence of other medications that interact with cytochrome P450 3A4 and 2D6 enzymes, among others. While starting with modest doses is a good strategy for an older and medically ill population, you may also find that antidepressants are continued by other medical providers at sub-therapeutic doses despite ongoing symptoms.

While tricyclic antidepressants and monoamine oxidase inhibitors (MAOIs) can be used safely in medically ill patients, they probably should be avoided in patients with active cardiac disease due to QT prolongation, postural hypotension, and risk of hypertensive crisis. Seizure threshold is reduced by most antidepressants in overdose (less so at normally prescribed doses), though MAOIs are safe in epilepsy. Duloxetine and bupropion can be problematic in both renal and hepatic failure.

Mania has received less attention in this chapter because manic symptoms are significantly less common than depressive symptoms in the

Table 3.4 Medication Options for Depression, Organized by Somatic Symptoms

Insomnia	SSRIs, melatonin, trazodone, mirtazapine, temazepam, zolpidem, zaleplon, ramelteon, eszopiclone, gabapentin, antihistamines
Anorexia	Mirtazapine, second generation antipsychotics (as augmentation strategy)
Fatigue and apathy	SSRIs, bupropion, venlafaxine, duloxetine, methylphenidate, amphetamines, atomoxetine, modafinil
Pain	venlafaxine, duloxetine, nortriptyline, desipramine, doxepin, amitriptryline

medical setting, and because there is less symptom overlap with medical problems; however, many of the drugs, hormones, and medical disorders that cause depression are also associated with secondary mania (see Table 3.2). As with depression, treatment options are tailored to the desired side-effect profile and pharmacokinetic/pharmacodynamic changes associated with the patient's condition. For example, while lithium may not be a first choice in patients with progressive renal insufficiency, it is the preferred mood stabilizer in the setting of acute liver disease, as all of the anticonvulsants are dependent on hepatic metabolism, and valproic acid and carbamazepine can independently cause liver failure. In a patient with no oral access, an antipsychotic with IV and/or IM formulations (such as haloperidol, olanzapine, or ziprasidone) may be preferred, or a benzodiazepine. Risperidone, olanzapine, aripiprazole, and asenapine are all available in dissolving tablets, which is convenient when a bleeding risk prevents IV or IM medication administration and a patient is uncooperative with tablets or capsules (see Tables 6.1–6.10 in Chapter 6).

Psychotherapeutic approaches are covered in detail in Chapter 8. Mood disorders have been successfully treated with interpersonal psychotherapy, cognitive behavioral therapy, and psychodynamic psychotherapy, either alone or with medications. For many patients, psychotherapy should be the first-line treatment, especially those who are apprehensive about psychiatric medications. General strategies involve helping a patient overcome a sense of demoralization and making sense of his or her life, up to and including the medical illness. Always ensure that a patient's spiritual needs are addressed, as a minister, priest, or other clergy may play an essential part in the patient's physical and emotional recovery.

Insomnia

Insomnia deserves special mention, not only as a symptom of mood and medical disorders frequently encountered in the medical setting, but also as its own unique clinical entity due to its impact on prognosis and treatment. Insomnia involves difficulty with initiating or maintaining sleep at least three nights per week with resultant daytime dysfunction.

Already a commonly encountered problem in the general population, insomnia is even more common among the hospitalized, who are likely to have sleep disruption due to pain, worsening of respiratory disorders, side effects of medications, increased stress, and the loss of a sleep-conducive environment at night. The presence of insomnia is also now recognized as a risk factor for suicidal ideation and completed suicide, independent of a comorbid mood disorder. Furthermore, residual insomnia is a predictor for recurrence of depressive symptoms; some studies have found that cotreatment of depression and insomnia yields better depression outcomes.

An important initial aspect in the diagnosis of insomnia is the differentiation between acute, transient insomnia arising in the medical wards versus a chronic insomnia that the patient brought with him to his inpatient stay. This requires the consultant to inquire about the quality of the patient's sleep in the hospital, his bedtime and wake time, and the amount and quality of sleep prior to the patient's admission.

The differential diagnosis for the new complaint of insomnia in the inpatient medical setting includes delirium, with its disruption of sleep-wake cycles; insomnia resulting from withdrawal from substances, especially sedative/hypnotic and alcohol withdrawal; medication effects, including disrupted sleep related to corticosteroids; and akathisia caused by antipsychotic medications.

In the evaluation of chronic insomnia, other common sleep disorders should be considered. In particular, obstructive sleep apnea can present with a complaint of insomnia, restless sleep, and frequent nocturia. This disorder should be screened for in patients older than 50 and in the obese by asking the patient and his or her family about snoring and nocturnal awakenings associated with gasping and choking sensations. This is especially important as sedative/hypnotics commonly used in the treatment of insomnia can worsen obstructive sleep apnea and can delay the diagnosis of this disorder, which is associated with significant neurocognitive, cardiovascular, and cerebrovascular morbidity. If this is suspected, further clinical and laboratory evaluation by a sleep specialist is warranted, and the appropriate referral should be made.

The treatment of insomnia often involves the use of medication, as described in detail in Table 3.5. It is recommended to use the lowest effective dose for the shortest possible duration, while monitoring for common side effects. These include residual daytime sedation, cognitive impairment, and impaired motor coordination, which increases the risk of falls. These effects tend to be more common and severe in elderly populations. Additionally, caution should be used in all patients with active respiratory disease since sedative/hypnotics may cause respiratory suppression.

Table 3.5 Pharmacologic Treatment of Insomnia

Treatment	Considerations of Use	Recommended Use
Short- to intermediate- acting benzodiazepines (lorazepam, triazolam, temazepam, etc.)	Tolerance and abuse potential, risk of falls and cognitive impairment; may worsen delirium	Short-term management of acute insomnia, especially with comorbid anxiety; avoid in active lung disorders, substance abuse, and the elderly
Non-benzodiazepine GABA receptor agonists (zaleplon, zolpidem, eszopiclone)	Tolerance and abuse potential, less anxiolytic effects than benzodiazepines, risk of falls and cognitive impairment, hallucinations, and complex sleep-related behaviors	Short-term management of acute insomnia; avoid in active lung disorders, substance abuse, and the elderly
Melatonin agonists (ramelteon, melatonin)	Smaller effect size limited to sleep onset, generally more benign side-effect profiles, preferable in elderly patients, may not be on formulary	Chronic initiation insomnia, preferred in the elderly, children, and substance abuse populations; may prevent and treat delirium
Mirtazapine	Metabolic side effects, may cause activation at doses > 30 mg	Comorbid MDD or GAD, when weight gain is desired; generally tolerated in the elderly, though may cause delirium
Trazodone	Shown effective short-term (< 2 weeks)	Comorbid MDD and substance abuse populations, usually tolerated in the elderly

(continued)

Table 3.5 (Continued)

Treatment	Considerations of Use	Recommended Use
Tricyclic antidepressants (doxepin, amitriptyline)	Overdose risk, anticholinergic side effects, doxepin specifically approved for insomnia at 3 mg and 6 mg dosages	Comorbid pain or migraine prophylaxis, doxepin few interactions and well tolerated at low doses; cautioned in patients with suicide attempt history
Sedating antipsychotics (quetiapine, olanzapine, etc.)	Little documented benefit, significant adverse effects	Reserve for psychosis, mania, or delirium.
Antihistamines (diphenhydramine, hydroxyzine)	Little documented benefit, risk of cognitive dysfunction and delirium	Useful for people with intermittent anxiety and insomnia, avoid in elderly

MDD = major depressive disorder; GAD = generalized anxiety disorder

Finally, the need for continued treatment of acute insomnia beyond the inpatient medical setting should be carefully re-evaluated prior to discharge. If these medications are continued, the patient should be cautioned not to consume alcohol and should be educated about potential occupational hazards such as impaired motor vehicle operation.

Conclusions

Mood disorders are commonly encountered in the medical setting. While it is not always easy to distinguish depressive symptoms from normal reactions to medical illness and treatment, psychiatric intervention can improve both psychiatric and medical outcomes. Insomnia is important both as an independent phenomenon as well as a key factor in episodes of depression and mania.

Key Points

- A wide array of etiological factors may underlie mood symptoms in the medical patient.
- Treatment of mood symptoms may improve medical outcomes.
- Insomnia is widespread and can be a symptom of and a trigger for mood episodes.

Disclosures

Dr. Severance has no conflicts of interest to disclose.

Dr. Hope has no conflicts of interest to disclose.

Further Reading

Berman AL, Pomili M (Eds.) (2005). *Medical Conditions Associated with Suicide Risk*. Washington, DC: American Association of Suicidology.

Berkman LF, Blumenthal J, et al. (2003). Effects of treating depression and low perceived social support on clinical events after myocardial infarction: The Enhancing Recovery in Coronary Heart Disease Patients (ENRICHD) randomized trial. *JAMA.*, *289*, 3106–3116.

Cohen BJ (Ed.) (2003). *Theory and Practice of Psychiatry*. New York: Oxford University Press.

Kendler K, Gardner C, et al. (2006). Toward a comprehensive developmental model for major depression in men. *Am J Psychiat.*, *163*(1), 115–124.

Kleinman A (1991). *Rethinking Psychiatry: From Cultural Category to Personal Experience*. New York: The Free Press.

Mackinnon RA, Michels R, et al. (2006). *The Psychiatric Interview in Clinical Practice*. Arlington: APP.

Ohayon MM (2002). Epidemiology of insomnia: What we know and what we still need to learn. *Sleep Med Rev.*, *6*(2), 97–111.

Young JS, Bourgeois JA, et al. (2008) Sleep in hospitalized medical patients, Part 1: Factors affecting sleep. *J Hosp Med.*, *3*(6), 473–482.

Young JS, Bourgeois JA, et al. (2009) Sleep in hospitalized medical patients, Part 2: Behavioral and pharmacological management of sleep disturbances. *J Hosp Med.*, *4*(1), 50–59.

Anxiety in the General Medical Setting

Robert Hudak and Rolf G. Jacob

Introduction

Anxiety is exceptional among psychiatric symptoms in that it also presents in the absence of overt pathology and can occur in virtually everyone. As a result, complaints of anxiety are common among patients hospitalized in the medical setting and are frequently cited as reasons for psychiatric consultation. Psychosomatic medicine physicians need to identify the etiology of the anxiety in order to appropriately address it. In a C-L setting, psychiatrists will be asked to diagnose and differentiate anxiety arising from multiple causes, including the following:

- Anxiety related to a primary anxiety disorder (e.g., panic disorder or generalized anxiety disorder);
- Anxiety as a symptom of a medical disorder (e.g., hyperthyroidism);
- Situational anxiety in response to the stress of medical illness and hospitalization (e.g., fear of a pending surgery, fear of pending test results, stress from difficulties at home); or
- Anxiety arising from current stressors triggering symptoms of a pre-existing psychiatric disorder (e.g., agitation in a patient with autism spectrum disorder in an unfamiliar setting).

The treatment of these various causes of anxiety will differ greatly and require the clinician to approach these patients, and the medical treatment team, in different ways. For example, the treatment of a patient suffering from anxiety associated with ventilator weaning is markedly different from the treatment of a patient presenting with chest pains secondary to panic disorder. Careful diagnosis is critical in making appropriate treatment decisions, as anxiety tends to be under-diagnosed and inadequately treated in the medical setting. Potential reasons for under-treatment of anxiety include time pressure, knowledge deficits, and lack of focus on psychiatric symptoms in patients with complex medical problems (Wise, 2008).

Anxiety can also be a risk factor for the onset and progression of medical symptoms. This relationship has been studied to the greatest extent for cardiovascular disorders, given the impact of anxiety on adrenergic systems, and the direct role that catecholamines play in modulating cardiac function. In several prospective studies, a positive relationship was found between anxiety and later myocardial infarctions (reviewed in Thurston et al., 2013). Less consistently, anxiety has also been shown to precede the occurrence of cardiac arrhythmias (Peacock & Whang, 2013). Recent evidence also suggests that anxiety may be a risk factor for the later development of stroke (Lambiase, 2013). Given this emerging evidence, early treatment of anxiety disorders can be advocated as an effort toward "primary prevention" of cardiovascular disorders.

As part of the consultation process, the psychiatrist should ensure that an adequate workup for anxiety has been performed. While this may not be necessary in cases where there is a clear and recent precipitant for the anxiety symptoms, such as acute onset of nervousness and panic upon learning of a cancer diagnosis, it should be considered in most patients, including those with premorbid anxiety disorders. In order to rule out medical issues posing as anxiety, tests should include a physical exam; complete blood count; electrolyte panel with blood urea nitrogen (BUN), creatinine, and fasting glucose; liver function tests; TSH and calcium levels; urinalysis; electrocardiograph (EKG); and a urine drug screen. Further testing can be ordered if clinical suspicion warrants.

Anxiety can be dysphoric, and a patient's chief complaint may be "depression" and not anxiety.

Anxiety Disorders in the Medical Setting

Anxiety disorders are markedly under-diagnosed in the medical setting, with as many as 50% of patients not being diagnosed or receiving inadequate treatment (Wise, 2008). This is particularly salient for C-L psychiatry due to the fact that almost 90% of patients with symptoms of anxiety present with physical symptoms as opposed to psychiatric symptoms (Roy-Byrne & Wagner, 2004). When patients present to primary care physicians (PCPs) with psychiatric symptoms, most PCPs readily recognize and address these issues. However, when patients present with predominantly physical symptoms of an underlying psychiatric disorder with no other psychiatric symptoms, these disorders are infrequently recognized and treated (Culpepper, 2003). According to Culpepper, there are four ways that patients with anxiety disorders typically present in the medical setting:

- Somatic complaints, which can include a variety of physical symptoms ranging from fatigue to insomnia to pain or gastrointestinal complaints;
- Exaggeration of underlying medical symptoms that typically would not be as distressing to other patients;
- Specific psychiatric complaints, although this presentation is less common;
- Normalization of behavioral health symptoms, that is, acknowledging psychiatric distress but blaming their symptoms on physical illness, stress, or lack of exercise.

A psychiatrist will often be consulted on somaticizing patients, not for help with the treatment of underlying psychiatric distress, but simply in response to frustration from the referring physician, family members, or other members of the primary team. A careful history can help determine if the underlying issue is a so-called "difficult" patient or a primary anxiety disorder as described in the following sections.

Generalized Anxiety Disorder

Generalized anxiety disorder (GAD) is a psychiatric disorder that is characterized by excessive anxiety and worry present on most days for at least a 6-month period, with the individual finding it difficult to control the worry. The worry is generally age appropriate and centers on everyday concerns and routine life circumstances. Often the worry takes the form of catastrophizing, in which the person imagines events in a worst-case scenario. Physical complaints such as pain or insomnia are typical presentations. Proper diagnosis is critical in the C-L setting, as this is a chronic condition that necessitates appropriate treatment and referral.

People with GAD will often report that they have always been a worrier, or that they have been anxious much of their life.

Panic Disorder

Panic disorder is defined as recurrent unexpected panic attacks, which are characterized by an abrupt surge of intense fear or intense discomfort that reaches a peak within minutes. This is accompanied by physical symptoms such as palpitations or GI distress. While panic attacks can be normal and non-pathological, patients with panic disorder will have persistent worry about further attacks or maladaptive changes due to the attacks.

Patients with panic disorder will frequently present to emergency medical settings with a rule-out diagnosis of acute myocardial infarction. Anecdotally, many cardiologists report that they see more panic attacks in the emergency setting than cardiac events. Due to the fact that people with panic disorder have a greater utilization of healthcare resources and health-related disability than people without panic, appropriate intervention is vital.

People with medical disorders often will have physical symptoms that mimic panic symptoms, such as shortness of breath experienced by patients with asthma or COPD. This can be difficult to distinguish from panic symptoms, as it is a natural reaction to experience anxiety when breathing is compromised. In order to make an appropriate diagnosis, the C-L psychiatrist should review the patient's history of anxiety prior to his or her illness and look for other emotional and physical symptoms unrelated to the medical condition (e.g., paresthesias in the asthma patient) and the fear of dying or going crazy. The psychiatrist should also ensure that the underlying medical condition is adequately treated.

- In panic disorder, panic attacks will often wake patients from their sleep.
- The symptom of feeling that one is suffocating or needing to consciously remember to breathe as one is falling asleep is pathognomonic for anxiety disorders.
- In cases of tachycardia with abrupt offset, suspect cardiac arrhythmia.

Obsessive-Compulsive and Related Disorders

Obsessive-Compulsive Disorder

While obsessive-compulsive disorder (OCD) is no longer classified as an anxiety disorder, anxiety can be a prominent consequence of obsessional content (e.g., a person with obsessions about germs may feel anxiety after touching a restroom doorknob), and these patients often present in the medical setting. The diagnosis of OCD is made by noting the presence of obsessions and compulsions that are time-consuming, or that cause clinically significant distress or impairment. OCD is a chronic condition affecting about 2.5% of the population. People with OCD are often ashamed or embarrassed by their symptoms and may go to great lengths to avoid talking about them. They are frequently high utilizers of medical services, particularly if the focus of their illness is somatic obsessions, or if the symptoms of their illness lead to medical complications (e.g., dermatitis in chronic hand washers or medication non-adherence in people afraid of poisoning). It is common for people with OCD to have markedly increased anxiety levels in the unfamiliar environment of a hospital.

Body Dysmorphic Disorder

Body dysmorphic disorder (BDD) is an obsessive-compulsive-related disorder that is characterized by an intense preoccupation with an imagined or slight defect in personal appearance. The illness is associated with a high level of distress and anxiety, as well as impaired psychosocial functioning, poor quality of life, poor insight, and a high rate of suicidality. Initial contact with psychiatry often occurs in the medical/surgical setting, where patients may seek numerous and inappropriate cosmetic surgical procedures. In some cases, patients with BDD will perform self-surgeries in order to relieve the distress associated with the illness; it is vital that the consulting psychiatrist distinguish this from self-mutilation secondary to a psychotic or personality disorder. The psychiatrist should encourage the surgical team not to perform cosmetic procedures on BDD patients who are not in active treatment.

> The role of the psychiatrist in working with patients with BDD should not be to reassure the patient that he or she looks normal or that no defects are apparent; instead, the psychiatrist should offer the suggestion that there is different treatment for the defect other than surgery, and should refer the patient to an expert in BDD.

Anxiety as a Symptom of Medical Conditions

In *DSM-5*, medically-induced anxiety conditions are categorized as "Anxiety Disorders Due to Another Medical Condition" (293.84), or if the anxiety is medication-induced, "Substance/Medication-Induced Anxiety Disorder with onset after medication use." The assumption is that the anxiety symptoms are a physiological effect of the medical condition (e.g., hyperthyroidism), rather than just cognitive worry regarding the meaning or consequence of the disorder (e.g., cancer diagnosis). If the anxiety is triggered by an acute stressor, *DSM-5* would suggest a diagnosis of "Adjustment Disorder With Anxiety" if the "adjustment" is considered to be maladaptive, but would not consider it pathological if the patient has a "normal" anxiety reaction to the catastrophic news; see discussion of "situational anxiety" later in this chapter).

Anxiety symptoms can present as symptoms of many medical conditions, including the following:

- Endocrine: for example, hyperthyroidism, pheochromocytoma, hypoglycemia;
- Cardiac: for example, angina, arrhythmia;
- Pulmonary: for example, COPD, asthma, weaning from respirators;
- Neurological: for example, migraines, vestibular dysfunction, balance disorders, stroke;
- Metabolic: for example, porphyria.

Substance-Induced Anxiety Disorders

In patients with substance-induced anxiety disorders, panic attacks and anxiety develop after exposure to or withdrawal from a medication or substance (see Table 4.1). Using *DSM-5* diagnostic criteria, the substance must be one that is capable of producing panic or anxiety, and the disturbance cannot be better explained by an independent psychiatric or anxiety disorder or occur solely in the presence of a delirium (e.g., delirium tremens). Anxiety disorders suppressed by substance use may re-emerge after use is stopped, but this would not be considered a substance-induced anxiety disorder. Urine and blood toxicology screens can be vital in making a diagnosis of substance-induced anxiety disorder. A broad range of prescribed medications can commonly cause anxiety symptoms as well, and these can include the following:

- Anesthetics and analgesics;
- Anticholinergics;
- Anticonvulsants;
- Antidepressants (may occur in the context of akathesia), including SSRIs, SNRIs, and others;
- Antiemetics, especially metoclopramide, promethazine, and prochlorperazine (usually in the context of akathesia);
- Antihistamines;
- Antihypertensives, including beta blockers and ACE inhibitors;
- Antiparkinsonian medications (especially compounds with levodopa);
- Antipsychotics (usually in the context of akathesia);
- Asthma medications, such as albuterol and theophylline;
- Benzodiazepines (seen as a paradoxical reaction);
- Corticosteroids;
- Lithium;
- Nasal decongestants, including phenylephrine and pseudoephedrine;
- Sympathomimetics, which includes amphetamines and methylphenidate;
- Thyroid medication.

Situational Anxiety

Anxiety is a normal and appropriate emotional response that is experienced by virtually everyone. It can be triggered by stresses in the environment, such as relationship problems or an important examination. In the medical setting, people are more likely to experience significant anxiety due to health concerns, financial strain, and being in unfamiliar and uncomfortable surroundings. In some cases, the symptoms of anxiety due to situational circumstances can mimic medical conditions. (e.g., pulmonary or cardiac conditions). If the patient experiences situational anxiety that that leads to maladaptive behavioral symptoms, a diagnosis of adjustment disorder might be warranted.

Table 4.1 Common Causes of Substance-Induced Anxiety

Substances Capable of Producing Anxiety with Use or Intoxication	Substances Capable of Producing Anxiety upon Withdrawal
Alcohol	Alcohol
Caffeine	Opioids
Cannabis	Barbiturates
Phenylcyclidine	Benzodiazepines
LSD and other hallucinogens	Non-benzodiazepine sedatives (e.g., zolpidem)
Stimulants/amphetamines/cocaine	Stimulants/amphetamines/cocaine
Inhalants	

Treatment

Treatment of anxiety in the medical setting involves different facets. See Figure 4.1 for a basic approach to managing and treating anxiety. During the evaluation process, the clinician needs to keep in mind both the current needs of the patient while in the hospital as well as post-discharge. Initiating a psychiatric medication on a medical/surgical inpatient may do more harm than good if there is not a trained provider available for follow-up after hospitalization.

Cognitive behavioral therapy (CBT) should be considered a first-line treatment for situational anxiety as well as anxiety disorders.

Collaborative Care and Education

The use of a collaborative care model, in which the psychiatrist and primary care provider (PCP) co-manage patients, and the PCP is educated about psychiatric illness and treatment guidelines, has led to improved outcomes for patients suffering from mood and anxiety disorders (Tylee & Walters, 2007). The psychiatrist should educate both the medical team and the patient regarding the impact of the patient's anxiety and effective treatments in order to improve outcome.

Medication Management

Medication is the most commonly used treatment of anxiety in the medical/surgical setting. Diagnosis is critical in this area, because the decision of whether to use medication and then the choice of which medication are dependent upon the etiology of the anxiety. If the anxiety is secondary to a different psychiatric disorder, medication treatment should be focused upon treating the primary disorder (e.g., antipsychotics in the case of an anxious schizophrenic patient or mood stabilizers for anxiety associated with bipolar depression). Benzodiazepines may play a role, if medically appropriate, as an adjunct treatment for anxiety in these patients. Patients with anxiety or obsessive-compulsive and related disorders will typically require antidepressant therapy.

Situational anxiety, including panic symptoms, that are appropriate responses to stressful circumstances can also be treated with short-term benzodiazepine therapy. If the patient is having anxiety secondary to a medical condition, treatment should focus on the underlying medical condition. If adjunct anxiolytic treatment is needed, the choice of medication would be dependent upon the medical condition. For example, anxiety associated with hyperthyroidism may linger during ablation treatment and would be appropriately treated with benzodiazepines; however, if agitation and anxiety are secondary to delirium, treatment with antipsychotics could be appropriate, as they may improve the course of delirium and benzodiazepines may worsen confusion.

In contrast to situational anxiety where benzodiazepine treatment would be appropriate, the presence of an anxiety disorder would necessitate the use of antidepressants or other anxiolytics such as buspirone. Benzodiazepine treatment of primary anxiety disorders should be used with caution. The use of benzodiazepines in anxiety disorders can actually worsen the response to antidepressant therapy, making the

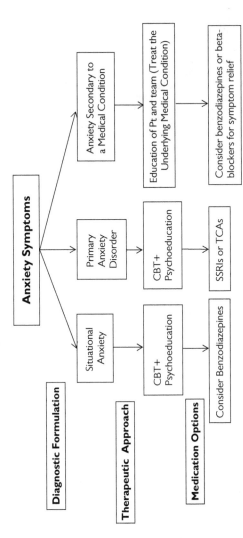

Figure 4.1 Treatment of Anxiety in a Medical Setting

antidepressants less effective than when used alone (Pollack et al., 2003). While benzodiazepines can help improve primary anxiety in the short term, the consulting psychiatrist will most often not be seeing the patient outside the medical hospital; therefore, any recommendations made for benzodiazepine use should be made with caution, as clinical experience shows that benzodiazepines are often continued long after discharge. Thus a proposed bridge course of benzodiazepines becomes long-term treatment with a less favorable risk/benefit ratio.

If antidepressants are to be initiated while the patient is in the hospital, selection of a proper agent is vital. Patients with OCD or obsessive-compulsive-related disorders often find SSRI treatment more effective than SNRI treatment or other atypical antidepressants (e.g., buproprion or mirtazapine; Denys et al., 2004). Therefore, patients with OCD should be treated with SSRIs exclusively. For patients with anxiety disorders such as GAD, personality disorder, or anxiety disorder NOS, the use of SSRIs is also recommended as first-line treatment, as SNRI therapy is not as effective for these illnesses (Andrisano et al., 2013).

Conclusion

When consulted on patients for anxiety in the medical setting, proper diagnosis is critical in determining the cause of the anxiety that the patient is experiencing, whether it is normal and appropriate anxiety or whether the anxiety is secondary to a medical or psychiatric disorder. Proper treatment of anxiety in the medical setting includes education of both the patient and the medical team, with SSRI treatment preferred for patients with primary anxiety disorders, and benzodiazepine therapy being used for appropriate patients with anxiety due to medical conditions or situational anxiety. In combination with CBT, patients can experience improved outcomes and quality of life, not just for their mental and emotional health, but for their medical conditions as well.

Key Points

- Anxiety is found in normal individuals as well as in individuals with pathology.
- Numerous medical conditions can mimic anxiety symptoms.
- Anxiety disorders are common in the medical setting; the medical setting can even induce anxiety issues.
- Excessive anxiety places the patient at greater medical risk.
- Benzodiazepines can be used to treat normal, appropriate anxiety (e.g., fear of a pending surgery).
- SSRIs and TCAs are more appropriate medications to treat primary anxiety disorders.

Disclosures

Dr. Hudak has no conflicts of interest to disclose.

Dr. Jacob has no conflicts of interest to disclose.

Further Reading

American Psychiatric Association (2013). *Diagnostic and Statistical Manual of Mental Disorders,* 5th ed. Arlington, VA: American Psychiatric Publishing.

Andrisano C, Chiesa A, et al. (2013). Newer antidepressants and panic disorder: A meta-analysis. *Int Clin Psychopharmacol., 28*(1), 33–45.

Culpepper L (2003). Use of alogorithms to treat anxiety in primary care. *J Clin Psychiat., 64*(suppl 2), 30–33.

Denys D, van Megen HJ, et al. (2004). A double-blind switch study of paroxetine and venlafaxine in obsessive-compulsive disorder. *J Clin Psychiat., 65*(1), 37–43.

Peacock J, Whang W (2013). Psychological distress and arrhythmia: risk prediction and potential modifiers. *Prog Cardiovasc Dis., 55,* 582–589.

Pollack MH, Simon NM, et al. (2003). Combined paroxetine and clonazepam treatment strategies compared to paroxetine monotherapy for panic disorder. *J Psychopharmacol., 17*(3), 276–282.

Roy-Byrne PP, Wagner A (2004). Primary care perspectives on generalized anxiety disorder. *J Clin Psychiat., 65*(suppl 13), 20–26.

Thurston RC, Rewak M, et al. (2013). An anxious heart: Anxiety and the onset of cardiovascular diseases. *Prog Cardiovasc Dis., 55,* 524–537.

Tylee A, Walters P (2007). Underrecognition of anxiety and mood disorders in primary care: Why does the problem exist and what can be done? *J Clin Psychiat., 68*(suppl 2), 27–30.

Wise TN (2008). Update on consultation-liaison psychiatry (psychosomatic medicine). *Curr Opin Psychiat., 21*(2), 196–200.

Exercises

1. Examples of non-pathological anxiety may include all of the following EXCEPT:
   a. Panic attacks in anticipation of a pending surgery
   b. Hyper-vigilance in a patient with schizophrenia who believes the government is spying on him
   c. Pulling out lines in the ICU after cardiac surgery in a patient who is not oriented to time
   d. Worries that not successfully treating an addiction problem will lead to loss of employment and spouse leaving

2. First-line medications to treat generalized anxiety disorder would include:
   a. Clonazepam
   b. Venlafaxine
   c. Mirtazapine
   d. Fluoxetine
   e. Trazodone

3. People with panic disorder will often be woken from their sleep with a panic attack.
   a. True
   b. False

4. People with anxiety disorders will often report depression as their primary complaint instead of anxiety.
   a. True
   b. False

5. Substances that can induce or contribute to anxiety include all of the following EXCEPT:
   a. Cannabis
   b. Diazepam
   c. Theophylline
   d. Mirtazapine
   e. Diphenhydramine
   f. All of the above can

Answers: (1) c (2) d (3) a (4) a (5) f

Somatic Symptom and Related Disorders

Christopher R. Dobbelstein

Introduction

Medical teams often consult psychiatric consultation-liaison (C-L) teams to provide guidance for patients who appear excessively concerned about medical illnesses or who report subjective symptoms that do not correspond with objective presentation or with known patterns of disease. This chapter will describe a general approach to interacting with these patients and will provide guidance on the diagnosis and management of somatic symptom disorder, illness anxiety disorder, conversion disorder, factitious disorder, and malingering.

General Approach

Patients with excessive medical concern or disproportionate symptoms often have known or undiagnosed medical illness, but the degree of dysfunction that they experience exceeds what is normally expected for patients with their objective findings.

Primary medical teams may feel angry that patients who they believe are not "really" sick are wasting their valuable time and expertise. The patients, too, may feel angry if they believe that their primary teams consulted psychiatry because they think that they are "fakers" and that their symptoms are "all in their heads." The patients may be guarded when interviewed by psychiatrists, as they may be fearful of what the psychiatrists will conclude and how this will influence their medical care in the future. In order to effectively diagnose and treat these patients, it is critical for psychiatrists to start with a solid working relationship with both the medical teams and the patients.

Start by asking the medical team what their concern is. If the problem is "symptoms out of proportion to objective findings," find out specifically what symptoms and findings are discordant. Ask about the patient's medical illness and how the patient's symptoms appear excessive. If the concern is for excessive anxiety about the course of the patient's medical illness, find out what the most likely prognosis is so that you understand what an appropriate patient response would be. If the medical team is feeling frustrated, encourage them to share this with you, and empathize with their feelings. Listening to their concerns can relieve some of their frustration and help them to be more empathic with the patient.

Next, interview the patient. He or she has likely been suffering profoundly, so it is crucial to express empathy from the beginning of the interview. Even deceptive patients are often in difficult situations and need help finding relief from their distress. If the patient appears guarded, ask how he feels about psychiatry having been consulted and if he fears that his medical team may undertreat his problems based on your assessment. Tell the patient that the medical team consulted psychiatry because they want to better understand his situation and that you will do your best to help him get better. Ask what physical symptoms the patient is having and how these symptoms are affecting his life. Reinforce that you believe that he is truly experiencing his symptoms. Ask what he thinks may be causing the symptoms—this can provide insight into his cognitions and behaviors. In order for the patient to feel heard, it may be necessary to listen to a long account of the various symptoms, tests, procedures, and diagnoses that he has endured, as well as a description of how the healthcare system may have let him down. Inquire about any other stressors in the patient's life and how he is coping with them. Screen for other psychiatric disorders, since these may be associated with physical symptoms. With the patient's consent, obtain collateral history from family and friends in order to accurately understand the patient's functional ability and social stressors. At the conclusion of the assessment, tell the patient what your diagnosis is (see the following section) and what you will be telling the medical team. The patient may disagree with your opinion, but being truthful with him will improve communication between him and the medical team.

Diagnosis and Management of Specific Disorders

The fifth edition of the *Diagnostic and Statistical Manual of Mental Disorders* (*DSM-5*) fundamentally changed the way that abnormal illness behavior is conceptualized, compared with *DSM-IV-TR*. Unlike the somatoform disorders of *DSM-IV-TR*, which were grouped together because they all required ruling out medical illness, the somatic symptom and related disorders of *DSM-5* are grouped based on the patients' excessive distress and impairment regarding physical symptoms or illness. This diagnostic grouping includes somatic symptom disorder (SSD), illness anxiety disorder (IAD), conversion disorder (CD), psychological factors affecting other medical conditions, factitious disorder, other specified somatic symptom and related disorder, and unspecified somatic symptom and related disorder (see Table 5.1). SSD replaces *DSM-IV-TR*'s somatization disorder, pain disorder, and undifferentiated somatoform disorder and also includes approximately 75% of those previously diagnosed with hypochondriasis (the other 25% who do not have physical symptoms are now diagnosed with IAD).

Epidemiology

Since SSD and IAD were only recently defined, epidemiologic data are extrapolated from studies using *DSM-IV-TR* diagnoses (Abbey et al., 2011; American Psychiatric Association, 2013; Haase, 2006; Strain & Loigman, 2006; Straker & Hyler, 2006; Yutzy, 2006) (see Table 5.2).

Table 5.1 Overview of Disorders and Conditions Associated with Abnormal Illness Behavior

Disorder/ Condition	Physical Symptom?	Rule Out Medical Cause?	Intentional Deception?	Primary External Benefit?
Somatic Symptom Disorder	Yes	No	No	No
Illness Anxiety Disorder	No	No	No	No
Conversion Disorder	Yes	Yes	No	No
Factitious Disorder	Yes	Yes	Yes	No
Malingering	Yes	Yes	Yes	Yes

Table 5.2 Epidemiology of Somatic Symptom and Related Disorders

Diagnosis	Prevalence	Male:Female	Age of Onset
Somatic Symptom Disorder	General population: 4%–19%	1:10 for somatization, likely more equal for SSD	Teens to 20s, maybe older
Illness Anxiety Disorder	General population: 0.25%–1% Medical or psychiatric settings: 1%–2%	1:1	Teens to 20s
Conversion Disorder	General population: 0.04%–0.3% Neurology patients: 4.5%–15%	1:1 to 1:10	Teens to 20s
Factitious Disorder	7.5% in medical setting in one study	More female	Unknown

Somatic Symptom Disorder

Diagnosis

A diagnosis of SSD as described in *DSM-5* requires that a patient experience excessive distress as the result of one or more somatic symptoms, with persistently dysfunctional thoughts, feelings, or behaviors surrounding the symptoms. It does not matter how many symptoms a patient has or what the symptoms are. Patients can be diagnosed with SSD even if their physical symptoms have a physiologic basis if their distress is excessive (e.g., paralyzing fear of another heart attack after the first one occurs). The question of whether the symptom is caused by physiologic dysfunction is left to the medical providers to answer; the psychiatrist's role is to help patients decrease their excessive distress. Also, some patients have medically unexplained symptoms, but this does not mean that they have a psychiatric disorder; it could be that a cause will be discovered in the future. SSD, factitious disorder, and malingering are not mutually exclusive, as patients can have aspects of all three conditions.

Typical Course and Clinical Features

Patients with SSD suffer profoundly from their symptoms, often seeking care from numerous medical providers because the treatments that they receive do not adequately treat their suffering. They are usually not reassured by negative test results because these do not validate their experience. Providers often order unnecessary or duplicates of tests and procedures; they may be fearful of missing medical problems or may be unaware that the tests were already performed at other institutions. Submitting to so many tests and procedures increases the risk of side effects and complications, thus compounding the patient's suffering. Providing patients with an accurate diagnosis of SSD not only guides useful treatment (see the following section), but spares unnecessary medical burdens and costs. The course is usually chronic or remitting and relapsing, but some patients do experience permanent remission of symptoms.

Treatment

As noted above, it is essential to cultivate a good working relationship with the patient and the medical team. Positive relationships can be therapeutic if they help the patient to feel more understood, and can also improve his willingness to engage in treatment planning. The patient may not see his concern or behavior as excessive, but if the clinician demonstrates to him an understanding of the details of all of his medical concerns, the patient will be more willing to try suggestions to improve his functioning despite those medical problems.

The most effective treatment for patients with excessive somatic distress and dysfunction is cognitive behavioral therapy (CBT). Studies have shown that CBT improves function, relieves psychological distress, decreases care utilization, and occasionally decreases physical symptoms (Abbey et al., 2011). While CBT is usually provided in the outpatient setting, it can be helpful to introduce some CBT concepts while the patient is seen in the medical hospital. Cognitive behavioral theory (see Figure 5.1) posits that abnormal cognitions cause patients to interpret physical sensations (which can be due to mental distress, normal physiologic processes, or minor physical disease) as "symptoms" of severe disease and to respond to these symptoms emotionally and behaviorally. Various harmful cycles then perpetuate these cognitions. Becoming upset about a symptom can sometimes worsen that very symptom as patients become hypervigilant and experience autonomic arousal. The health system may cause the patient to undergo diagnostic tests that can increase anxiety. Those who overreact to symptoms tend to assume that any symptom must mean that disease is present. This assumption can be due to prior experiences of the patient or other people in his life. The goal of the cognitive behavioral therapist is to discern what specific feedback loops are occurring in a particular patient and to use cognitive and behavioral strategies (e.g., exposure and response prevention, behavioral experiments, etc.) to gradually stop these cycles by substituting dysfunctional thoughts with more balanced ones.

For example (see text in *italics* in Figure 5.1), if a patient experiences epigastric discomfort, his beliefs and assumptions will influence his assessment of this discomfort. A man who just consumed a spicy meal may interpret the discomfort as heartburn, but a man with a history of diagnosed coronary artery disease may interpret it as angina. If a patient who has ruled out heart disease continues to fear that he is having angina despite appropriate reassurance, it may be because his beliefs and assumptions lead him to assume that all chest pain must

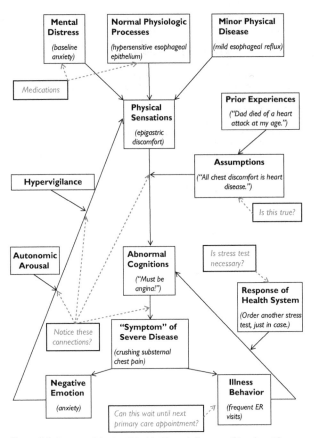

Figure 5.1 Cognitive Behavioral Model of Somatic Symptom Disorder with *examples in italics* and possible interventions in dashed arrows.

mean heart disease. Perhaps this is because he has a strong family history of heart disease or because someone he knew had a particularly tragic cardiac death. He could be hypersensitive to normal amounts of stomach acid in his distal esophagus, or he could have mild esophageal reflux. It is also possible that anxiety is causing this symptom directly. If his concern is excessive for his medical problem, then he can be diagnosed as having SSD. He might manifest his excessive concern by frequenting medical providers in order to be reassured that he is not having a heart attack. The effects of this reassurance may be short-lived if his sensations, cognitions, and assumptions persist. His concern may cause him to be especially vigilant to his epigastric area so that he notices minute sensations, even those that would normally go unnoticed, thus perpetuating the cycle. A goal of therapy would be for him to notice his sensations but not assume that he is having a heart attack, perhaps by helping him to remember that his prior investigations have been negative. If he finds himself spending an excessive amount of time monitoring himself for symptoms, then the therapist may ask him how useful spending time in this way has been. Naming his disorder as SSD could also help the healthcare system to do less testing, which would both decrease costs and side effects and show him that he is not sick enough to need all this testing—a form of exposure and response prevention. While the patient may never be completely free of his concern, therapy can help him to live a richer life nevertheless. For a more thorough description of specific strategies for doing CBT in these populations, see articles in the Further Reading section (Salkovskis, 1992; Sharpe et al., 1992).

Antidepressant medications may also be helpful for SSD. They can decrease anxiety about the patient's symptoms, even if the sensations still persist, and they may decrease neuropathic pain and gut hypersensitivity (Fass & Dickman, 2006).

Illness Anxiety Disorder

Diagnosis

Patients who have excessive anxiety about being or becoming ill but who do not have any signs or symptoms of the feared illness may be diagnosed with IAD. In *DSM-IV-TR*, these patients, along with a subset of patients with SSD who have excessive concern about their physical symptoms, were diagnosed with hypochondriasis. The difference between IAD and SSD is that patients with IAD have no physical symptoms, while those with SSD do. If there is legitimate reason for concern, such as a rich family history of the feared illness, the patient's fear must be clearly excessive. Beyond the concern regarding a specific illness, these patients tend to be overly preoccupied with their health in general, checking themselves for signs of illness or visiting medical providers frequently. Often these patients' concerns change from one illness to another over their lifetimes. Some patients refuse to seek any medical care out of intense fear of what will be discovered, and these patients can suffer from lack of timely care of medical problems.

Typical Course and Clinical Features

Patients with IAD often spend a large amount of time monitoring their bodies for signs of illness and doing research on feared medical diagnoses. This preoccupation can cause profound dysfunction in the patient's life, interfering with relationships and with work. Some patients use a large amount of medical resources but are not reassured by negative results of diagnostic tests.

Treatment
Like SSD, the doctor-patient relationship is of paramount importance. CBT can improve anxiety-related cognitions and behaviors. Antidepressants can decrease preoccupation but may not completely remove the idea that something is wrong.

Conversion Disorder

Diagnosis
According to *DSM-5*, CD is diagnosed when patients experience distressing neurological symptoms that are incompatible with known pathologic processes. Unconscious production and association with psychological factors are no longer required, as they were in *DSM-IV-TR*, since neither of these criteria can be empirically proven. Clinically, these patients do not appear to intentionally cause their symptoms, and stress does tend to exacerbate them. In SSD, it is the excessive concern about physical symptoms that is the disorder, but in CD, it is the pseudo-neurological symptom itself that is the disorder.

   Diagnosis can often be difficult, especially since 5%–15% of patients with CD also have a neurological disease (Haase, 2006). A thorough history and physical examination are usually sufficient to make the diagnosis, but other diagnostic tests are occasionally required, such as video electroencephalography (EEG) for non-epileptic seizures, electromyography for conversion paralysis, or MRI for pseudo-multiple sclerosis. Table 5.3 lists tests that help to distinguish true neurological diseases from CD and contrasts these with tests that do not help make this distinction.

Typical Course and Clinical Features
Patients with CD can have symptoms that mimic any kind of neurological dysfunction, including seizures, paresis, numbness, or movement disorders, and symptoms tend to worsen with stress. Episodes usually start abruptly and dramatically, last two to three months, and then resolve, but relapse is common. People are more likely to have CD if they live in a culture or family in which other ways of expressing emotion are not acceptable. Conversion symptoms tend to disappear when the patient believes that she is not being observed, perhaps because the symptoms serve as a way of communicating distress. Patients tend to be especially suggestible or hypnotizable, to come from poorer or rural areas, and to have less formal education. They often have a history of childhood trauma and may have comorbid PTSD, SSD, mood disorder, dissociative disorder, or personality disorder. Having a neurological disease increases the risk of having a conversion symptom that mimics it. Some patients appear to be surprisingly unconcerned about their symptoms (this has been termed *la belle indifférence*). Dissociative symptoms (e.g., depersonalization, derealization, and dissociative amnesia) are common features but are not necessary for the diagnosis. Of note, dissociative pseudo-neurological phenomena that do not cause any distress or dysfunction (e.g., trances as part of cultural rituals) are not considered to be CD.

Table 5.3 Helpful Signs (Occur with CD but not with Neurological Disease) versus Unhelpful Signs (Can Occur with Both CD and with Neurological Disease) for Distinguishing CD from Neurological Disease

Helpful Signs (CD only)	Unhelpful Signs (CD or neurological disease)
Weakness	Weakness
Hoover's sign (see Stone et al., 2002)	Collapsing weakness
Dragging gait	Midline splitting
Weak ankle plantar-flexion on exam but can walk on tiptoes	Split vibration across the forehead
Seizures	Seizures
Eyes shut during episode	Tongue biting
Resistance to having eyes pulled open	Incontinence
Episode lasting more than 2 minutes	Pelvic thrusting
Interacting with examiner during episode	Injuries
"Post-ictal" crying	
Video-EEG without epileptic activity	
Movement Disorders	Movement Disorders
Tremor disappears when distracted	Worsening with anxiety
Tremor matches rate of oscillation of opposite extremity	
Visual Symptoms	General
Tubular field defect	*La belle indifference*
Spiraling visual fields	Looking depressed

Psychosomatic Medicine Pocket Cards, ©2014, University of Pittsburgh and UPMC. Reprinted and used with permission; all rights reserved.

Treatment

Start by telling the patient that these symptoms are not caused by any neurological disease and are most likely due to stress. Some patients respond favorably to this news and welcome interventions to relieve stress, but others feel dismissed by the diagnosis and insist that the symptoms are not "all in their heads." In this case, tell the patient that you know that the symptom is real to her and that you believe that she is not producing it voluntarily. Tell the patient that you have seen many patients like this get better and that you expect her to get better as well; this reassuring statement, coming from a person with authority, can produce remarkable results in these typically suggestible patients. Give patients a face-saving way to regain functioning, such as recommending physical therapy for strengthening. If hospital staff feel annoyed by the patient because the symptoms are inconsistent or fluctuate according to who is watching, tell them that the patient is likely using the symptom to express feelings that are verbally inexpressible. Since the symptoms serve to communicate distress, it would not be logical for the patient to have the symptom unless someone is there to observe it. This explanation, while perhaps not true in all cases, can help to strengthen staff's empathy toward patients with CD.

For many patients, conversion serves as a maladaptive mechanism for coping with stress. Using techniques such as relaxation, CBT, or psychodynamic therapy, the therapist can decrease the need for conversion by helping the patient to find more adaptive coping strategies. Definitive treatment usually occurs in the outpatient setting, but as in SSD, introducing the patient to some concepts while hospitalized can be helpful. See Chapter 8 for more strategies to improve patients' coping skills. Be sure to screen for comorbid psychiatric disorders and treat those as well.

Factitious Disorder Imposed on Self and on Another

Diagnosis

Factitious disorder (FD) imposed on oneself is a psychiatric disorder in which the patient seeks care for a medical or psychiatric disorder that is either feigned or caused by the patient without any clear external reward for being ill. This is done by pretending to have symptoms, exaggerating symptoms, or harming one's own body in order to create medical or psychiatric problems that would not otherwise exist.

FD imposed on another is diagnosed when the patient harms his children or other vulnerable dependents (such as elders or physically or intellectually handicapped people) in order to present the victim as ill and in need of care. This is not done for monetary gain or other tangible benefit.

Typical Course and Clinical Features

The diagnosis of FD is suspected when a patient's clinical course does not progress as expected by the medical team. These patients appear to gain something psychologically from playing the sick role or presenting others as ill. They may enjoy the attention that they receive, welcoming diagnostic tests and procedures. It is likely that these patients consciously produce the symptoms but are unaware of their motivation for doing so, but this is challenging to prove. Many appear to have no recollection of causing the illness or falsifying data, as if they did so in a dissociative state. The most extreme form of this disorder has been called Munchausen syndrome after an eighteenth-century German soldier known for traveling from place to place and telling fanciful untrue stories about his accomplishments. Patients with extreme FD similarly travel from place to place, receiving large amounts of medical care and potentially dangerous interventions, moving again once their habits are discovered. Their self-destructive behavior can cause severe morbidity and even mortality due to the direct effects of their behavior or from complications from the resulting tests or treatment.

Diagnosing FD requires proving that a patient is being deceptive (to distinguish it from SSD or CD) and that there are no external benefits (to distinguish it from malingering). The psychiatric consultant must discuss the case extensively with the patient's medical team to discover if there is any way that the patient's symptoms and signs could be physiological. Once the diagnosis is suspected, 1:1 supervision or video monitoring is necessary to prevent the patient from inflicting any further harm. This can help with confirming the diagnosis as well, since the patient or victim may start to recover once illness is no longer being imposed. It may be necessary to search the patient's room and belongings to discover hidden medications or paraphernalia used to feign illness, and collateral history from family or friends can be crucial. Special lab studies can sometimes detect drugs that have been taken surreptitiously.

Patients often feel insulted by these investigations because they feel accused of lying. The psychiatrist should empathize with these feelings but insist that the investigations are necessary to keep the patient safe. It can be helpful to tell the patient that some people have a disorder in which they harm themselves for unconscious reasons, and the medical team is just being thorough in making sure that the patient does not have this disorder. If the patient refuses the investigations, then it may be necessary to inform him that the hospital cannot continue to safely provide care unless he agrees to them. It may be necessary to discuss the situation with hospital legal personnel or risk management team and to present the patient with a formal letter describing the conditions under which treatment can continue.

Treatment

Treatment of FD is even more difficult than diagnosis, and no treatment has been found to be consistently effective. Still, it is possible to try to avoid or minimize harm. One-on-one supervision or video monitoring must be continued while the patient is in the hospital. Medications for any comorbid psychiatric disorders may help. Medical staff might feel extremely frustrated and even angry at patients with FD, but reminding them that a person must be extremely ill in order to behave in this way can increase their empathy and help them to treat the patient in a more caring way. If possible, find ways to satisfy the patient's need for attention (e.g., by arranging for regular appointments with a medical provider even in the absence of physical symptoms) so that the patient does not need to manufacture reasons for seeking care. Patients who are imminently at risk of causing harm to themselves may require involuntary inpatient psychiatric evaluation in order to temporarily keep them safe and to treat any comorbid psychiatric disorders, but it usually takes months or years of outpatient psychotherapy to adequately treat the root causes of this illness. Unfortunately, however, even intensive treatment often fails to prevent death in many of these patients.

Malingering

Diagnosis

When a patient deliberately feigns a psychiatric or medical illness in order to receive an obvious external benefit (such as disability benefits, relief from military duty, substances of abuse, lawsuit settlements, a warm place to sleep, etc.), it is termed malingering. This is not a psychiatric disorder, but it is a condition worth noting while treating patients. Similar to SSD, CD, and FD, malingering is suspected when the patient's subjective statements are discrepant from the objective findings or when the patient's group of symptoms does not fit any known pattern of disease. As in CD and FD, it is necessary to confirm with the medical team that no medical diagnosis can explain the symptoms. Also similar to CD, the behavior of patients who are malingering often differs when observed than when not observed, but those with CD lack the obvious external gain. As in FD, it is necessary to prove deception (see earlier discussion), but unlike FD, malingerers tend to be resistant to medical exams and tests because they fear that their deception will be exposed.

Management

Some malingerers have antisocial traits and are just trying to gain whatever they can for themselves, but many others are truly in need of help. For the latter, ask social services to help the patients find what they really need, such as a warm place to stay, appropriate financial assistance, and so on, and treat them with the respect they deserve. Be sure to screen for any psychiatric illnesses that may be increasing the patient's distress as well.

For those with antisocial traits, it is necessary to be respectful but firm. Controlled substances should only be prescribed for objective dysfunction. Paperwork for disability should be deferred to an outpatient provider who has a relationship with the patient. The patient should only remain in the hospital long enough for evaluation and treatment of any medical problems. Once malingering patients realize that they cannot obtain what they want from a particular facility, they usually move on to another one. For more information on interacting with hostile patients, see Chapter 8.

Conclusion

When a patient's physical findings and subjective experience do not fit the patterns that medical providers expect, both providers and the patient can feel extremely frustrated. A psychiatric consultant can relieve some of this frustration by clarifying the diagnosis and providing guidance on ways to improve the patient's functioning and relationship with the medical team.

Key Points

- Patients with somatic symptom and related disorders suffer profoundly and often seek care from medical rather than psychiatric providers.
- Patients with somatic symptom disorder have excessive concern or dysfunction due to a physical symptom.
- Patients with conversion disorder experience distressing neurological symptoms that are incompatible with known pathologic processes.
- Patients with illness anxiety disorder have excessive anxiety about being or becoming ill, but do not have any signs or symptoms of the feared illness.
- Patients with medically unexplained physical symptoms do not necessarily have a psychiatric disorder.
- Treatment of somatic symptom and related disorders requires an excellent relationship with both the patient and the medical team.
- Psychotherapy can be started in the medical hospital both to reduce distress and to introduce important concepts to the patient.
- Reducing medical harm and unnecessary utilization are key benefits to accurately diagnosing and treating somatic symptom and related disorders.

Disclosures

Dr. Dobbelstein has no conflicts of interest to disclose.

Further Reading

Abbey SE, Wulson L, et al. (2011). Somatization and somatoform disorders. In Levenson JL. (Ed.), *The American Psychiatric Publishing Textbook of Psychosomatic Medicine: Psychiatric Care of the Medically Ill.* (2nd ed., pp. 261–289.) Arlington, VA: American Psychiatric Publishing.

American Psychiatric Association (2013). *Diagnostic and Statistical Manual of Mental Disorders*, 5th ed. Arlington, VA: American Psychiatric Association.

Dimsdale JE, Creed F, et al. (2013). Somatic symptom disorder: An important change in DSM. *J Psychosom Res., 75*, 223–228.

Eastwood S, Bisson JI (2008). Management of factitious disorders: A systematic review. *Psychother Psychosom., 77*(4), 209–218.

Fass R, Dickman R (2006). Non-cardiac chest pain: An update. *Neurogastroent Motil., 18*, 408–417.

Haase E (2006). Conversion disorders. In Blumenfield M, Strain JJ (Eds.), *Psychosomatic Medicine* (pp. 555–564). Philadelphia: Lippincott, Williams and Wilkins.

Kroenke K (2007). Efficacy of treatment for somatoform disorders: A review of randomized controlled trials. *Psychosom Med., 69*, 881–888.

McDermott BE, Feldman MD (2007). Malingering in the medical setting. *Psychiat Clin N Am., 30*, 645–662.

Salkovskis PM (1992). Psychological treatment of noncardiac chest pain: The cognitive approach. *Am J Med., 92*, 114–121.

Sharpe M, Peveler R, et al.(1992). The psychological treatment of patients with functional somatic symptoms: A practical guide. *J Psychosom Med., 36*, 515–529.

Strain JJ, Loigman M (2006). Hypochondriasis. In Blumenfield M, Strain JJ (Eds.), *Psychosomatic Medicine* (pp. 565–569). Philadelphia: Lippincott, Williams and Wilkins.

Straker D, Hyler S (2006). Factitious disorders. In Blumenfield M, Strain JJ (Eds.), *Psychosomatic Medicine* (pp. 571–578). Philadelphia: Lippincott, Williams and Wilkins.

Stone J, Zeman A, et al. (2002). Functional weakness and sensory disturbance. *J Neurol Neurosur Ps., 73*, 241–245.

Stonnington CM, Barry JJ, et al. (2006). Conversion disorder. *Am J Psychiat., 163*(9), 1510–1517.

Yutzy SH (2006) Somatization. In Blumenfield M, Strain JJ (Eds.), *Psychosomatic Medicine* (pp. 537–543). Philadelphia: Lippincott, Williams and Wilkins.

Exercises

1. A patient presents to the medical hospital with abdominal pain, nausea, and vomiting for which no physiological cause can be found. She complains about her symptoms, wanting relief from her pain and nausea/vomiting. She uses a normal amount of analgesic and antiemetic medication. She has some underlying anxiety but generally functions well in the community, with no past psychiatric history, substance use history, or psychiatric medications. She denies any body image problems and is not trying to lose weight. She has lost a few pounds over the past two weeks and is mildly dehydrated. Nursing staff report that she is pleasant but withdrawn, is not overly demanding or needy.

   What is her most likely psychiatric diagnosis?

   a. Somatic symptom disorder
   b. Factitious disorder
   c. Anxiety disorder NOS
   d. Malingering

2. The same patient as in exercise 1 presents to the hospital several more times over the following weeks. She has become more demanding, using more analgesics and less antiemetics. Sometimes she appears almost obtunded by the high doses of opioids that she is using. She appears to enjoy the attention of nursing staff and invites as many procedures as needed to find an answer to her pain. A nursing aid happens to notice her inducing vomiting with her finger.

   What additional diagnosis(es) are now most likely?

   a. Opioid use disorder
   b. Malingering
   c. Factitious disorder
   d. All of the above

3. For the past three weeks, a patient has been in and out of the hospital with right lower extremity paralysis. During physical exam, he cannot move his hip, knee, ankle, or toes, but nursing staff have noticed him using that leg to adjust his position in bed. Labs, spine imaging, and nerve conduction studies are normal. He has a history of depression, fairly well-treated on medication. He notes that he and his wife are having some financial stress, but fortunately his father is helping out substantially. He later notes that his father is extremely controlling and manipulative.

   After providing empathic support and an explanation of his diagnosis, what is the most appropriate next step in his treatment?

   a. Referral to acute physical rehabilitation
   b. Increase dose of antidepressant
   c. Administrative discharge from the hospital
   d. Referral to psychotherapy

4. A 50-year-old man whose father died of a myocardial infarction at age 51 has been presenting to the ED every few weeks with chest pressure on exertion. He is in excellent physical shape except for some

mild hyperlipidemia, treated with a statin. He is very anxious about his chest pain but denies any other psychiatric symptoms. He easily passed an exercise nuclear stress test, which did replicate some of his typical chest sensation. He insists that there is no link between his diet and his symptom. His cardiologist is certain that this is non-cardiac chest pain. A trial of proton-pump inhibitor is not helpful, and he is referred to a cognitive therapist for treatment.

What is the primary goal of his psychotherapy?

a. Relief of his abnormal chest sensation
b. Resolution of his dysfunctional relationship with his deceased father
c. Decreased concern about his chest sensations
d. Prevent his abuse of the medical system

Answers: (1) c (2) d (3) a (4) c

Psychopharmacology in the General Medical Setting

Robert H. Howland and Kurt D. Ackerman

Introduction

We will review pharmacokinetic and pharmacodynamic processes relevant to drug use in medical patients, including drug-drug interactions and administration routes. Special considerations with psychopharmacology in the medical setting will be reviewed, including adjustment of dosing of psychotropic medications based on liver injury, pancreatitis and hyperammonemia, hepatic insufficiency, gastric bypass, renal insufficiency, cardiovascular toxicity, hematologic effects, and fall risk.

Pharmacokinetic Processes

Pharmacokinetics—the absorption, distribution, metabolism, and excretion of drugs—is influenced by age, sex, pharmacogenetic variability, medical comorbidity, and concurrent drug use.

Drug Absorption

Most drugs are mainly absorbed in the small bowel. Food can slow the absorption rate, but the extent of absorption is unaffected. Malabsorption syndromes (Crohn's disease, coeliac disease), previous GI surgery (gastric bypass surgery, surgical removal of the small intestine), or conditions associated with decreased GI blood flow impair or delay orally administered drug absorption. Antacids may decrease drug bioavailability (by chelation or altered gastric pH). Patients should take drugs one to two hours before or after an antacid.

Drug Distribution

Volume of Distribution

Volume of distribution depends on total body mass (muscle and fat) and total body water, both of which are decreased in debilitated patients and the elderly. Most psychotropic drugs are lipophilic and stored in fat, with lithium as a notable exception. Drug elimination from fat is slow and accumulation occurs with chronic dosing, resulting in prolonged effects after discontinuation.

Higher water-soluble drug concentrations such as lithium concentrate as body water decreases. Dehydration increases adverse effects associated with water-soluble drugs. Edematous states increase the volume of distribution, resulting in lower concentrations. Efficacy and toxicity monitoring is essential when patients' fluid status shifts or when their relative proportion of lean muscle mass to total body fat changes.

Protein Binding

Psychotropic drugs are mostly highly protein-bound. Some have lesser degrees of protein-binding. Lithium, gabapentin, and pregabalin are not protein-bound. The protein-bound fraction exists in reversible equilibrium with the unbound free fraction. Only the free fraction has therapeutic or adverse effects, undergoes liver metabolism, and is excreted. Plasma proteins are decreased with age, in liver or renal failure, and in debilitated or undernourished patients. Protein-bound drugs have a higher free fraction in such patients, with increased adverse effects unless lower doses are used.

When the free fraction is increased because of decreased binding proteins, the total concentration (bound plus free fraction) will not reflect the pharmacologically active amount. Under this circumstance, a "therapeutic" total drug concentration may be associated with increased adverse effects in patients with decreased binding proteins.

Drug-drug interactions may occur based on protein-binding competition. Narrow therapeutic index drugs such as warfarin should be monitored closely when starting or stopping highly protein-bound psychotropic drugs.

Drug Metabolism

Most psychotropic drugs are metabolized in the liver. Two metabolic pathways utilize Phase I and Phase II reactions. Cytochrome P-450 (CYP450) system is a Phase I process. Glucuronide conjugation is a Phase II process. Many drug metabolites undergo Phase II conjugation after their parent undergoes initial Phase I metabolism. Lorazepam, oxazepam, temazepam, lamotrigine, valproate, haloperidol, olanzapine, and other drugs are largely metabolized by glucuronidation.

Glucuronidation is greater in men than women, increased in overweight patients and cigarette smokers, and decreased with alcohol use, in underweight or malnourished patients, and with hepatitis, cirrhosis, hypothyroidism, and HIV infection. Age-related decreases in liver blood flow and the activity of some metabolic enzymes may result in decreased drug metabolism.

Drug-drug interactions occur when metabolic enzyme inhibitor or inducer drugs are combined with drug substrates for that enzyme. Stopping such drugs will reverse their enzyme effect.

Drug Excretion

The kidneys are the principal organ for water-soluble drug excretion. Liver metabolism often increases water solubility, but glucuronidation facilitates biliary excretion. The ratio of renal to GI excretion varies from drug to drug, which is relevant to drug dosing in renal insuffiency (see discussion later in this chapter).

Increased lithium concentrations and toxicity can occur when potassium-sparing and thiazide diuretics, ACE inhibitors, or NSAIDs are co-prescribed.

Pharmacodynamic Processes

Pharmacodynamics refers to the action of a drug at its particular target(s), including therapeutic and adverse effects.

Adverse effects are more likely in elderly than in younger patients, and more likely in medically ill or debilitated patients. Pharmacodynamic drug-drug interactions can involve psychotropic and non-psychotropic drugs when they have additive or antagonistic effects at the same site. Anticholinergic toxicity (Chapter 15), serotonin syndrome (Chapter 14), and QTc prolongation (Chapter 13) are examples of adverse effects resulting from additive pharmacodynamic drug-drug interactions. As another example, anticholinergic drugs can antagonize acetylcholinesterase inhibitor drug efficacy.

Drug Administration Routes

See Tables 6.1 and 6.2 for available psychotropic drug formulations. Dissolvable tablets are used when swallowing is difficult. Liquid formulations and crushed tablets can be given through nasogastric and jejunum tubes. Delayed-, controlled-, sustained-, or extended-release formulations should not be used with small intestine disorders or following gastric bypass surgery, and should not be crushed for use with nasogastric or jejunum tubes.

Rectal (suppository) formulations are rare, but most oral tablet or capsule drug formulations can be compounded and given rectally.

Table 6.1 Psychotropic Medication Options for Limited GI Access (I)

Available in Rapid-Dissolve Formulation	Alprazolam (*Xanax*), Aripiprazole (*Abilify Discmelt*), Clonazepam (*Klonopin Wafer*), Clozapine (*Fazaclo*), Donepezil (*Aricept ODT*), Mirtazapine (*Remeron SolTab*), Olanzapine (*Zyprexa Zydis*), Risperidone (*Risperdal M-Tab*)
Available in Liquid Form	Alprazolam (*Xanax*), Aripiprazole (*Abilify*), Carbamazepine (*Tegretol*), Chlorpromazine (*Thorazine*), Citalopram (*Celexa*), Dextroamphetamine (*Liquadd*), Diazepam (*Valium*), Diphenhydramine (*Benadryl*), Doxepin (*Sinequan*), Escitalopram (*Lexapro*), Fluoxetine (*Prozac*), Fluphenazine (*Prolixin*), Haloperidol (*Haldol*), Hydroxyzine HCl (*Atarax*), Levetiracetam (*Keppra*), Lithium, Lorazepam (*Ativan Intensol*), Methylphenidate (*Methylin*), Nortriptyline (*Pamelor*), Phenytoin (*Dilantin*), Risperidone (*Risperdal*), Valproic Acid (*Depakene*)
Available Intravenously	Benztropine (*Cogentin*), Chlorpromazine (*Thorazine*), Diazepam (*Valium*), Diphenhydramine (*Benadryl*), Levetiracetam (*Keppra*), Lorazepam (*Ativan*), Phenytoin (*Dilatin*), valproate sodium (*Depacon*)
Available Intramuscularly (IM, Acute)	Aripipriazole (*Abilify*), Benztropine (*Cogentin*), Chlorpromazine (*Thorazine*), Diazepam (*Valium*), Diphenhydramine (*Benadryl*), Fluphenazine HCl (*Prolixin*), Haloperidol (*Haldol*), Lorazepam (*Ativan*), Olanzapine (*Zyprexa IntraMuscular*), Ziprasidone (*Geodon*)

Table 6.2 Psychotropic Medication Options for Limited GI Access (II)

Available in Intramuscular (IM) Depot Formulation	Aripiprazole (*Abilify Maintena*), Haloperidol Decanoate (*Haldol Decanoate*), Fluphenazine Decanoate (*Prolixin Decanoate*), Naltrexone (*Vivitrol*), Olanzapine (*Zyprexa Relprevv*), Paliperidone Palmitate (*Invega Sustenna*), Risperidone (*Risperdal Consta*)
Available in Transdermal Patch Formulation	Clonidine (*Catapres*), Methylphenidate (*Daytrana*), Nicotine (*Nicotrol*), Rivastigmine (*Exelon Patch*), Selegiline (*Emsam Patch*), Fentanyl, Buprenorphine, Scopolamine, Estrogen, and Testosterone
Available in Sublingual (SL) Formulation	Asenapine (*Saphris*), Buprenorphine/ Naloxone (*Suboxone*), Buprenorphine (*Subutex*) Fluoxetine (*Prozac*), Methylphenidate (*Ritalin*), and Mirtazapine (*Remeron*) may demonstrate some buccal or sublingual absorption but are not available in SL dosage forms.
Available in Suppository Formulation	Diazepam Gel (*Valium*), Prochlorperazine (*Compazine*). TCAs, Trazodone, Citalopram, Carbemazepine, Lamotragine, and Topiramate have been used with some success. Most crushable medicines can be compounded into suppositories, although absorption may be variable.
Medications That Should Not Be Crushed (e.g., into enteral tubes)	Any dissolving tablet or sustained/ extended-release formulation

Antipsychotic IM formulations are short-acting or long-acting. Short-acting IM or IV antipsychotic and benzodiazepine drug formulations are intended for urgent use or when oral use is not possible. Long-acting IM antipsychotic formulations are intended for maintenance use in patients who struggle with adherence. An inhalational formulation of loxapine is used for acute agitation (caution regarding risk of bronchospasm).

Sublingual, rectal, and injectable administration bypasses first-pass liver metabolism, leading to greater bioavailability and higher concentrations compared to oral doses. Doses should be adjusted accordingly when switching between oral and non-oral forms.

Special Considerations with Psychopharmacology in the Medical Setting

Liver Injury

Anticonvulsant, antidepressant, and antipsychotic drugs are associated with significant liver injury or failure (see Chapter 13), but this is rare compared to other non-psychotropic drugs. Mild asymptomatic liver function elevations (less than 3 times the upper limit of normal for alanine transaminase or less than 2 times the upper limit of normal for alkaline phosphatase) are more common and do not predict progression to severe liver injury. Severe liver toxicity associated with valproic acid and carbamazepine occurs primarily in pediatric populations, often when multiple anticonvulsants are used. Monitoring liver function before and during treatment is recommended with valproic acid and carbamazepine, but not for other psychotropic drugs. Laboratory testing alone is not a reliable method for detecting or preventing severe liver injury. Clinical monitoring (fatigue, poor appetite, abdominal pain, nausea, vomiting, dark urine, jaundice) is necessary, together with laboratory testing.

Pancreatitis and Hyperammonemia

Valproic acid and some antipsychotic drugs (clozapine, olanzapine, risperidone, haloperidol) have been rarely associated with pancreatitis. Clinical monitoring is warranted, but routine pancreatic enzyme testing is not needed. Valproic acid inhibits the conversion of ammonia to urea, resulting in elevated ammonia levels that sometimes cause confusion or encephalopathy. Monitoring ammonia levels is not necessary, but should be done if confusion develops.

Hepatic Insufficiency

Drug-metabolizing enzyme activity is generally reduced with increasing liver disease severity. Chronic liver diseases are associated with variable and non-uniform reductions in CYP450 enzyme activity. Glucuronidation is affected to a lesser extent than CYP450-mediated reactions.

Liver function tests do not correlate with drug-metablizing enzyme capacity. Low doses and slower dose titration of most drugs should be used with severe liver disease. Usual dosing strategies can be safely followed for mild to moderate liver disease. Avoiding the use of nefazodone, duloxetine, and valproic acid is recommended with pre-existing liver disease. Lorazepam, oxazepam, and temazepam are preferred benzodiazepine drugs as they are metabolized by glucuronidation and have no active metabolites. Drugs metabolized mainly by conjugation are preferred in older patients and patients with severe liver disease (see Tables 6.3–6.5).

Gastric Bypass and Feeding Tubes

In certain gastric bypass procedures, the stomach is attached to a distal portion of the small intestine such that the duodenum (or the duodenum

Table 6.3 Hepatic Adjustment of Psychotropic Medications (I)

General

Primary factors affecting drug availability include

1. Decreased liver blood flow, leading to greater bioavailability of drugs with first-pass metabolism
2. Change in volume of distribution due to ascites/edema
3. Decreased protein production, affecting drugs with high protein binding (e.g., warfarin)
4. Change in liver clearance; relative loss of CYP450 before glucuronidation
5. Concurrent loss of renal function; decreased effectiveness of prodrugs requiring conversion to active form; greater pharmacodynamic effects of certain drugs (e.g., benzodiazepines)
6. Choose drugs with high therapeutic index, renal clearance, few active metabolites, and measurable levels.

Antidepressants	
Bupropion	*Mild-Moderate Hepatic Impairment*: Reduce dose and/or frequency *Severe Hepatic Impairment*: Caution. Max 75 mg/day IR, 100 mg SR daily or 150 mg XL every other day.
Mirtazapine	Clearance reduced by 30% in hepatic disease.
Nefazodone	Not recommended in hepatic disease; associated with liver failure.
Venlafaxine	Generally safe; use lower doses (approx. 50%) for mild-moderate hepatic disease.
Desvenlafaxine	Dose adjustment required for moderate-severe hepatic impairment.
Duloxetine	Not recommended in hepatic disease.
Vortioxetine	Not recommended in severe hepatic impairment.
SSRIs	Generally safe. Use lower doses (~50% initial and final dose), longer intervals between dose adjustments in hepatic disease. Watch for bleeding due to platelet inhibition. **FDA recommends citalopram doses no more than 20 mg/day (risk for QTc-prolongation).**
TCAs	Caution; limited therapeutic index; rarely precipitates hepatic injury. No dosing guidelines.

Table 6.4 Hepatic Adjustment of Psychotropic Medications (II)

CNS Stimulants and Related Medications	
Amphetamines	Little data available; use cautiously with hepatic disease.
Atomoxetine	↓ dose by 50% with moderate hepatic disease, 75% with severe hepatic disease.
Methylphenidate	Relatively safe, with ~80% renal clearance.
Modafinil	Reduce dose by 50% with severe hepatic disease.

Antipsychotics	
Aripiprazole	No adjustment necessary with hepatic disease.
Chlorpromazine	Avoid with severe hepatic impairment.
Clozapine	Can cause hepatitis; monitor levels and discontinue with marked liver disease or jaundice.
Haloperidol	Limited data. Use cautiously with hepatic disease; adjust dose slowly; monitor side effects.
Olanzapine	Limited data. No dosage adjustment needed, per manufacturer. Monitor transaminases.
Perphenazine	Dose reduction recommended (but not specified).
Quetiapine	Clearance decreased with hepatic disease; start 25 mg/day, increase 25–50 mg/day.
Paliperidone	Relatively safe (largely renally cleared); no dose adjustment for mild-moderate disease.
Risperidone	Free risperidone increased by ~35%. Start and increase dose by no more than 0.5 mg bid, no more quickly than weekly.
Iloperidone	Hepatic impairment: mild (no dose change); moderate (dose adjustment); severe (not recommended).
Asenapine	Not recommended with severe hepatic impairment.
Lurasidone	Hepatic impairment: Moderate (dose ≤ 80 mg/day); severe (dose ≤ 40 mg/day).
Thioridazine	Limited data supports avoiding thioridizine and other phenothiazines with liver disease.
Ziprasidone	No adjustment necessary for mild-moderate disease, per manufacturer.

Antiparkinsonian/Anticholinergic Medications	
Benztropine	Little data available. Use with caution. Risk of sedation.
Diphenhydramine	Little data available. Use with caution. Risk of sedation.

Table 6.5 Hepatic Adjustment of Psychotropic Medications (III)

Anxiolytics and Hypnotics	
Alprazolam	Start dosing at 0.25 mg 2–3 times/day; titrate gradually if needed and tolerated.
Buspirone	Higher plasma levels and longer half-life noted. Avoid with severe hepatic impairment.
Clonazepam	Relatively poor choice with hepatic disease, given half-life, potency, and potential for sedation.
Diazepam	↓ dose by 50% with mild-moderate hepatic impairment. Avoid with severe or acute liver disease; long half-life with active metabolites makes diazepam a poor choice in liver disease.
Lorazepam	Relatively safe. Largely metabolized by glucoronidation, bypassing most CYP effects. Dose adjustments may be needed with severe impairment.
Midazolam	↓ dose by approx. 50% with hepatic disease.
Oxazepam	Relatively safe; largely metabolized by glucoronidation, bypassing most CYP effects.
Temazepam	Relatively safe; largely metabolized by glucoronidation, bypassing most CYP effects.
Zolpidem	Reduced dose (2.5–5 mg QHS) recommended for hepatic impairment; lower doses recommended in women (max recommended dose = 5 mg); do not use with severe impairment.
Mood Stabilizers	
Carbamazepine	Caution with hepatic impairment; consider decreased dose. Avoid with hepatic porphyria. Rare cases of hepatic failure reported. Discontinue with acute liver disease.
Lamotrigine	Mild disease: no adjustment. Moderate-severe disease without ascites: decrease initial and escalating doses by 25%–50%. Moderate-severe disease with ascites: ↓ dose by 50%–75%.
Lithium	Relatively safe with hepatic disease, given renal clearance.
Oxcarbazepine	No adjustment needed for mild-moderate impairment. No data available for severe impairment. Extended release products should be avoided.
Topiramate	Clearance may be reduced in hepatic disease; limited data.

(continued)

Table 6.5 (Continued)	
Valproic Acid	Avoid if possible; can cause hepatic failure. Reduce dose in liver disease, given decreased clearance and greater unbound (active) drug with lower albumin, despite normal total levels.
Cognitive Enhancers	
Donepezil	No specific recommendations. Mildly reduced clearance, active metabolites and long half-life.
Memantine	Relatively safe with hepatic disease (60%–80% renal clearance). Caution with severe impairment.
Tacrine	Avoid with liver disease; can induce hepatotoxicity.

and jejunum) is bypassed. Decreased drug absorption occurs when the stomach or proximal small intestine is an important site of absorption. Absorption of drugs given through feeding tubes in the jejunum can be affected because the stomach and duodenum are effectively bypassed. Drugs with extensive first-pass hepatic metabolism can have increased concentrations and greater systemic effects if given into distal segments of the jejunum. Lower initial doses and slower titrations should be used when drugs are given through jejunum tubes. Delayed-, controlled-, sustained-, or extended-release formulations depend on extended intestinal exposure, and their absorption is decreased in small intestine disorders, gastric bypass procedures, or jejunum-tube administration. Immediate-release formulations should be used.

Renal Insufficiency

The clinical relevance of renal impairment varies between drugs. Reduced renal function is important for lithium and certain other drugs largely excreted through the kidneys (see Tables 6.6 and 6.7).

Renal failure is characterized by proteinuria, hypoalbuminemia, accumulation of protein-binding inhibitors, and an increased free fraction of drugs. Decreased renal clearance can result in higher drug and active metabolite concentrations.

Most psychotropic drugs can be used safely in renal disease. Low starting doses, slow titration, and close monitoring are necessary in moderate-severe renal insufficiency. Most psychotropic drugs are highly protein-bound and are not dialyzable, but can be used safely in dialysis because they are fat-soluble, metabolized mainly by the liver, and excreted in bile. Dialyzable drugs can often be used by dosing during or after dialysis sessions.

Table 6.6 Renal Adjustment of Psychotropic Medications (I)

Antidepressants	GFR 50–70	GFR 10–50	GFR < 10	Hemodialysis
Amitriptyline, citalopram, desipramine, doxepin, escitalopram, fluoxetine, nefazodone, mirtazapine, nortriptyline, sertraline, trazodone	None	Mirtazapine (CrCl < 40) increase slowly	Mirtazapine ↓ dose by 50%	Avoid Mirtazapine
Bupropion (CrCl < 90: consider reduction of dose and/or frequency)				Caution
Duloxetine	Caution	Avoid < 30	Avoid	Avoid
Paroxetine: maximum recommended dose = 40 mg	None	Plasma levels ↑ x2 with CrCl 30–60	Plasma levels ↑ x4 with CrCl < 30	10–30 mg/day
Venlafaxine	↓ dose by 25–50%	↓ dose by 25–50%	↓ dose by 50%	↓ dose by 50%
Desvenlafaxine		CrCl 30–55; dose < 50 mg/day	CrCl < 30; dose 50 mg every other day	Dose 50 mg every other day
Levomilnacipran	None	CrCl 30–59; dose < 80 mg/day	CrCl 15–29; dose < 40 mg/day	Not recommended in ESRD
Vortioxetine, vilazodone	None	None	None	None

(continued)

Table 6.6 (Continued)

Sedatives-Hypnotics	GFR 50-70	GFR 10-50	GFR < 10	Hemodialysis
Alprazolam, chlordiazepoxide, clonazepam, lorazepam, oxazepam, temazepam, zolpidem	None	None	Chlordiazepoxide ↓ dose by 50%	None
Diazepam (active long-acting metabolites)	None	Caution	Caution	Avoid

Mood Stabilizers	GFR 50-70	GFR 10-50	GFR < 10	Hemodialysis
Carbamazepine	None	None	Give 75% of dose	Give 75% of dose pD
Gabapentin (renal clearance only)	Reduce in proportion to GFR			100-300mg pD
Lamotrigine	May need to decrease maintenance dose; use with caution			
Lithium (renal clearance only)	None	↓ dose by 50%-75%	↓ dose by 25%-50%	Dose pD
Oxcarbazepine	None	CrCl < 30: initiate at 50% of usual starting dose	↓ dose by 50% of usual starting dose	Use immediate release products
Topiramate: < 70 administer 50% of dose	CrCl < 70—administer 50% of dose	None	None	Dose 100% pD
Valproic acid	None	None	None	Dose pD

Percentages signify proportion of typical therapeutic dosing; pD = after dialysis
Psychosomatic Medicine Pocket Cards, ©2014, University of Pittsburgh and UPMC. Reprinted and used with permission; all rights reserved.

Table 6.7 Renal Adjustment of Psychotropic Medications (II)

Antipsychotics	GFR 50–70	GFR 10–50	GFR < 10	Hemodialysis
Aripiprazole, clozapine, haloperidol, olanzapine, perphenazine, quetiapine, thioridazine, ziprasidone PO (not IM), iloperidone, asenapine	None	None	None	Limited data; monitor for side effects
Risperidone (renal active metabolite)	None	Starting dose for CrCl < 30: no more than 0.5 mg bid	Caution	Caution
Paliperidone (renal clearance only)	CrCl 50–79: 3mg daily; max dose = 6mg	CrCl 10–49: 1.5mg daily; max dose = 3mg	Not recommended	Not recommended
Lurasidone	None	CrCl < 50: dose 20–80 mg/day	Caution	Caution

Anticholinergics	GFR 50–70	GFR 10–50	GFR < 10	Hemodialysis
Benztropine (accumulates in renal failure)	None	Caution	Caution	Caution
Diphenhydramine	increase dosing interval to q6hr	increase dosing interval to q6–12hr	increase dosing interval to q12–18hr	Unknown
Hydroxyzine	None	Lower by 50%	Lower by 50%	Lower by 50%

(continued)

Table 6.7 (Continued)

Cognitive Enhancers	GFR 50–70	GFR 10–50	GFR < 10	Hemodialysis
Donepezil	None	None	None	None
Memantine	None	CrCl 5–29: 5mg daily; can titrate after 1 week to 5 mg bid	Caution	Unknown

Stimulant Medications	GFR 50–70	GFR 10–50	GFR < 10	Hemodialysis
Methylphenidate	None	None	None	None
Adderall/Amphetamines (renal clearance influenced by urine pH and GFR)	None	Caution	Not Advised	Avoid
Modafinil	None	None	Insufficient data	Insufficient data

Opioid Agonists	GFR 50–70	GFR 10–50	GFR <10	Hemodialysis
Methadone	None	None	↓ dose by 50%	↓ dose by 50%
Buprenorphine	Caution	Caution	Caution	Caution

Percentages signify proportion of typical therapeutic dosing

Cardiovascular Toxicity of Psychotropic Drugs

Many non-cardiac drugs can prolong the QTc interval, increasing the risk of Torsade de Pointes (see Chapter 13).

Older patients are more sensitive to drug effects on cardiovascular function, including heart rate, blood pressure, and rhythm changes. Cardiac effects are magnified with concurrent use of non-psychotropic drugs affecting cardiac function (see Tables 6.8–6.10).

Hematologic Effects of Psychotropic Drugs

SSRI and SNRI drugs are associated with bruising and prolonged bleeding times. SSRIs are associated with an elevated risk of stroke, but the absolute magnitude of the elevated risk is very small and the validity of this finding is debatable because of study methodologies. Serious upper GI bleeding can occur with SSRI/SNRI drugs, primarily among elderly patients also taking NSAIDs. Bruising or bleeding should be assessed in patients taking NSAIDs or other drugs affecting platelet function or coagulation (heparin, fish oil supplements, vitamin E). Valproic acid is associated with thrombocytopenia. Selecting a non-SSRI non-SNRI antidepressant or mood stabilizer other than valproic acid should be considered in the early post-stroke phase, post-surgery, or for patients with liver disease and coagulopathies.

Leukocytosis occurs with lithium. Leukopenia/agranulocytosis is associated with some antipsychotics (clozapine, quetiapine, risperidone, paliperidone, lurasidone), anticonvulsants (carbamazepine, oxcarbazepine), and antidepressants (nefazodone, mirtazapine). These drug effects may affect white cell count interpretation. They should be used cautiously in patients with bone marrow suppression or undergoing immune-suppressing therapies. White cell count monitoring is required with the use of clozapine, but is not routinely necessary with other psychotropic drugs.

Fall Risk and the Use of Psychotropic Drugs

Falls are the single most important serious complication associated with prescription and non-prescription drugs. No particular drug or drug class should be considered risk-free. Falls are caused by various mechanisms, including sedation, confusion, cognitive impairment, vision changes, blood pressure changes, cardiac rhythm changes, balance problems, and neuromuscular incoordination. Fall risk is increased in elderly patients, patients taking multiple drugs, and patients with comorbid medical conditions.

Table 6.8 Cardiovascular Effects of Psychotropic Medicines (I)

Antidepressants	
TCAs	Sinus tachycardia (typically benign). Postural hypotension (increases with age), least likely with nortriptyline, desipramine. AV block. EKG changes: T-wave flattening, ST depression, QT prolongation (especially in overdose), PR/QRS prolongation (quinidine-like effect).
	Effects vary by drug; secondary amines (e.g., desipramine, nortriptyline) tend to be less cardiotoxic. Avoid with conduction block, prolonged QT, and after myocardial infarction (MI).
	Risk of QTc prolongation or Torsades de Pointes is elevated with advanced age, female sex, heart disease, congenital long QT syndrome, hypokalemia, hypomagnesemia, hypocalcemia, elevated serum drug concentrations (drug overdose, interacting drugs, organ failure) and combination of drugs with QTc prolonging effects.
MAOIs	Postural hypotension. Hypertensive crisis (with tyramine or sympathomimetic exposure). Serotonin syndrome when used with other serotonergic agents.
SSRIs	For most SSRIs, minimal direct cardiovascular effects at therapeutic dosing **FDA Safety Announcement: Dose-dependent QTc prolongation with citalopram** (recommends dosing ≤ 40 mg/day or 20 mg/day if hepatic impaired, age > 60, poor 2C19 metabolizers, or taking cimetidine). All SSRIs may prolong QTc, particularly in overdose. From SADHART study: sertraline safe for use soon (2 weeks) after acute MI; use associated with 20% fewer serious cardiovascular events, including death and nonfatal MI.
SNRIs	Tachycardia. Hypertension: benign, transient with duloxetine, dose-dependent with venlafaxine (HTN in 3% of patients receiving < 100 mg/day, up to 13% if > 300 mg/day).
Trazodone/ nefazodone	Postural hypotension (≤ 7%), Syncope (≤ 5%, less with food). Edema (3%–7%), hypertension (1%–2%), conduction abnormalities, ventricular ectopy (< 1% overall, higher with pre-existing ectopy). Priapism (< 1% of men).
Bupropion	Tachycardia (11%), palpitations (2%–6%), arrhythmia (5%), flushing/hot flashes (1%–4%). Hypertension (2%–4%)—can be severe, may exacerbate baseline hypertension and induce high BP when combined with nicotine patch (6%). Caution with concurrent use of β-Blockers or type Ic antiarrhythmics (levels may be increased by bupropion).
Mirtazapine	Mild cardiac effects: Tachycardia, postural hypotension, vasodilation, peripheral edema (reported in 1%–7%).

Table 6.9 Cardiovascular Effects of Psychotropic Medicines (II)

Mood Stabilizers	
Lithium	**At therapeutic levels (< 1.2 mEq/L):** Usually well tolerated. Flattened/inverted T waves, SA-node dysfunction, edema, bradycardia, and syncope have been reported (frequency unknown). **At toxic levels (> 1.5mEq/L):** Complications include 1st degree AV block to complete heart block, bradycardia, ventricular arrhythmia, hypotension, and peripheral circulatory collapse.
Valproic Acid	Tachycardia, palpitations
Carbamazepine	Prolongation of QT, PR, QRS (quinidine-like effect). Arrhythmias, AV block, bradycardia, chest pain, CHF, edema, hypotension, syncope (all at unknown frequency except where noted).
Lamotrigine	Peripheral edema (2%–5%).

CNS Stimulants and Cognitive Enhancers	
Amphetamines Atomoxetine Methylphenidate Modafinil	Mild tachycardia and HTN are common. Chest pain, palpitations, vasodilation, and edema also described. Sudden cardiac death, CVA, MI, and other cardiovascular events have been reported with use, particularly with family history of arrhythmia or sudden cardiac death, or personal history of cardiac defects or disease. Consider baseline VS, screening for family and personal cardiac history, and ongoing VS monitoring. Consult medicine/cardiology if risk factors present. Modafinil may be less likely to cause cardiac symptoms at doses < 600 mg.
Donepezil	Hypertension (3%), syncope (2%). Atrial fibrillation, bradycardia, EKG changes, edema, and hypotension each noted (at least 1%).
Rivastigmine	Hypertension (3%), syncope (3%), hypotension.
Tacrine	Hypertension, hypotension, bradycardia, tachycardia.
Memantine	Hypertension (4%), hypotension, syncope.

Table 6.10 Cardiovascular Effects of Psychotropic Medicines (III)

Benzodiazepines	
All Benzodiazepines	Minimal direct cardiac effects. Hypotension (baseline and postural) reported in elderly patients, those taking propofol, midazolam, temazepam, and concurrent antipsychotic use.

Antipsychotics	
Class Effect (FDA Black-Box Warning)	**Increased mortality in patients with dementia treated with all antipsychotics, attributed in part to cardiovascular, cerebrovascular causes. Metabolic syndrome also contributes to cardiovascular risk.**
First-Generation Antipsychotics	Postural hypotension and tachycardia (particularly with low-potency FGAs). Prolonged QTc (particularly with thioridazine, parenteral haloperidol, pimozide, droperidol).
Second-Generation Antipsychotics*	Postural hypotension (CLZ 9%, QUE 2%–7%, RIS < 4%, OLA 1%–10%, ZIP 5%, PAL 2%–4%, ILO 3%–5%, LUR 1%–2%) syncope (QUE < 5%, ILO, LUR < 3%) Tachycardia (CLZ 25%, QUE 1%–11%, RIS < 4%, OLA 1%–10%, ZIP 2%, PAL 3%–14%, ILO 3%–12%, LUR) Hypertension (CLZ 4%, OLA 1%–10%, ZIP 1%, QUE 1%–2%, RIS <3%, ZIP 2%–3%, ASE 2%–3%) Prolonged QTc (ARI < CLZ < OLA < RIS < QUE < ZIP; PAL, ILO, ASE limited data) Decreased HR variability, angina, atrial fibrillation, CHF, ventricular extrasystole, and stroke with variable reports (< 1% each).
Clozapine	In addition to general SGAs: myocarditis (0.3%–1.2%), possible acutely in first 2 months of use; cardiomyopathy with chronic use (usually after 8 weeks of treatment); EKG ST- and T-wave changes that mimic ischemia; dose should be re-titrated with brief interval (≥ 2 days) off clozapine.

Anticholinergic/Antiparkinsonian Medications	
Benztropine Biperiden Diphenhydramine	Anticholinergic medications are associated with tachycardia and, less frequently, hypertension. Diphenhydramine effects are more variable, with reports of tachycardia, hypotension, palpitations and extrasystole.

ARI = aripiprazole, ASE = Asenapine, CLZ = clozapine, ILO = Iloperidone, LUR = Lurasidone, OLA = olanzapine, PAL = Paliperidone, QUE = quetiapine, RIS = risperidone, ZIP = ziprasidone

Key Points

- Practical information on drug absorption and bioavailability, protein binding, major and minor metabolic pathways, renal and GI clearance, and drug-drug interactions are readily available through online electronic resources.
- Because of the potential for drug-drug interactions in medical settings, psychiatric consultants should review all other non-psychotropic drugs and be familiar with their pharmacological properties and expected side effects.
- Active collaboration with other medical services ensures that psychotropic drugs are used safely, appropriately, and optimally in medical settings.
- Drug selection should be based on age, gender, intended use, expected side effects, known medical comorbidities, current drug regimen, patient preferences, dosing schedule, administration routes, and factors unique to a patient.
- All prescription and non-prescription drugs (including vitamins, supplements, and herbal products), alcohol, nicotine, and illicit drugs should be noted.
- Selecting a drug with the least expected "unsafe" profile is preferred when multiple drugs are available. Drugs with short half-lives and no active metabolites are preferred.
- Drugs sometimes are stopped on medical admission because a patient is seriously ill. This usually is not necessary. Abrupt discontinuation can cause or contribute to psychiatric and medical symptoms. Psychiatric consultants should review the appropriateness of continuing, tapering, or stopping home medications.
- Drug regimens should be simplified when possible, in collaboration with other physicians, including the number and types of psychotropic and non-psychotropic drugs, the timing of drug doses, eliminating unnecessary drugs, and avoiding potential drug-drug interactions.
- Efficacy and adverse effects should be monitored during dose titration. White cell counts, electrolytes, ammonia levels, liver function, renal function, EKG, drug levels, or other laboratory testing before or during treatment may be a useful adjunct for monitoring pharmacotherapy.
- During the transition of care from an inpatient setting, it is critically important to ensure that drug indications, target doses, planned dose titration schedules, and requisite clinical monitoring are clearly communicated.

Disclosures

Dr. Howland has no conflicts of interest.

Dr. Ackerman has no conflicts of interest.

Further Reading

Baghdady NT, Banik S, et al (2009). Psychotropic drugs and renal failure: Translating the evidence for clinical practice. *Adv Ther.*, 26(4), 404–424.

Hilmer SN, McLachlan AJ, et al (2007). Clinical pharmacology in the geriatric patient. *Fund Clin Pharmacol.*, 21, 217–230.

LiverTox. *Clinical and Research Information on Drug-Induced Liver Injury.* US National Library of Medicine. Retrieved from http://livertox.nih.gov/index.html.

Mackin P (2008). Cardiac side effects of psychiatric drugs. *Hum Psychopharm Clin.*, 23(Suppl 1), S3–S14.

Matzke GR, Aronoff GR, et al. (2011). Drug dosing consideration in patients with acute and chronic kidney disease—a clinical update from Kidney Disease: Improving Global Outcomes (KDIGO). *Kidney Int.*, 80(11), 1122–1137.

Micromedex®. Truven Analytics. Retrieved from http://www.micromedexsolutions.com/micromedex2/librarian/.

Miller AD, Smith KM (2006). Medication and nutrient administration considerations after bariatric surgery. *Am J Health-Syst Ph.*, 63(19), 1852–1857.

UpToDate®. Wolters Kluwer Health. Retrieved from http://www.uptodate.com/contents/search.

Verbeeck RK (2008). Pharmacokinetics and dosage adjustment in patients with hepatic dysfunction. *Eur J Clin Pharmacol.*, 64, 1147–1161.

Williams NT (2008). Medication administration through enteral feeding tubes. *Am J Health-System Ph.*, 65(24), 2347–2357.

Exercises

1. Potentially important drug-drug interactions can occur at which site?
   a. Liver
   b. Plasma proteins
   c. Kidneys
   d. a and c
   e. All of the above

2. An example of a pharmacodynamic drug-drug interaction is the following:
   a. Increased bruising when taking sertraline and acetaminophen
   b. Increased tremors when taking lithium and ibuprofen
   c. Increased bruising when taking valproic acid and acetaminophen
   d. Increased cognitive impairment when taking benztropine and donepezil
   e. Increased confusion when taking valproic acid and gabapentin

3. Which statement is accurate?
   a. Lithium extended release should not be used in renal dialysis.
   b. Venlafaxine extended release should not be used after gastric bypass surgery.
   c. Gabapentin extended release should not be used with warfarin.
   d. All of the above
   e. None of the above

4. Which statement is true?
   a. Switching from an oral to a non-oral drug formulation generally does not require a dose adjustment.
   b. Liquid drug formulations generally should be used with nasogastric or jejunum tubes.
   c. Long-acting intramuscular antipsychotic and benzodiazepine formulations are generally preferred for urgent or emergency use.
   d. All of the above
   e. None of the above

Answers: (1) e (2) d (3) b (4) e

Management of Agitation in the General Medical Setting

Ghennady V. Gushchin

Introduction

Management of behavioral disturbance is one of the most common reasons for urgent psychiatric consultation in general hospitals. This chapter is intended to guide the reader through assessment and management of agitated patients in medical settings.

Clinical Presentation

The term "agitation" in medical settings is used to describe disruptive, or threatening behavior indicating a distressing health condition and/or psychopathology. A psychosomatic physician may be asked to evaluate patients who exhibit behavior such as constant moaning, repetitive loud outcries, restlessness, "fighting" the vent, attempting to get out of bed or discontinue life-preserving treatment, wandering, punching, hitting others, and so on.

The diversity of these behaviors can be organized into four clusters based on the predominant type of behavior (verbal/vocal or physical), and degree of aggression (non-aggressive or aggressive). Physical aggression or violence may be directed against property, self, or others. An experienced clinician is aware that the verbal and non-aggressive behaviors may easily transform from verbal to physical and escalate to violence.

Characteristics of agitation include the following:

- Disproportionate, tumultuous emotions;
- Fierce or excessive gestures/movements;
- "Emotional contagiousness" (powerful disruptive effect on the observer/caregivers).

"Emotional contagiousness" is a key feature/element of agitation that is a major challenge for caregivers. The key for a clinician who is involved in the management of an agitated patient is to stay calm and focus on the goals of care. A psychiatrist should recognize and master his or her countertransference and help other professionals not to become entangled in the emotional turmoil.

Evaluation of Agitated Patients

The main goal in the management of agitation is to identify and treat the reversible medical/psychiatric causes of behavioral disturbance. The assessment of an agitated patient begins immediately as part of the discussion with the consulting clinician. The small details gathered from this conversation not only can provide significant clues about the problem, but also can aid greatly in its resolution.

From the narrative of the requesting physician, a psychiatrist can receive information about:

- **Chief complaints** such as uncontrollable pain, anxiety, urges for excretion (inability to express desires), sleep deprivation (disturbed by care), boredom (lack of progress or activity or stimulation, removal from familiar environment), frustration (failed expectations, poor coping skills, isolation), hallucinations, delusions;
- **Substance use** and symptoms of withdrawal (due to underreported substance use at home, it is safe to consider all nonverbal ICU patients at risk for drug or alcohol withdrawal unless proven otherwise);
- **Current medical problems** from inquiry about reasons for admission (trauma, surgery, infection) and ongoing treatment;
- **Psychiatric/medical history** will help to focus clinical attention on the most likely cause of the behavior disturbance.

If time permits, a quick review of vital signs, labs (e.g., metabolic panel, toxicology screen), brain imaging, and EEG data could be essential for understanding the underlying medical condition.

A list of current medications can be helpful, as many antibiotics (acyclovir, amphotericin B), cardiac drugs (digoxin, dopamine), steroids, narcotics, and additional medications (hydroxyzine, ketamine, metoclopramide, theophylline) are associated with agitation, particularly in intensive care units.

Rushing to the floor, a psychiatrist can mentally review the data already obtained to make a preliminary differential diagnosis for an agitated patient. This initial list should be as extensive and inclusive as possible since the correct diagnosis could be easily missed if never considered. The following conditions are roughly ranked in a descending order of frequency of agitation (based on personal experience in the university hospital setting):

- **Delirium** (constitutes a majority of psychiatric urgent/stat consults, see Chapter 10);
- **Drugs** (or substance-induced disorders including intoxication/ withdrawal from alcohol, illicit drugs such as cocaine, heroin, phencyclidine (PCP), or medications such as benzodiazepines, hypnotics, anesthetics);
- **Dementia** (or neurocognitive disorders often comorbid with delirium);
- **Adjustment disorder** with disturbance of conduct (including non-adherence to treatment);
- **Personality disorders** (borderline, antisocial, histrionic, schizotypal);
- **Anxiety disorders**, especially panic disorder with agoraphobia;

- **PTSD** (including iatrogenic PTSD related to hospitalization);
- **Mania** (as bipolar disorder or medication-induced mood disorders);
- **Psychoses** (in the context of mania or depression, schizophrenia, or delusional disorder);
- **Catatonia** related to either psychiatric disorders (mania or psychosis) or general medical condition (excitatory state with automatism and repetitive actions);
- **Akathisia** (substance-induced movement disorder), which occurs in a diverse group of patients exposed to neuroleptics/antiemetics, antipsychotics, SSRIs/SNRIs, and presents with restlessness, pacing, and dysphoria;
- **Intellectual disabilities** and **autism spectrum disorders** (can present a challenge in management because these patients have a tendency to act out when they are taken out of a nurturing environment and placed in an unfamiliar and foreign environment);
- Other behavioral disorders (**disruptive, impulse-control, conduct disorders, and attention deficit hyperactivity disorder**) combined with poor coping skills;
- **Epilepsy**, especially complex partial seizures (including status epilepticus, interictal, and postictal delirium/psychosis).

Management of Agitation

Coming to the floor, a psychosomatic physician should feel confident that the challenge of managing a disturbed patient will always find an appropriate resolution and should bring this aura of confidence to the floor (remember the staff is watching you!).

Management of an agitated patient requires high levels of concentration and the ability to manage one's own anxiety and countertransference in situations that are sometimes very challenging. Personal safety is of paramount importance. Clinicians should always maintain a safe distance and position themselves near an unrestricted exit. It is critical to recognize signs of escalation: the patient gets louder, making belligerent statements, avoids eye contact, hides hands, assumes aggressive postures with clenching fists, "plays" with masticators, or increases pacing in search of a weapon. If a clinician feels unsafe for any reason, he or she should terminate the interview, leave the room immediately, and call for help from trained security/safety officers. A clinician should always respect a patient's needs and rights, using the least restrictive measures possible to maintain safety. Keep in mind that the patient's inability to control his or her behavior is due to a treatable medical/psychiatric condition.

To treat an agitated patient, a clinician should use behavioral techniques and medication management appropriate for the particular behavior.

Behavioral Approaches to Agitation Management

Despite the common expectation that a psychiatrist will come and give the patient something to calm him or her down, an emphasis should be made on behavioral techniques (safer, reversible), depending on patient's ability to communicate and cooperate. Behavioral approaches include verbal de-escalation, environmental modifications, boundary-setting and rule-reinforcement strategies, education of medical staff (to resolve patient-staff conflict), and physical restraints.

The main strategic goal of behavioral techniques is to engage the patient in the process of identifying the troublesome issue and finding a mutually accepted solution to the patient's concerns. In interaction with the patient, a clinician must master nonverbal communication through position and posture (body language): maintain a safe distance (important for both patient and clinician) with a clear view of the exit, and a neutral posture (hands are visible to the patient) with appropriate eye contact (do not stare!).

It is important to convey sincerity. A clinician should explicitly show that he or she is ready to listen.

A clinician should avoid sudden movements and touching the patient (except introductory handshaking). Verbal communication should focus on remaining calm, and speaking with a clear tone, in a personalized manner, and avoiding confrontational statements or threats.

Verbal de-escalation is essential for actively engaging the patient in problem-solving and working toward patient and staff goals. Appropriate techniques include the following:

- Deflating the tension (acknowledging the patient's grievance and frustration, and shift the focus to discussion of how to solve the problem);
- Aligning goals, with emphasis on common ground (desire to get well and out of the hospital), focusing on the big picture (goal for admission and stage of recovery), and finding ways to make small concessions from both sides to get the best care for the patient ("choose your battle," and protect the patient from him or herself);
- Monitoring the progress and recognizing when to disengage (do not insist on having the last word, give the patient time to process, and keep in mind that you do not need the patient's acknowledgment that she or he was wrong; remember that your goal is what is best for the patient in long term).

Environmental modifications as a result of discussion of the patient's concerns include adjustment of lighting and noise, room temperature, sleep protection, and addressing concerns regarding roommates and visitation policies.

Boundary-setting and rule-reinforcement strategies include maintaining expectations regarding following hospital rules (in neutral, matter-of-fact manner), including clarification of reasons for limitations based on concerns regarding the patient's medical condition or behavior. Controversial smoking arrangements could be a topic of discussion, depending on the hospital's policies.

Education of medical staff who are involved with management of the agitated patient usually includes the following:

- Presentation/interpretation of the patient's behavior in the context of the patient's medical and psychiatric illness with identification of current stressors and potential triggers;
- Discussion of techniques that were previously helpful for this patient to regain control or that might be used for patients with this condition/diagnosis (see also Chapter 8).

With medical staff at times becoming overwhelmed by the demands of patient care, patient-staff dynamics pose a potential threat to the therapeutic alliance and may trigger conflict, with both sides spiraling up their "emotional temperature." It may be helpful to provide suggestions/directions to medical personnel to extract themselves from the ongoing conflict by focusing on the big picture and setting limits, rather than responding to a patient's provocative behavior.

Use of restraints is a behavioral technique used when a clinical situation requires immediate action to help a patient regain control of their behavior and when less intrusive behavioral measures or pharmacological treatment are not effective or appropriate.

The purpose of restraints is to ensure the safety of patients and caregivers (not staff's convenience). They should only be used when the patient is unable to maintain his or her safety, and must be discontinued as soon as the patient regains control. The patient should always be asked to stop the disruptive behavior prior to implementing the restraints. Physical restraints should be left to those who are specifically trained to use them. Physical restraints may have advantages over medication in addressing specific behaviors and being quickly reversible when patients are able to calm down, regain control, and engage in treatment; however, they do not address the underlying cause of agitation.

Pharmacological Treatment of Agitated Patients

Medications can be used as the primary treatment of agitation when the cause of the agitated behavior is identified or known, such as pain, anxiety, psychosis, or mania. Introducing the medication, a C-L psychiatrist should try to involve the patient in decision-making by asking, "Can I get you something to feel better (to calm down)? What works for you?" The response, "Oh doc, I'd like to have Valium!" should be regarded as a good outcome because for some patients it would be the choice of the physician (benzodiazepine or alcohol withdrawal); in some cases, it is a starting point for involving the patient in his or her care ("There is a problem with Valium, it may suppress your breathing, how about some haloperidol?").

The term "chemical restraint" should be avoided at all times because it undermines the very purpose of the pharmacological treatment. The use of a medication is based not on the goal of immobilizing the patient, thereby making him incapable of posing a danger to self or others, but rather to address the core problem (or in uncertain cases, to be close to the possible nature of the problem). Therefore, physicians have an arsenal of pharmacological agents to choose from in the attempt to relieve the patient's symptoms and address the underlying cause of agitation: antipsychotics, benzodiazepines, sedative-hypnotics, anticonvulsants, opioids, antihistamines, trazodone, beta-blockers, and so on. Patient consent should be obtained, when possible, prior to treating with medication. Treatment over objection should be reserved for emergency situations in which the patient lacks capacity, or presents a danger to himself or others.

Besides the choice of medication class, physicians also may choose the dosing strategy (loading vs. titration). Loading techniques are considered as standard in the setting of emergency departments when the priority is to get violent behavior under control quickly and gain time for the collection of necessary information from all available sources. Titration is more laborious since it consists of frequent dosing of the chosen medication in escalating doses to achieve cumulative doses that produce sustained relief of symptoms while at the same time allowing the patient to cooperate with evaluation and care.

Antipsychotics are the most frequently used medications for agitated patients because they can provide symptom relief for many of the causes of agitation (delirium, psychosis, mania) with a relative lack of respiratory depression. Risks of antipsychotics include EPS, akathisia, NMS, tardive dyskinesia, seizures, and QTc prolongation with an increased chance of cardiac arrhythmias.

Haloperidol (Haldol) can be administered orally, intramuscularly, and (off label) intravenously. As a loading technique, consider haloperidol 5 mg IM/PO (2.5 mg IV) administered every 60 minutes until an appropriate level of symptom relief is achieved. In titration mode, begin with 0.5–1 mg IV and continue administration every 30 minutes in increasing doses, for example, 2–3–5–10 mg, until the patient is comfortable and

Table 7.1 Antipsychotic Medications for Treatment of Agitation. Maximal doses and ranges provided according to PDR reference; consider lower doses in elderly and debilitated patients

Name	Route	Dose	Max/24h	Risks
Haloperidol *Haldol*	IV* IM PO	0.5–10 mg q30 min 5 mg q1h 0.5–5 mg q1–4h	20 mg	EPS, NMS, tardive dyskinesia (TD), akathisia, arrhythmias, seizures
Chlorpromazine *Thorazine*	IV IM PO	10–25 mg q 1–4h 25 mg q1–4h 25–100 mg q4h	400 mg	Hypotension, EPS, NMS, TD, seizures
Loxapine *Loxitane* Abusive**	IM PO Inhalant	10–50 mg q4h 25 mg q4h 10 mg/ application	250 mg	EPS, NMS, TD, akathisia, seizures, hypotension
Olanzapine *Zyprexa*	IM PO	2.5–10 mg q2–4h*** 2.5–20 mg q2–4h	30 mg	Hyperglycemia, akathisia, EPS, NMS, hypotension
Ziprazidone *Geodon*	IM PO	10 mg q2h 40 mg	40 mg 80 mg	QT-prolongation, EPS, NMS, TD, akathisia, hypertension
Aripiprazole *Abilify*	IM PO	5.25–9.75 mg q2h 5–10 mg	30 mg 15 mg	NMS, TD, hypotension, seizure
Quetiapine *Seroquel*	PO	12.5–50 mg bid	200 mg	Hypotension, NMS, TD
Risperidone *Risperdal*	PO	0.25–2 mg daily	6 mg	Hypotension, EPS, NMS, TD (avoid with renal and severe liver disease)

* Not FDA approved
** Limited to designated facilities
*** Avoid IM Zyprexa within 2 hrs. of parenteral lorazepam

slightly sedated but easily arousable. With both techniques, the cumulative dose can serve as a reference to calculate the most effective dose if administration of haloperidol will be required in the future to manage the patient's agitation. Usually, this total dose is divided by three for administration every 8 hours. Intravenous haloperidol is less likely to cause EPS compared with oral haloperidol, but may be associated with higher incidence of cardiac side effects, including Torsades de Pointes. Maximum cumulative daily dose of haloperidol should not exceed 20 mg, as according to *in vivo* binding studies virtually all D_2 receptors of the human brain are blocked at that dose. If the maximum dose of haloperidol is not effective, reconsider the etiology of agitation. In cases when antipsychotics are still the best choice, switch to another antipsychotic (see Table 7.1), or add benzodiazepines or other hypnotics.

Benzodiazepines, the second most frequently used group of medications to treat agitation, would be first choice when the agitated patient is treated for alcohol/benzodiazepine withdrawal as well for patients with most toxidromes, brain injury, and unknown etiology of agitation. Benzodiazepines can have prolonged elimination, and IV loading of benzodiazepines should be done cautiously because of the substantial risk of respiratory depression, particularly when combined with narcotics and other sedative medications. Lorazepam (Ativan) is used widely in medical settings as it may be administered by mouth, IM, or IV. It is also relatively safe for patients with liver injury. Loading doses of 0.5–2 mg every 10 minutes may be administered IV until symptom relief and the patient is drowsy with periods of sustained wakening. In rare cases, for example delirium tremens, a continuous IV infusion of lorazepam (0.05 mg/kg/hr) may be necessary and requires continuous monitoring for possible respiratory depression and propylene glycol diluent toxicity. Diazepam (Valium) can be used for detoxification in complicated benzodiazepine/alcohol withdrawal delirium using a loading strategy, for example, 10 mg diazepam IV every 10 minutes until the patient is drowsy but arousable, and then observing patient's vital signs until recovery. In some cases, midazolam (Versed) can be used as a loading dose (5 mg IM) or for titration with continuous IV infusion (0.12 mg/kg/hr), most often for patients on a ventilator.

In some cases, when antipsychotics and benzodiazepines (alone or in combination) are not effective, propofol (Diprivan) or dexmedetomidine (Precedex) may be effective for severe agitation in ICU or ED settings while ensuring airway protection. Recovery from propofol sedation may be complicated by agitation and could require cross tapering with other sedatives/anxiolytics.

Anticonvulsants may be the first choice of medications for management of agitation in patients with seizures and head trauma. They also may be used as a supplement when antipsychotics and benzodiazepines are ineffective and sedation is undesirable. Valproate (Depakote) has an advantage of serving as a mood stabilizing medication for patients with severe mood dysregulation who have limited response to other agents, or for traumatic brain injury (TBI) patients (as it does not slow cognitive rehabilitation). Risks include liver and fetus toxicity (particularly Depakote). Among anticonvulsants, phenobarbital can be clinically useful for management of severe risk of complicated alcohol/benzodiazepine withdrawal with a loading dose of 10–20 mg/kg IV or titration by 10–40 mg PO/IM/IV every 8 hours.

For patients with poorly controlled pain resulting in agitation, opioid medications are the first choice. The benefit of opioids is that they treat both pain and anxiety; the primary risk is respiratory depression. Particular choice of narcotics and dosages should be left to the primary medical team. Consultation of a Pain Service (where available) can be advisable for patients with high tolerance to opioids and when patients with pain may benefit from utilization of both opioids and non-opioid modalities. Among opioids, fentanyl (Sublimaze) is most frequently used in acute settings, followed by hydromorphone (Dilaudid) as well as oxycodone and OxyContin. In some cases, methadone (Methadose, Dolophine) is used for management of chronic pain (see Chapter 20).

On many occasions, antipsychotics, benzodiazepines, hypnotics, anticonvulsants, and opioids are contraindicated or clinically inappropriate. A miscellaneous group of medications may be useful to manage agitation, depending on the underlying etiology.

- Antihistamines: diphenhydramine (Benadryl): 25–50 mg PO/IM/IV every 4–6 hours; hydroxyzine (Vistaril): 25–100 mg IM PO/IM every 4–6 hours (patients with anxiety, as alternatives to benzodiazepines);
- Trazodone: 12.5–200 mg (as an alternative to antipsychotics and benzodiazepines in elderly patients; can be given in low doses during the day);
- Propranolol (Inderal): 20–40 mg PO twice a day (severe anxiety, restlessness, thyroid crisis),
- Memantine (Namenda): 5 mg daily–10 mg twice a day (as an alternative to antipsychotics in patients with dementia);
- SSRIs (sertraline, citalopram), SNRIs (venlafaxine XR, duloxetine), TCAs (nortriptyline, clomipramine) in regular or smaller doses as an alternative to antipsychotics in patients with dementia;
- Buspirone (Buspar): 5–15 mg twice a day (bruxism, restlessness, anxiety).

Conclusion

Overall, the evaluation and management of an agitated patient is a significant part of a psychosomatic physician's responsibilities in hospital settings. This work has a direct impact on improvement of quality of care for the patients and assists the other medical professionals to do their job in an optimal environment.

Key Points

- Behavioral disturbances may occur in the course of a variety of medical conditions that require hospitalization.
- Agitation in medical settings is considered as a sign of distress and/or psychopathology and one of the most common reasons for urgent psychiatric consultation.
- Management of an agitated patient requires high levels of concentration, professional knowledge/training, and the ability to manage the clinician's own anxiety and countertransference.
- This work has a direct impact on improvement of quality of care for the patients and assists the other medical professionals to do their job in an optimal environment.

Disclosures

Dr. Gushchin has no conflicts of interest to disclose.

Further Reading

Levenson, JL (Ed.) (2005). *Textbook of Psychosomatic Medicine*. Washington, DC: American Psychiatric Publishing, Inc.

Wise MG, Rundell JR (2005). *Clinical Manual of Psychosomatic Medicine*. Washington, DC: American Psychiatric Publishing, Inc.

Wyszynski AA, Wyszynski B (2005). *Manual of Psychiatric Care for the Medically Ill*. Washington, DC: American Psychiatric Publishing.

Exercises

1. The psychiatrist is interviewing a patient who begins to make threatening statements and becomes more agitated. The psychiatrist begins to feel uneasy. The most appropriate next step is to:
   a. Tell the patient to calm down.
   b. Ask the patient more direct questions.
   c. Interrupt the interview to get help.
   d. Place a reassuring hand on the patient's shoulder.
   e. Offer the patient lorazepam.

2. Medications can be administered without a patient's consent under which of the following circumstances?
   a. The patient is in an emergency setting, such as a fully accredited hospital ED.
   b. The patient is judged to be psychotic.
   c. The patient is clearly delusional and has been on an inpatient unit for greater than 1 month without receiving any type of pharmacological treatment.
   d. An emergency situation exists and can be documented.

3. The psychiatrist has been called to evaluate a 58-year-old patient who is threatening to leave the hospital against medical advice, complaining of poor care. The patient was admitted for elective foot amputation. He has no psychiatric history and no history of substance abuse. The previous day, he was switched from patient-controlled analgesia (PCA) to PO opioids. What medication would be helpful to treat his agitation?
   a. Haloperidol 5 mg IM
   b. Hydromorphone 0.4 mg IV
   c. Lorazepam 2 mg IM
   d. Cymbalta 30 mg PO

4. A 25-year-old Malayan man suddenly reacts with unprovoked rage and begins aimlessly attacking people and animals. When finally subdued, he claims to have no memory of the incident. Which of the following culturally related syndromes is most likely responsible for his actions?
   a. Amok
   b. Ataque
   c. Koro
   d. Spirit possession
   e. Falling-out

Answers: (1) c (2) d (3) b (4) a

Strategies to Improve Coping and Manage Maladaptive Behaviors in the General Medical Setting

Christopher R. Dobbelstein and Mary G. Fitzgerald

Introduction

When patients cope poorly with the stress of their medical hospitalization, they can exhibit maladaptive behaviors and emotions. Medical staff may feel frustrated or saddened by these behaviors and emotions and may seek a psychiatric consultation to help improve the patient's coping. Examples of maladaptive behavior include refusing care, treating staff inappropriately, and seeking unnecessary care or medications. Anxiety, demoralization, and depression can also complicate patients' medical courses. This chapter explains why some patients respond to their stressors in maladaptive ways and provides practical strategies for helping these patients.

Strategies for the Initial Interview

In order to provide the best advice to the hospital staff and the optimal treatment for the patient, the consultation-liaison (C-L) psychiatrist must first understand why this particular patient is responding to this particular stress in this particular way. The following enhancements to the initial psychiatric consultation (see Chapter 2) will help you to accomplish this.

Before seeing the patient:

- Be sure that you understand the patient's medical situation: the diagnosis, prognosis, and physical symptoms; the treatments already received and those being proposed; and any important medical choices that the patient is facing.
- Are the patient's behaviors affecting his health or his medical care? If so, which ones, and in what way?
- How are staff members responding to his behaviors?
- What does the medical team want from the consultation?
- If the above information is not evident from the medical record, obtain it from the medical staff.

During the patient interview:

- Monitor your own emotions while interacting with the patient. If a particular emotion is elicited in you, it is likely that the patient is feeling something similar. You can thus use your emotions as a tool to better understand the patient's inner experience.
- Do not take patient's behaviors personally; assume that they are an expected reaction given the patient's circumstances, personality, and past experiences.
- Introduce yourself as a psychiatric consultant, and ask the patient if she knew that the psychiatric service was consulted. Ask her if she knew why you were consulted, and if not, tell her.
- Pay attention to the patient's initial reaction to your having been consulted. If he is suspicious or angry, ask him why he feels this way. This will show him that you are interested in his point of view and will give you valuable information about how he sees his situation. If either he or you have any misinformation, clear this up before moving on with your interview.
- Optimize the patient's physical comfort before asking any more questions. This is another way to demonstrate empathy.
- Sit in a chair near the patient if it is logistically possible and if the patient appears comfortable with this.
- If the patient does not start talking immediately, start by asking some non-threatening questions, such as how his medical course is going or how he feels today.
- If the patient is still hesitant to talk, tell him or her that you are an expert in helping people to cope with difficult circumstances.
- Ask what the patient understands about his medical illness—its name, cause, prognosis, and treatment options. If his understanding is different from what his medical team believes, gently explore this and explain the medical team's point of view.
- Ask what this illness experience means to the patient. What has he lost as a result of being ill?

- Ask what support he is receiving from his friends or family and how they are reacting to his illness.
- Ask how she feels her care team is treating her.
- Ask how things were going prior to the medical problem. This helps you to understand the context preceding the illness. Sometimes the illness is just one of many problems the patient is facing. In that case, ask what the most difficult aspect of his situation is; his response will show you his priorities and may surprise you.
- After you have built rapport with the patient, ask potentially uncomfortable questions, such as why she was having difficulty with staff or why she wanted to leave against medical advice (AMA). Bring up these concerns directly so that your dialogue is open and honest.
- If it is impossible to build rapport due to psychosis, paranoia, or personality problems, you should still be open and honest with the patient regarding your perspective. See Chapter 7 regarding management of agitated patients. See discussion later in this chapter regarding interacting with patients with difficult personality types.
- If necessary, gather more information from the patient's family or friends, especially if any aspect of his history does not fit together logically. Be sure to obtain consent from the patient.
- After you have gathered the necessary information to make your psychiatric diagnosis, ask the patient if she has any questions for you or any other information that she thinks is important to share.
- Conclude your interview by telling the patient your opinion and recommendations, and invite him to comment on whether they seem reasonable or helpful. If he disagrees with you, then discuss this. You may disagree, but at least he will know what recommendation you will be giving to the medical team. If he agrees with your assessment, his experience of feeling heard and understood can start the healing process, even before any medications or formal psychotherapy have been prescribed.
- Finally, let the patient know when you will be back to see him and how to contact you.

Understanding the Patient's Perspective

Appreciating an illness episode from the patient's perspective involves understanding various factors including the unique stress of the hospitalization and how it interacts with the patient's personality type, defense mechanisms, and culture.

Stress of Medical Hospitalizations

Medical staff who are accustomed to working in a hospital can easily overlook how stressful hospitalizations can be for patients. Box 8.1 describes factors that can cause stress during medical hospitalizations.

Personality Type

When people encounter stressful situations, they tend to revert to their core personality type, and this can be maladaptive. For example, a successful accountant whose obsessive-compulsive personality type is useful at work may become rigid and stubborn as a way to cope with the loss of control inherent in being a patient. Table 8.1 describes how patients with different personality types tend to react to the stress of hospitalization and gives suggestions of how to help them. Patients with previously diagnosed personality disorders can also benefit from these strategies but will likely have even more difficulty coping.

Defense Mechanisms

Defense mechanisms are automatic processes by which a person's mind unconsciously confronts a threat or intolerable conflict and makes the threat or conflict more manageable; they influence the patient's perception of reality so that reality is not as overwhelming. Some defense mechanisms are more adaptive than others, with mature defenses being the most helpful, followed by neurotic, then immature, then psychotic (see Table 8.2). In psychosomatic medicine, the most commonly encountered threats or conflicts involve the stress of a medical illness or its treatment. Identifying and explaining a patient's defense mechanisms can help the

---

Box 8.1 Factors That Can Cause Stress during Medical Hospitalizations

- Isolation from social supports
- Hospital gown can make the patient feel demeaned or vulnerable
- Lack of control and autonomy due to tests, procedures, or the illness itself
- Dependence on others for basic needs such as bathing, toileting, eating, etc.
- Physical symptoms such as pain, gastrointestinal distress, or fatigue
- Inability to do things that make the patient feel useful and valuable
- Loss of financial security, sexuality, roles, identity, or plans for the future.

Table 8.1 Descriptions of Common Personality Types and Suggested Interventions to Help with Coping

Type	Typical Behaviors	Interventions
Paranoid	Pervasive distrust; motives interpreted as malevolent; overreacts with anger	Explain everything in minute detail; involve trusted others
Schizoid	Detached; prefers to be socially isolated; emotionally restricted	Screen for depression; ensure that the patient is receiving sufficient information; involve trusted others
Borderline	Fears abandonment; impulsive; self-injurious behaviors; prone to rage and near-psychosis; affective lability; unstable and intense relationships; cannot appreciate ambiguity or uncertainty; tends to split staff	Acknowledge real stress of situation; avoid challenging patient—choose battles wisely; keep rigid boundaries to prevent impression of closeness; do not offer anything unless you are certain that you can provide it; be sure that the entire medical team communicates the same message to the patient in order to avoid splitting
Histrionic	Interpersonal interactions are inappropriately sexually provocative; exaggerated expression of emotion, which can change dramatically; uses appearance to draw attention to self	Provide positive reinforcement; communicate to the patient that you appreciate his intense suffering; avoid any words that can sound devaluing
Narcissistic	Needs to feel special; extremely entitled and grandiose; lacks empathy	Provide ample praise; use feeling of entitlement to motivate compliance; avoid becoming entangled in unnecessary debates

Antisocial	Lack of remorse; aggressive; recklessly impulsive; deceitful; pattern of irresponsibility	Avoid confrontations; do not attempt to change underlying motives; be honest about power differentials so that patient knows where he stands; recognize your own anger at patient and rechannel it
Avoidant	Fears rejection; reluctant to engage in new activities; believes self to be inferior and unappealing	Screen for depression; be careful to phrase advice to avoid appearing critical
Dependent	Feels unable to care for self; clinging behavior; difficulty making decisions for self; complains but rejects help	Gratify needs for nurturing but set limits early; recognize your own feeling of annoyance and rechannel it; avoid saying anything that can sound dismissive
Obsessive-compulsive	Perfectionism interferes with completing tasks; preoccupied with rules, schedules, details, order; rigid and stubborn	Remember that patient fears loss of control in the hospital; help patient to use intellectualization in order to feel like she has more control

Table 8.2 Summary of Common Defense Mechanisms

Defense	Description	Example
Psychotic		
Projection	Projecting one's own unacceptable impulses, affects, or desires onto another person and then reacting to that person accordingly. Can be psychotic or immature.	A patient who is unaware of unconscious racist beliefs inaccurately accuses African American staff of mistreating her.
Denial	Avoiding becoming aware of some painful aspect of reality. Can be psychotic or immature.	A patient ignores a clearly necrotic breast lump, which is only discovered when she presents to the hospital for another reason.
Immature		
Acting out	Gratifying unconscious desires with impulsive behaviors in order to avoid becoming conscious of the accompanying uncomfortable affects.	A lonely patient who craves attention shouts obscenities at staff when he is discharged in order to sooth his anger about having to leave.
Passive-aggressive	Expressing aggression through passivity and masochism.	A patient who is isolated from supports speaks extremely slowly when talking to her. They have to listen to her, which makes them angry and decreases their empathy for her, thus harming her in the end.
Projective identification	Causing others to feel one's own unacceptable feelings, then reacting to the others' resultant behaviors with fear or by trying to control them.	A patient who has repressed anger at her father is rude to staff, provoking them into feeling anger at her. When staff perform their duties professionally but without warmth, the patient feels horrified that they would treat her this way.

Regression	Returning to a previous stage of development to avoid the anxieties inherent in later stages, often seeking instinctual gratification by returning to earlier modes of gratification because later modes have failed.	A patient with many responsibilities is having financial and relationship problems despite usually making good decisions. She starts to overeat in order to soothe herself.
Splitting	Tending to experience oneself and others as either all good or all bad.	A patient adores her surgeon but despises the surgeon's housestaff.

Neurotic

Controlling	Excessively attempting to manage or regulate the environment in order to minimize anxiety and resolve internal conflicts.	A cancer patient insists on only having certain nurses, only eating certain foods, only seeing certain consultants in an excessively controlling way.
Displacement	Shifting affects from an unacceptable object to an acceptable one.	A patient who contracted HIV from her partner becomes enraged at nursing staff for minor problems.
Dissociation	Temporarily modifying one's personal identity in order to avoid emotional distress, including fugue states and conversion reactions.	A patient presents to the ED having forgotten who he is. Collateral history reveals that he is going through bankruptcy.
Intellectualization	Controlling affects and impulses by excessively thinking about them instead of experiencing them.	A patient with recently diagnosed pancreatic cancer avoids feeling fearful and sad by researching all possible treatments.
Repression	Unconsciously withholding from conscious awareness unacceptable ideas or affects.	A patient experiences depressive symptoms and is not aware that they stem from anger at her mother for favoring the patient's sibling when they were young.

(continued)

Table 8.2 (Continued)

Defense	Description	Example
Mature		
Altruism	Constructively serving others as a way to gratify normal instincts.	A transplant patient volunteers to help mentor patients awaiting transplant.
Anticipation	Overly planning for realistic future discomfort, worrying about possible terrible outcomes.	A woman makes plans for who will care for her children should she die prior to undergoing gall bladder surgery.
Humor	Expressing difficult affects overtly without personal discomfort and without distressing others.	A chemotherapy patient intentionally wears outlandish hats in order to cope with hair loss.
Sublimation	Gratifying an impulse by substituting a socially objectionable aim with a socially valued aim. Feelings are acknowledged and channeled such that gratification occurs to a modest degree.	An adolescent patient who believes that premarital sex is wrong derives sexual pleasure from kissing her boyfriend.
Suppression	Consciously deciding to postpone attention to an uncomfortable affect or conflict.	A patient with a rich family history of early colon cancer receives all necessary screenings and tries not to think about cancer between screenings.

Note that some terms may be used to describe normative behaviors (such as humor or altruism) in addition to categorizing a defense mechanism.
Adapted from Bromheim (2006) and Groves & Muskin (2011).

patient to understand the rationale behind behaviors that may at first seem to be irrational, thus helping him to feel more in control of himself. Explaining them to staff can also improve their empathy for the patient.

Culture

Patients' cultures profoundly shape their worldview surrounding health and illness. A thorough discussion of this is beyond the scope of this chapter, but it is worth noting that healthcare professionals must always keep culture in mind when caring for patients, especially when helping them to make meaning out of their illness experience. For example, some religions teach that if someone prays "enough," then God will heal him. If a patient is not healed, then he can interpret this to mean that he did not pray enough, which can cause feelings of guilt.

If you do not understand something about a patient's cultural background, consider looking up some basic information. Remember, though, that not every member of a culture or subculture has the same perspective as other members of that group. It is best to inquire about cultural beliefs directly, respectfully asking the patient what he believes about a situation, rather than assuming that he holds certain beliefs that represent a stereotypical characterization of his background.

Treating Patients Who Do Not Adhere to Medical Recommendations

Medical teams often ask psychiatric consultants to "fix" patients who are not participating in their care as expected. Some patients truly disagree with the medical recommendations, but others would comply if outside factors were not obstructing them. It is critical to understand the patient's perspective when evaluating non-adherence. Common causes of non-adherence, as well as strategies to overcome them, are listed in Table 8.3.

Evaluating Patients Who Ask to Leave Against Medical Advice (AMA)

When patients ask to leave the hospital AMA, medical teams often urgently consult psychiatry because leaving prematurely may be associated with imminent risk. The psychiatric consultant must first determine the capacity of the patient to make this decision (see Chapter 9), then explore the patient's reasons for leaving, attempting to remove any obstacles to staying. Finally, if the patient has capacity and is allowed to leave, help the medical team to understand why he left so that they can optimize his post-hospitalization care.

Possible reasons for wanting to leave AMA, and ways to respond, include the following:

- Overwhelming confusion, anxiety, or fear due to delirium, dementia, psychosis, or paranoid personality. Listen empathically to the patient; once he feels that you understand his reasons for leaving, he may be more open to productive problem-solving so that he can make the best choice for himself. If he lacks capacity to make the decision to leave AMA, detain him pending input from his surrogate decision-maker.
- A patient who feels unheard by medical staff may say that he is leaving AMA in order to get their attention. Listen to the patient and apologize for any actual wrongs that have been done to him.
- Craving for substances of abuse may cause a patient to put her health in danger in order to relieve this craving. Control all withdrawal symptoms (see Chapter 16), but keep in mind that some patients choose to leave despite excellent care.

Patients Who Seek Medical Care Inappropriately

Psychiatric consultants are frequently asked to evaluate patients who appear to seek and use more medical care than would be expected for their medical diagnosis. These patients may have somatic symptom and related disorders. See Chapter 5 for strategies to diagnose and treat these patients.

Improving Motivation to Change Behavior

The C-L psychiatrist is often asked to assist with the care of patients with substance use disorders (SUD; see Chapter 16) or other patients whose chronic behavior is adversely affecting their health (e.g., unhealthy diet).

Table 8.3 Common Causes of Medical Non-Adherence and Strategies to Overcome Them

Cause	Strategy
Practical limitations (e.g., cost, transportation, child/elder care, inflexible work schedules)	Social work consult, clinical pharmacy consult
Medication side effects or frequent dosing	Clinical pharmacy consult
Incomplete education about the medical problem	Inform primary team of this need; consider specialized educator consult (e.g., diabetes, nutrition, or congestive heart failure educator).
Shame/embarrassment (e.g., HIV, cancer)	Dynamic or cognitive therapy to treat dysfunctional thoughts and emotions
Need to demonstrate autonomy (e.g., adolescent with type I diabetes)	Cognitive therapy to find more adaptive ways of demonstrating autonomy
Unconscious desire to make medical providers experience the same negative feelings that the patient experiences (makes patient feel less alone or more powerful, common with cluster B personality traits)	Long-term psychotherapy is the best treatment, but in the meantime, explain this phenomenon to the medical team so as to improve their empathy.
Suicidality	If imminent, inpatient psychiatric admission; if not imminent, medications and psychotherapy
Amotivation/anergia due to depression	Antidepressant medications and psychotherapy
Memory impairment or executive dysfunction due to dementia	Improve social support or place patient in a facility that will manage medical care.
Psychosis/paranoia	Antipsychotic medications; inpatient psychiatric admission if imminent harm is likely
Substance use	See Chapter 16
Cultural beliefs	Clarify capacity; talk with family if patient allows.
Tendency to value immediate comfort more than long-term health	Clarify capacity; help medical team to appreciate patient's perspective.

Even if the focus of the consultation is on other matters such as intoxication, withdrawal, or depression, the C-L consultant can start the process of engagement in treatment so that the patient is more likely to follow up with specialized treatment after discharge (e.g., rehabilitation for SUD, bariatric treatment). Patients who are admitted to a medical hospital may be more motivated to make behavioral changes to improve their health, so they may be more open to motivational interviewing (MI).

The technique of MI is based on the assumption that patients considering behavioral change must first overcome ambivalence about the change. The goal of MI is to help the patient to examine and resolve this ambivalence by using the following strategies:

- Explicitly acknowledge that there are pros and cons to the behavior in question and invite the patient to discuss both of these. This can in itself demonstrate empathy.
- Elicit motivation to change from the patient; do not impose it on him or her.
- Do not jump ahead of the patient's readiness for change and thus generate resistance.
- Use reflective listening (repeating back to the patient what he or she has said by rephrasing and summarizing key points or ideas).
- Express acceptance and affirmation.
- Selectively reinforce the patient's own self-motivational statements.
- Teach the patient about the stages of change (pre-contemplation, contemplation, preparation, action, maintenance) and invite the patient to consider which stage best fits him.
- Challenge the patient to reflect on how his behavior is affecting his life with questions such as "What is a typical day like for you?" "What was life like before this behavior?" "How has your behavior impacted the lives of the people you value and care about?" "Who is your 'ideal (or best or true) self' and what are his values?" "What will your future be like if you continue this behavior vs. if you stop it?" "How important is it for you to change?" "How confident are you that you can change (have you had other such accomplishments in your life)?"
- If the patient is ready for change, make an action plan for quitting; if not, invite the patient to predict how his life will be as he continues his lifestyle.

Helping Patients to Cope with the Stress of Medical Hospitalization

Multiple theoretical approaches exist to explain why certain patients react to stress in a particular way, and each approach provides a method of psychotherapy that can help the patient to cope more effectively. These approaches include existential psychotherapy, psychodynamic psychotherapy, cognitive behavioral therapy, family therapy, interpersonal therapy, and problem-solving therapy. Specific psychotherapeutic interventions have been developed for different diseases (e.g., cancer, HIV, pain, and various organ system dysfunctions), but there are no evidence-based guidelines describing which specific method is best for each individual patient. Despite this limitation, the rich and extensive literature on bedside psychotherapy can guide your approach.

It is important to note that psychotherapy can have a very broad definition, including any way in which the patient-provider relationship intentionally provides symptom relief. Every sentence that you utter can be therapeutic if you are attuned to the patient's needs, even if you never sit down and do formal psychotherapy. You can relieve distress from the very first handshake and expression of genuine concern. Just acknowledging the suffering caused by being in the hospital can be therapeutic, as can listening empathically to the patient's illness narrative. If the psychiatrist allows the patient to linger on the painful details without feeling rushed, this will convey to him or her that the psychiatrist can tolerate being empathetic and that the situation, though difficult, is not completely overwhelming. An empathic understanding of the patient's situation lays a foundation for a good therapeutic relationship, which in itself gives the patient hope, knowing that she is not alone and that someone is confident that she can overcome her suffering.

If there is an opportunity for the psychiatrist to see the patient several times during the hospitalization, then it may be helpful to agree to come back to provide more extended psychotherapy. Keep in mind that psychotherapy in the hospital must be more flexible than in most other settings due to the patient's physical symptoms and interruptions from medical staff, other patients, and family members. The information provided in the following sections will help to inform bedside psychotherapy for those patients coping with stress, whether the psychotherapy lasts one session or several.

Treatment of Demoralization

Demoralization is generally defined as the helplessness, hopelessness, confusion, and subjective incompetence experienced by patients who are failing to fulfill their own expectations (or those of others) as they cope with a stressful situation, typically in isolation from their usual social supports. It often results from a severe life defeat that has caused the patient to feel ineffective, resulting in a change in self-image that makes him feel helpless.

While demoralization is similar to depression, it is pedagogically useful to delineate their differences so that the psychiatrist can be more attuned to demoralization and thus can recommend more precise treatment. "Depression" may be considered more biologic, with the patient *lacking the ability* to experience pleasure, while "demoralization" is more due to *external events causing the patient to lose hope* that pleasure could ever exist for him. Demoralized patients stop trying to find pleasure, which increases their suffering all the more. A psychiatric consultant can help relieve this suffering by taking the initiative to find pleasure for the patient (e.g., by asking the patient to call a friend or watch a funny TV show); the patient will likely be surprised by how good this makes him feel.

Similarly, "depressed" patients may know what to do in a given situation, but they lack the motivation to do it. By contrast, demoralized patients may feel like they do not know what to do, but might have plenty of motivation. If a psychiatrist provides direction to channel the motivation, the demoralized patient can in fact be productive, thus improving his confidence and self-image.

It can be useful to consider the needs of demoralized patients in a hierarchical way, addressing the more basic needs before attempting to meet the more complex ones. Table 8.4 is adapted from Griffith and Gaby (2005).

Dynamically Informed Bedside Psychotherapy

Patients are often distressed when they do not understand why they are reacting to a stressor in a particularly maladaptive way. They may feel "crazy" or may feel that they cannot control their affects or their behaviors. Dynamically oriented therapy can relieve this distress by identifying the unconscious conflicts and desires that are causing these maladaptive reactions and by sharing appropriate interpretations with the patient. Not every patient is ready to confront these repressed conflicts and desires, so the therapist must be sensitive as to whether the patient would be able to endure the extra stress that doing so would cause. Still, if a therapist can interpret a patient's current reactions to stress as being completely expectable given what he or she has been through in life, then this can help the patient to feel more in control and thus more confident.

In order to do this, the psychiatric consultant must listen to the patient's life story, attending especially to those aspects that helped form the patient's values and beliefs. For example, if a patient's parent shamed him when he showed signs of weakness as a child, the patient may later feel overly anxious while hospitalized due to feeling vulnerable and weak. The psychiatric consultant can relieve this anxiety by pointing out that feeling independent is extremely important to him, so of course he is feeling so anxious in the dependent role of a patient. There is no need for the patient to reconcile his conflicting emotions (love and anger) toward his parent at this time; this task can wait until the patient is ready to work through that conflict.

Bedside Cognitive Behavioral Therapy

The premise of cognitive behavioral therapy (CBT) is that depression and anxiety are caused by automatic thoughts that are either false or maladaptive. Replacing these thoughts with more balanced or adaptive

Table 8.4 A Hierarchical Approach to Treating Demoralization

Underpinnings of *Vulnerability*	Approaches to Maximize *Resilience*
Confusion: Medical (delirium, physical discomfort) or psychological (when the medical condition does not make sense to the patient or doctors).	**Coherence:** Treat delirium or physical discomfort. Lend your executive function to the patient (e.g., make a list of questions for the primary team with the patient).
Isolation: Inherent to the experiences of medical illness and hospitalization; associated with poor medical outcomes.	**Communion:** Find ways to support the patient's natural connections while in the hospital (e.g., video conferencing). *"Does anything help you feel connected when family and friends are not available?"* (e.g., faith)
Despair: Associated with poor medical outcomes.	**Hope:** *"What keeps you from giving up?"*
Meaninglessness: Illness/disability may make it impossible for the patient to do things that used to give life meaning (professional or recreational).	**Purpose:** *"How can you contribute to the world or enjoy yourself despite the limitations imposed by illness?"* Inquire about how spirituality may give the patient a sense of purpose.
Helplessness: Lack of control due to the course of illness or treatment environment; associated with poor medical outcomes.	**Agency:** Help the patient to make meaningful choices despite the lack of control, and to recapture his or her identity as a competent person: *"Describe a time when you were on top of your game."*
Cowardice: Cycle in which the patient sees himself as fearful, which diminishes self-esteem, leading to increased anxiety and further retreat from challenges.	**Courage:** Remind the patient of his courageous acts, no matter how small. This encourages him to maximize control over fear.
Resentment: Focused on their situation and the people around them.	**Gratitude:** *"Is there any good that has come out of these tragic events? For what in your life are you most deeply grateful?"*

thoughts results in less distress. The role of the cognitive therapist is to learn from the patient what situations trigger depressive or anxious feelings, to help the patient to link these feelings to the automatic thoughts that generate them, and to guide the patient to more balanced or adaptive thoughts. The unconscious is not a focus in this therapy.

In the hospital, situations that can trigger dysfunctional thoughts and emotions include those that remind patients of various losses (function, identity, physical attractiveness, independence, time with loved ones). The script presented in Box 8.2 demonstrates how CBT can be used in a medical setting.

Strategies to Relieve Pain or Anxiety (Deep Breathing, Progressive Muscle Relaxation, and Guided Imagery)

Medical inpatients frequently confront situations in which they must cope with physical discomfort or anxiety due to various causes (e.g., mechanical ventilation, pain, loneliness, boredom, immobilization, and bed rest in pregnancy). Deep breathing, progressive muscle relaxation, and guided imagery all provide opportunities for patients to disengage from the distress and to let their minds relax. This can decrease their need for analgesic and sedative medications (see Chapter 20 for additional information).

Psychotherapy for Grief

Medical inpatients frequently experience many losses. Grief therapy is a way to help these patients to confront and mourn these losses, ushering them through profound pain to acceptance. It involves the following techniques:

- Relate the patient's distress to his losses.
- Help the patient to anticipate the normal process of mourning by describing the stages of grief: disbelief, yearning, anger, depression, and acceptance.
- Explain the process of normal grief, which includes oscillation between "attending to the loss" and "restoring a new normal."
- For patients who have difficulty restoring a new normal:
  - If the patient appears ambivalent about moving on (e.g., believes that moving on might imply that the loss was not severe), use motivational interviewing (see earlier discussion) to explore reasons that moving on would be desirable or undesirable, selectively affirming how the patient will function better if he does successfully restore a new normal.
  - If the patient appears to be idealizing the past and catastrophizing the future, use cognitive therapy (see earlier discussion) to help replace cognitive distortions with more balanced views.
  - Help the patient to replace previously enjoyed activities with new ones, or plan for changes that need to be made upon discharge from the hospital.
- If the patient is having difficulty attending to the loss:
  - Refer the patient to an experienced therapist who can use exposure therapy to demonstrate to the patient that she can endure these painful emotions and not be crushed by them.

Box 8.2 Sample CBT Script

Psychiatrist: "In what situations do you feel angry or sad?"

Patient: "Every time I have to be helped to the darn commode."

Psychiatrist: "What goes through your mind when you feel angry or sad?"

Patient: "I'll be confined to a wheelchair for the rest of my life."

Psychiatrist: "If that's true, what does that mean for you?"

Patient: "I'm helpless so I'm not a real man, I'll never find a wife, I'll be lonely forever. . ."

Psychiatrist: "I can see how that'd be horrible. Let's look at the evidence for and against your thought that you'll be confined to a wheelchair for the rest of your life. Are there any other possibilities?"

Patient: [Looks at the evidence and articulates other possibilities.]

Psychiatrist: "What is the effect on your emotions if you believe your original thought vs. an alternative?"

Patient: [Articulates how his thoughts affect his emotions.]

Psychiatrist: "What is the worst that could happen? The best? The most likely?"

Patient: [Realizes that a realistic assessment of the situation shows that, while the future will likely have some difficulties, it is not hopeless.]

Psychiatrist: "Even if you are in a wheelchair, what's the evidence for your belief that you'll be helpless, not a real man, never find a wife, and will be lonely forever? What about the evidence against?" *Continue Socratic questioning for each maladaptive belief. Socratic questioning can also be used to help the patient decide whether to linger on a particular thought, since lingering on some true thoughts (e.g., "I'm missing out on so much during this hospitalization") can also affect mood.*

Conclusion

All patients have ways of coping with the unique stresses of medical hospitalization. By using the strategies discussed here, the psychiatric consultant can identify the reasons behind patients' maladaptive behaviors and emotions and then guide them to more positive ways of coping with these stresses.

Key Points

- If you pay attention to why a patient is acting maladaptively, you can attempt to make every interaction that you have with him or her therapeutic, from the first introduction to the last goodbye.
- A patient acts the way he does due to the way that his particular personality and background interact with his current particular situation.
- Sometimes you cannot change a patient's maladaptive behavior, but you can help the medical staff to feel less frustrated by it.
- You can use aspects of existential, psychodynamic, cognitive, and grief psychotherapy to better understand and treat many patients who have difficulty coping with the stress of medical hospitalization, even if you interact with the patient only once.

Disclosures

Dr. Dobbelstein has no conflicts of interest to disclose.

Mary G. Fitzgerald has disclosed no conflicts of interest.

Further Reading

Blumenfield M, Strain JJ (Eds.) (2006). *Psychosomatic Medicine*. Philadelphia, PA: Lippincott, Williams, & Wilkins.

Griffith JL, Gaby L (2005). Brief psychotherapy at the bedside: Countering demoralization from medical illness. *Psychosomatics*, 46, 109–116.

Levenson JL (Ed.) (2009). *The American Psychiatric Publishing Textbook of Psychosomatic Medicine: Psychiatric Care of the Medically Ill*, 2nd ed. Arlington, VA: American Psychiatric Publishing.

Rollnick S, Miller WR (1995). What is motivational interviewing? *Behav Cogn Psychother.*, 23, 325–334.

Stroebe M, Schut H (1999). The dual process model of coping with bereavement: rationale and description. *Death Stud.*, 23, 197–224.

Exercises

1. Which personality type is characterized by needing to feel special, acting extremely entitled and grandiose, and lacking empathy?
   a. Obsessive-compulsive
   b. Antisocial
   c. Narcissistic
   d. Borderline

2. What is a strategy that can optimize interactions with patients of the above personality type?
   a. Provide ample praise so that the patient feels special.
   b. Keep rigid boundaries to prevent impression of closeness.
   c. Help patient to use intellectualization in order to feel like he or she has more control.
   d. Ensure that the patient is receiving sufficient information.

3. A patient who works full-time but does not have health insurance is admitted for complications from recently diagnosed metastatic breast cancer. She is angry at her employer and at herself, believing that if she had received routine mammograms, she would not be in this situation. She becomes enraged at hospital staff because of a minor mistake on her dinner tray. In order to help the staff to feel less personally assaulted, you inform them that she has likely been manifesting which of the following defense mechanisms?
   a. Acting out
   b. Denial
   c. Projection
   d. Displacement

4. A patient with alcohol use disorder has nearly completed treatment for withdrawal and is considering substance use rehabilitation. Which of the following strategies is most likely to be useful?
   a. Lecturing him about how he will die if he does not stop drinking.
   b. Reflecting that his drinking may be a punishment due to excessive guilt.
   c. Explicitly acknowledging that there are pros and cons to his drinking and inviting him to discuss both of these.
   d. Referral to social work.

Answers: (1) c (2) a (3) d (4) c

Assessment of Decision-Making Capacity

Abhishek Jain and Kurt D. Ackerman

Overview

In 1914, Justice Benjamin Cordozo famously articulated, "Every human being of adult years and sound mind has a right to determine what shall be done with his own body" (*Schloendorff v. Society of New York Hospital*, 105 N.E. 92 [N.Y. 1914]).

While any physician can determine whether or not a patient is of "sound mind" to make medical decisions, psychiatrists are often consulted due to their expertise in understanding and diagnosing psychiatric disorders that may impact a person's decision-making capacity. In one study, 10% of psychiatric consultations were requested to determine a patient's medical decision-making capacity (Kornfeld et al., 2013). On our consultation service, an estimated 5% of requests are explicitly for capacity assessment (e.g., "Can the patient sign out of the hospital against medical advice?"), but many more cases either indirectly involve capacity or evolve into formal capacity assessments (e.g., a patient initially seen for delirium subsequently refuses placement in a skilled nursing facility).

When consulting on challenging or emotionally charged cases involving capacity determinations, psychiatric providers may also help medical teams manage their own expectations and countertransference. Such evaluations often involve balancing patient autonomy with beneficence (i.e., when should a patient be allowed to retain the right to make even an ill-advised medical decision, and when should a patient be deemed incapacitated and protected from making harmful choices?). Allowing a patient to make an ill-advised decision can be disquieting for medical providers and families, and seemingly places the patient at odds with the medical team, but this may also provide an opportunity for dialogue, education, and collaboration among providers, families, and patients.

Like other areas of medicine, understanding the concept of patients' decision-making capacity can be relatively straightforward, but applying the concept in clinical care can often be challenging. *A patient's capacity typically comprises four abilities: (1) communicating a choice, (2) understanding relevant information, (3) appreciating the current situation and the potential consequences of a decision, and (4) rationally manipulating information* (Appelbaum, 2007). Over the years, medical, legal, and bioethical perspectives have generally agreed that an individual retains the right to make medical decisions unless he or she has a significant deficit in at least one of these four abilities pertinent to the decision-making process.

Of note regarding terminology, although "competency" and "capacity" are often used interchangeably to refer to a person's ability to make decisions, "competency" is a legal determination and "capacity" is a clinical assessment. Additionally, the term "informed consent" incorporates "capacity" as one of its three components: (a) relevant medical information must be disclosed to the patient, (b) the patient must make his or her decision voluntarily, and (c) the patient must possess sufficient capacity.

Although a formal capacity assessment is not required in every clinical encounter, each clinical encounter involves some assessment of a patient's ability to consent or refuse, to understand medical information, to appreciate the consequences of a decision, and to demonstrate sound reasoning in the decision-making process. For example, if a patient were to refuse a routine blood draw, a clinician may naturally wonder, "Why is the patient refusing?" This inquiry is essentially a question about the patient's capacity and whether or not the patient understands the purpose of the blood draw, and further discussion with the patient may allow an opportunity for clarification and education.

In this chapter, we highlight (1) key concepts, (2) a proposed step-wise approach, (3) some frequently encountered challenges, and (4) documentation.

Key Concepts

- Capacity is generally presumed in adults.
  - Adult patients are presumed to have decision-making capacity unless a legal determination of incompetence or a court-ordered guardian has already been established, or if clinical evidence of impairment is present, as described in the previous section.
- Capacity is time-specific.
  - Certain chronic conditions, such as severe dementia, may render an individual unable to make most or all relevant future medical decisions. However, most clinical capacity determinations are specific to the current moment.
  - A patient's capacity may fluctuate over time (e.g., in medical delirium); thus a change in mental status may prompt reassessment.
- Capacity is decision-specific.
  - Unless the purpose of the evaluation is to pursue guardianship, focusing on the patient's capacity for one specific decision is more practical than addressing a general question of capacity.
  - A patient may have sufficient capacity to make a lower-risk decision, but the same patient may not have sufficient capacity to make a higher-risk decision. This concept of a "sliding scale" has been discussed in medical, legal, and bioethical literature, and can be clinically useful (see Table 9.1).
- Capacity determinations are rarely simply binary (i.e., just determining that a patient does or does not have capacity in a vacuum) and often involve multiple factors (e.g., social circumstances) and consideration of alternative solutions.
- The observation that patients are considered to have capacity only if they agree with medical recommendations is likely related to the idea that medical recommendations typically represent the choice with the most favorable risk/benefit ratio, and that it is human nature to favor mutually shared opinions. Similarly, clinicians should be cautious of the inverse: a patient who automatically acquiesces to medical recommendations may actually not have sufficient capacity to consent.
- The mere presence of mental illness, such as dementia, schizophrenia, or intellectual disability, is not sufficient to deem a patient incapacitated; clinical evidence of impairment in one of the four elements of capacity (communication, understanding, appreciation, or reasoning) relevant to the specific decision must still be demonstrated.
- Although patients may reasonably change their decisions, frequent and abrupt decision changes can raise a "red flag" about a patient's capacity. This is especially true when a patient has suddenly changed his or her initial decision to a decision that is no longer consistent with his or her previous value system.

- Once a patient is determined to have sufficient capacity to make a specific decision, the patient is entitled to make that decision, even if the choice is unwise or against medical advice. This situation is often unsettling for clinicians and families, but the focus of a capacity assessment is the "process" of reaching a decision rather than the decision itself. Of course, the capacity assessment also provides an opportunity to educate patients, discuss risks, and establish a safety plan for potential negative consequences.
- In complex situations, before meeting with the patient or family, it can be helpful for medical providers and consultants to collaborate and determine the proposed medical recommendations, any reasonable alternatives, and the likely risks and benefits of each. A team meeting can help quell complex, stressful, or emotionally charged medical situations (e.g., preterm cesarean delivery in a high-risk pregnancy). If patients are provided with conflicting information or observe disagreements among providers, they can become further confused and anxious in an already potentially anxiety-provoking situation.

Table 9.1 Sliding Scale of Capacity

Low-Risk/High-Benefit	High-Risk/High-Benefit
Lowest degree of capacity needs to be demonstrated *Example: consenting to a routine blood draw*	Higher degree of capacity needs to be demonstrated than for low-risk decisions *Example: consenting to coronary artery bypass grafting (CABG)*
Low-Risk/Low-Benefit	**High-Risk/Low-Benefit**
Usually not consulted on these decisions but would require a relatively low degree of capacity *Example: splinting a broken toe*	Highest degree of capacity needs to be demonstrated *Example: consenting to a Phase I chemotherapy trial*

Proposed Step-Wise Approach to Capacity Assessment

In this section we offer a systematic process to evaluate capacity in a hospital setting.

1. Clarify the exact medical decision that the patient is being asked to make. For example, a consult request of "Does the patient have capacity to refuse a peripherally inserted central catheter (PICC)?" is generally more practical than the nonspecific question "Does the patient have capacity to make medical decisions?"

2. Gather the relevant background medical and psychosocial information from medical records and the primary team.

3. Determine the urgency of making the medical decision. Generally, in a medical emergency, medical providers can proceed with necessary intervention, unless clear advanced directives exist. The legal role of a surrogate decision-maker in these circumstances may vary by jurisdiction.

4. Clarify with the medical team the current medical recommendation, the risks and benefits to the patient of refusing or consenting to the recommended treatment, the risks and benefits of reasonable alternatives, what the medical team has actually told the patient, and what makes the medical team concerned about the patient's decision-making capacity.

5. When evaluating the patient, consider bringing along a medical team representative to help explain and clarify any specific medical information or questions that arise during the capacity assessment.

6. Although clinicians' styles of engaging patients may reasonably differ, a helpful strategy is to explain the psychiatric consultant's role to the patient, expressing that part of this role involves conveying the patient's wishes to the medical team, and attempting to align with any common interests (e.g., "We want to make sure you have all the information you need to make your decision to sign out of the hospital").

7. As outlined previously, the key focus of a capacity evaluation typically involves assessing the four elements (communication, understanding, appreciation, and reasoning) listed above. Elicit the following, and document exact quotes where possible:
   a. The patient's expressed medical decision;
   b. The patient's understanding of current medical issues relevant to the decision;
   c. The patient's appreciation of the severity and consequences of the available choices;
   d. How the patient arrived at his or her decision and what factors played an important role;
   e. Any thought, mood, or cognitive disturbance that may impair the patient's decision-making capacity;
   f. The patient's desired surrogate decision-maker.

8. Consider using a semi-structured interview such as the Aid to Capacity Evaluation, which, along with its instructions and scoring guide, is available online. This evaluation may be copied for non-commercial use, takes 10–20 minutes to administer, has been standardized in medical inpatients, and has a 93% inter-rater agreement (Dunn et al., 2006).

9. If the patient demonstrates sufficient capacity, recommend that the medical team allow the patient to make his or her expressed decision. However, to help minimize any potential negative outcomes of the patient's decision, consider educating patients and families regarding foreseeable risks and outlining a safety plan.

10. If the patient does not have sufficient capacity, look for opportunities to build a consensus and pursue another course that would still maintain safety (e.g., if a patient does not have sufficient capacity to refuse nursing home placement, but still adamantly demands to be discharged home, consider whether home healthcare nursing aides or moving in with a relative would maintain safety and be agreeable to the patient). Consider deferring non-urgent decisions until reversible causes of incapacity are addressed and the patient can regain capacity. Also, enlisting the patient's surrogate decision-maker may help facilitate communication with the patient. The proposed algorithm in Figure 9.1 outlines further considerations when a patient is found to not have sufficient decision-making capacity.

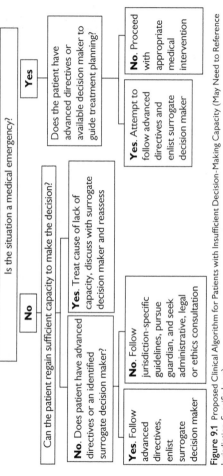

Figure 9.1 Proposed Clinical Algorithm for Patients with Insufficient Decision-Making Capacity (May Need to Reference Jurisdiction-Specific Laws)

Is the situation a medical emergency?

No

Can the patient regain sufficient capacity to make the decision?

No. Does patient have advanced directives or an identified surrogate decision maker?

Yes. Treat cause of lack of capacity, discuss with surrogate decision maker and reassess

Yes. Follow advanced directives, enlist surrogate decision maker

No. Follow jurisdiction-specific guidelines, pursue guardian, and seek administrative, legal or ethics consultation

Yes

Does the patient have advanced directives or available decision maker to guide treatment planning?

Yes. Attempt to follow advanced directives and enlist surrogate decision maker

No. Proceed with appropriate medical intervention

Some Frequently Encountered Challenges

What if the Patient Refuses an Interview?

Similar to other patient encounters, capacity evaluations often require an "art" of engaging patients and building rapport. Considerations when assessing a patient's decisional capacity include the following:

- Clearly explain to the patient the reason for the consult and the primary team's concerns (e.g., the primary team wants to ensure the patient has sufficient information to make a decision).
- Acknowledge that the patient has the right to refuse the evaluation, but due to the concerns raised by the primary team (e.g., patient's recent confusion, etc.), if the patient does refuse the interview, then the team will have to rely on what others (e.g., providers, family, medical records) report to determine if the patient has sufficient capacity.
- While refusing an interview is not sufficient grounds to deem a patient incapacitated, the inability to understand concerns regarding his or her capacity and not appreciating the consequences of refusing the interview would raise concerns about the patient's capacity.
- Although patients are generally assumed to have capacity, if there is evidence that the patient's capacity is likely impaired (e.g., recent hallucinations, memory impairment, etc.), the "burden of proof" could be thought of as shifting to the patient having to demonstrate that he or she has capacity (especially in higher-risk decisions).

What if the Patient Lacks Capacity and Does Not Have Clear Advanced Directives?

In non-emergencies, and depending on the jurisdiction, medical decisions would generally be turned over to the identified durable power of attorney or the legal surrogate decision-maker. For example, Pennsylvania law outlines the order of priority (e.g., spouse, adult child, or parent) if a healthcare representative has not been previously designated (20 Pa. C.S.A. Chapter 54).

Typically, a patient requires a relatively lower degree of capacity to identify a desired surrogate decision-maker (usually a relatively low-risk/high-benefit decision). In situations in which a dispute or concern about the surrogate decision-maker exists, consultation from the hospital's legal department or an ethics committee may be helpful.

Documentation

The following is an example of documentation of a case involving an elderly man with schizophrenia who wants to postpone a non-urgent CABG surgery to attend his daughter's wedding. Key words are bolded for illustration purposes:

> Although Mr. Smith has a history of schizophrenia and is at a moderate medical risk by declining surgery, he currently demonstrates the necessary capacity to make this decision. The patient has clearly and consistently **communicated a choice** to decline surgery at this time. He **understands** and communicates his current medical condition, the medical team's recommendations, benefits of surgery, and risks of postponing the surgery. He demonstrates insight into his medical and psychiatric illnesses, and he **appreciates** the potential consequences (including death) of delaying surgery. He is able to **rationally manipulate** the necessary medical information and compare risks and benefits of the relevant options. Despite the patient's history of schizophrenia, his current **reasoning** is sound and not impaired by cognitive, psychotic, or emotional symptoms. His reasoning is consistent with previously held **values** (i.e., importance of not missing his daughter's wedding) and prior decisions regarding his medical condition.

Additionally, outlining specific recommendations in the treatment plan can be helpful. For example:

- If the patient is assessed to have capacity and thereby is entitled to make a relatively high-risk decision, the consultant can recommend ongoing steps for education, safety planning if the patient's condition continues or worsens (e.g., call 911 or seek immediate medical attention), and, with appropriate consent, discussion with family members.
- If the patient lacks capacity, the consultant can specify the reasonable next steps (e.g., appropriate to treat over the patient's objection, or contact the surrogate decision-maker to develop a care plan until the patient regains capacity), can provide treatment recommendations to help restore capacity (e.g., continue treating underlying medical causes of delirium while using low-dose antipsychotic medications to target agitation and reassess capacity as condition improves), and can address disposition planning and immediate safety concerns (e.g., the patient may require inpatient psychiatric hospitalization, a guardian, close family monitoring, or oversight by the Department of Aging).
- It is important to reinforce that decisional capacity is time-specific and that ongoing decisions, such as consent for hemodialysis, should be reassessed over time.

Key Points

Although psychiatric consultation requests for patients' decision-making capacity can be complex and time-consuming, they are important components of medical care. These evaluations often involve the confluence of art (patient engagement and problem-solving), science (understanding and clarifying the medical issues), and law (jurisdiction-specific legalities of surrogate decision-making), and can provide an opportunity to work as a collaborative interdisciplinary team.

The mnemonic "SCURVIES" (adapted from CURVES; Chow et al., 2010) outlines the key points to consider in capacity assessments:

Specific question: What is the exact medical decision the patient is being asked to make?

Communicating a choice: Is the patient able to communicate a clear and consistent choice?

Understanding and appreciating information: Is the patient able to understand the relevant information and appreciate the potential consequences of consenting or refusing?

Rationally manipulating information: Does the patient have any disturbance of thought or mood that would impair his or her ability to weigh relevant risks and benefits?

Values: Is the patient's medical decision consistent with his or her previously expressed values and wishes?

Intervention: Can medical or psychiatric intervention help the patient regain capacity?

Emergency: Is this a medical emergency? Generally, for medical emergencies, a medical team can reasonably proceed with a necessary intervention unless there is a clear advanced directive.

Surrogate decision-maker: Is there an identified durable power of attorney? Does the patient have sufficient capacity to identify a surrogate decision-maker? Clarify any jurisdiction-specific laws regarding identifying a surrogate decision-maker or appointing a court-ordered guardian.

Disclosures

Dr. Jain has no conflicts of interest to disclose.

Dr. Ackerman has no conflicts of interest to disclose.

Further Reading

Appelbaum PS. (2007). Clinical practice: Assessment of patients' competence to consent to treatment. *N Engl J Med.*, *357*(18), 1834–1840.

Chow GV, Czarny MJ, et al. (2010). CURVES: A mnemonic for determining medical decision-making capacity and providing emergency treatment in the acute setting. *Chest*, *137*(2), 421–427.

Dunn LB, Nowrangi MA, et al. (2006). Assessing decisional capacity for clinical research or treatment: A review of instruments. *Am J Psychiat.*, *163*(8), 1323–1334.

Ganzini L, Volicer L, et al. (2005). Ten myths about decision-making capacity. *J Am Med Dir Assoc.*, *6*(3 Suppl), S100–104.

Kornfeld DS, Muskin PR, et al. (2009). Psychiatric evaluation of mental capacity in the general hospital: A significant teaching opportunity. *Psychosomatics*, *50*(5), 468–473.

Exercises

1. The four components of decision-making capacity typically include:
   a. Communication, understanding, appreciation, and reasoning
   b. Expertise, knowledge, ability, and execution
   c. Communication, reasoning, ability, and psychometric testing
   d. Communication, expertise, paternalism, psychometric testing

2. A patient disagreeing with medical advice:
   a. Is legally presumed to lack decision-making capacity until proven otherwise
   b. Is legally presumed to have decision-making capacity until proven otherwise
   c. Is legally required to undergo a guardianship evaluation
   d. Is legally required to undergo psychometric testing

3. In the United States, who can perform capacity assessments?
   a. Only psychiatrists
   b. Only physicians with Competency Assessment Certification
   c. Any physician
   d. Any court-appointed lawyer

4. Using the theory of a "sliding scale" in capacity determinations, which of the following would generally require the most extensive evaluation?
   a. Consenting to a high-benefit, low-risk life-saving procedure
   b. Consenting to a low-benefit, high-risk experimental surgery
   c. Consenting to a low-benefit, low-risk meal item
   d. Consenting to a high-benefit, high-risk medication

5. Who among the following would be automatically deemed incapacitated to make medical decisions?
   a. Patient with borderline intellectual functioning
   b. Patient with active auditory hallucinations
   c. Patient with recurrent self-injurious behaviors
   d. None of the above
   e. All of the above

Answers: (1) a (2) b (3) c (4) b (5) d

Psychiatric Presentations Associated with Neurologic and Other Medical Conditions

Delirium

Ghennady V. Gushchin

Delirium (from Latin *de* ["out"] and *lira* ["furrow or track"], i.e., "out of the furrow") is one of the "D" conditions (along with drugs, depression, dementia, dissociation, and deception) that require a psychiatrist's expertise in medical/surgical settings. Delirium is a clinical syndrome, which may occur in the course of serious medical illness, or substance intoxication or withdrawal. It is characterized by a relatively sudden onset of altered mental status and fluctuating intensity of disturbances of patient's awareness and arousal, deficits in attention, cognitive impairment, behavioral disturbances (hypoactive or hyperactive), and sleep/wake cycle alteration. In psychosomatic medicine, delirium is dubbed as "a great imitator" because it can mimic a wide range of mental disorders including psychosis, mania, depression, anxiety, sleep disorders, and dementia. See Box 10.1 for a sample case presentation.

Box 10.1 Clinical Vignette

A woman in her late seventies underwent elective hip replacement surgery. In the post-op room, her caregivers did not recognize that she regained some awareness of her environment and self and continued to treat her as a patient in a coma (moving from stretcher to bed, placing an indwelling catheter without interacting with her). When the patient was brought back to her room, she told her husband a passionate and convincing story that she was raped in the post-op room by a nursing staff member. The couple barricaded themselves in the room to prevent medical personnel from entering, and demanded a lawyer. A psychiatrist was called, who was allowed to enter the room, probably by mistake (did not wear a white lab coat that day). The psychiatrist quickly determined that the patient was delirious, but spent considerable time diffusing the critical situation, mostly by working with the patient's husband, appealing to his common sense (patient needs pain medications, food, PT/OT), and persuading the couple to cooperate with care. Even a week later, at discharge to a rehabilitation facility, the patient told the psychiatrist that "something wrong happened that day in the post-op room."

Epidemiology

Older age, severe medical illness, and substance use (in combination with immobility, sleep deprivation, visual and hearing impairment, dehydration, and dementia) are among the most recognized risks for delirium (see Table 10.1 for incidence among patients and the general population).

Undiagnosed and untreated delirium is a culprit for increased morbidity (bed sores, aspiration pneumonia, nosocomial infections, and cardiovascular events) and is one of the leading causes of an extended stay in the hospital, prolonged rehabilitation, and admissions to nursing facilities. There are data to suggest that patients with delirium are two times more prone to die in the next six months compared with patients with similar medical problems but without delirium.

Surprisingly, only 10% of patients with delirium will receive a psychiatric consultation in the hospital setting. In 32%–81% of the cases, delirium (especially the hypoactive subtype) goes unrecognized, underestimated, or misdiagnosed by both doctors and nurses. When nurses are asked, they usually explain that they are not accustomed to taking the lead in making diagnoses. Physicians' reluctance to recognize delirium and make a diagnosis has an apparently more complex nature. At best, physicians can put "altered mental status" or "metabolic encephalopathy" on the problem list, but in most cases they will just ignore any diagnostic category and will focus on the evaluation of clinical features pertinent to their specialties. They will call a C-L psychiatrist if the patient "looks crazy" or "severely depressed." It is not rare that a C-L psychiatrist will be asked to see a patient for "depression (anxiety, mania, or psychosis)" when the patient is floridly delirious. Unfortunately, this "hospital culture" may result in delay of the medical workup for delirium, can cause additional suffering for patients, and definitely compromises health information/statistics by underreporting a huge health problem.

Table 10.1 Incidence of Delirium

Postsurgical patients	75%
Terminal stages of cancer	25%–85%
ICU patients	12%–50%
All hospitalized patients	9%–30%
General population (older than 55)	1.1%
General population	0.4%

Etiology

Delirium is associated with a wide variety of medical conditions. Several mnemonic tools have been introduced to identify main causative factors of delirium; one is listed here (Wise et al., 2005):

I WATCH DEATH

I: Infections (encephalitis, meningitis, HIV, syphilis, sepsis, typhus, malaria)

W: Withdrawal from the substance of the abuse (alcohol, sedative-hypnotics, barbiturates)

A: Acute metabolic (acidosis, alkalosis, liver/kidney failure)

T: Trauma (closed head trauma, heatstroke, recent surgery, severe burns)

C: CNS pathology (abscess, tumor, seizures, hydrocephalus)

H: Hypoxia (anemia, hypoperfusion due to heart/lung failure, CO poisoning)

D: Deficiencies of Vitamins (B_{12}, folate, thiamine, niacin)

E: Endocrinopathies (hyper/hypoglycemia, hypo/hyperadrenocorticism, hyperparathyroidism)

A: Acute vascular (hypertension, stroke, TIA, arrhythmia)

T: Toxins (medications, illicit drugs, pesticides, solvents)

H: Heavy metal (lead, manganese, mercury).

Pathophysiology of Delirium

The exact pathophysiological mechanisms of delirium remain obscure. Several existing hypotheses are based on clinical observations, effects of certain medications, and studies of neurotransmitter, neuropeptide, cytokine, and hormonal mechanisms (Maldonado, 2013):

- Neurotransmitter dysregulation (dopamine vs. acetylcholine, GABA, serotonin)
- Neuro-inflammation (cytokines IL-1, IL-2, TNF, IL-6)
- Oxidative stress
- Neuro-aging (homeostenosis)
- Neuro-endocrine (aberrant stress)
- Sleep/wake dysregulation (melatonin)
- Network disconnectivity.

Currently, most experts in the field acknowledge that the pathophysiology of delirium cannot be explained by any of the existing hypotheses alone, and that these mechanisms could contribute collectively to this complicated condition. It is likely that future studies will reveal heterogeneity of the conditions that present as delirium, and more specific mechanisms will be elucidated.

Brain imaging studies on delirium are in their infancy.

Clinical Features

The use of multiple names for delirium in the peer-reviewed literature still causes confusion across medical disciplines. Reviewing the existing synonyms/aliases of delirium may help to emphasize some important clinical features of this condition. "Organic brain syndrome" indicates the presence of identifiable medical illness. "Acute brain failure" stresses the lack of brain reserves and puts the condition in the same category of emergency as acute renal, respiratory, and heart failure. "Acute confusional state" reflects such important clinical features as a rapid onset and disorientation. "Reversible dementia" points at the reversible character of cognitive impairment (in contrast to dementia). "Toxic/metabolic encephalopathy" refers to the failure of general metabolism as an underlying cause of brain dysfunction. "ICU psychosis" points out the setting associated with increased incidence. "Sundowning" indicates diurnal fluctuation of mental status.

Delirium is often associated with a disturbance in the sleep-wake cycle. Using the Delirium Rating Scale (DRS-98R), Meagher et al. (2007) have presented evidence that attention impairment and sleep-wake cycle disturbance are the most prevalent symptoms of delirium. Surprisingly, impairment of orientation was registered in only three-quarters of cases. Delusions/hallucinations, abnormalities in thought processes, and language abnormalities were present in 31%–57% of patients (see Table 10.2).

Table 10.2 Symptoms of Delirium

Symptom	Presence at any Severity of Delirium (%)
Attention impairment	97
Sleep-wake cycle disturbance	97
Long-term memory impairment	89
Short-term memory impairment	88
Visuospatial ability impairment	87
Orientation	76
Motor retardation	62
Motor agitation	62
Language	57
Thought process abnormalities	54
Lability of affect	53
Perceptual abnormalities	50
Delusions	31

Assessment of the Patient with Delirium

The diagnosis of delirium is usually easy to make based on history (sudden onset, fluctuating mental status changes, sleep/wake cycle disturbance) collected from caregivers and mental status examination (with obvious confusion, poor attention, disorganized thinking). Nevertheless, in some cases, especially in the absence of caregivers' input, only repetitive assessments provide the information necessary to make the diagnosis and distinguish delirium from other conditions such as dementia. It makes it very important that clinicians use the standardized assessment instruments (scales), which allow documenting the result of assessment in the chart and monitoring the progression and resolution of delirium.

Standardized Assessment Scales for Delirium

The Confusion Assessment Method (CAM-ICU; Ely et al., 2001) is the most frequently used delirium scale, especially in intensive care units. The clinician needs to complete a review in four areas of assessment: onset/course, presence of inattention, disorganized thinking, and altered level of consciousness, i.e. awareness and arousal. If three of these areas are positive, a diagnosis of delirium is established.

The CAM-ICU has several advantages as a delirium screening tool: it is quick to administer, easy to use (important for busy ICU nurses), and it does not require skilled mental health professionals. It may be used in nonverbal patients, and can be repeated. Its disadvantages include the following: the CAM-ICU does not reflect sleep-wakefulness cycle abnormalities, does not specify the abnormal behavior (characteristics of altered mental status), and does not determine severity of impairment.

Delirium Rating Scale (DRS-R98, a revision of the original 1998 version; Trzepacz et al., 2001) is considered a "gold standard" for the diagnosis of and assessment of the severity of delirium. It comprises 16 areas of assessment: sleep-wake cycle disturbance, perceptual disturbance and hallucinations, delusions, lability of affect, language, thought process abnormalities, motor agitation, motor retardation, orientation, attention, short-term memory, long-term memory, visuospatial ability, temporal onset of symptoms, fluctuation of symptom severity, and presence of physical disorder. Each area is scored from 0 (normal) to a maximum of 2 or 3, yielding a maximum score of 46 for the most severe delirium and 19 as cutoff score for diagnosis. The advantages of the DRS-R98 are its comprehensiveness and ability to determine severity of delirium. As disadvantages in everyday clinical settings, it requires a trained examiner for scoring and is time-consuming.

Assessment of Nonverbal Patients

Additional difficulties in assessment of the patients with delirium may arise if the patient is not able to speak (intubated) or has sensory limitation (poor vision, hard of hearing). For nonverbal patients, it is important first to establish the patient's ability to comprehend and communicate by making an agreement with patient to answer "yes" by nodding and "no" by shaking their head (or raising gaze up as "yes" or lowering gaze down as "no" in patients with locked-in syndrome). At times, it could be prudent to rephrase a simple question so the patient will answer "yes" and "no" to comment on the same topic (e.g., "Are you anxious?" and "Are you relaxed?").

Once the communication mode is established, a clinician may inquire if the patient has difficulty sleeping or staying alert, which the patient may report spontaneously or may give indirect indication by being much too sleepy during the day and excessively excited during the night. The inquiry about sleep problems makes it easier to transition to testing attention span. A clinician may use the different tools (depending on the patient's sensory deficiencies). Auditory testing is usually preferable (the patient may not have his or her glasses available). The choice of specific testing tasks is up to the clinician. For example, one can use a letter "H" cancellation test (the same test can be used in verbal patients).

Orientation and memory can also be assessed in nonverbal patients using a similar approach: the patient is given a task and then is asked to indicate the correct answer (by nodding his or her head or pointing his or her index finger at the ceiling) from a few choices. For example, the patient is asked "What is today's date?" and is given a choice of three options (separately for year, season, month, weekday, and day) with instruction to indicate the correct answer. Then the patient is asked about the current location with three choices for building, room number, city, county, state. Further orientation could be checked by asking to point at the door (window, ceiling). Immediate memory could be assessed by request to memorize three words (e.g., cat-apple-blue, or tuna-coat-penny, or sparrow-table-red, one word per second) and then recall five minutes later by choosing from three options (e.g., "Choose from three animals: dog-cat-hamster" where "cat" would be the correct answer).

Diagnostic Criteria

The fifth edition of the *Diagnostic and Statistical Manual of Mental Disorders* (*DSM-5*; APA, 2013) provides generic diagnostic criteria for delirium, which essentially duplicate the diagnostic criteria of delirium from the previous edition (*DSM-IV*). The criteria are based on changes in attention, awareness, description of time of onset and the clinical course, presence of relevant medical conditions, and exclusion criteria.

DSM-5 fell short of recognizing disturbance of arousal and, in particular, sleep-wake cycle disturbance as diagnostic features of delirium. Meanwhile, studies on neurotransmitter circuits promoting arousal—NE (N. ceruleus), Histamine (tuberomammillary nucleus), Acetylcholine (lateral tegmental and pedunculopontine tegmental, basal forebrain nucleus), Orexin/Hypocretine (lateral hypothalamus, perifornical area), Serotonin (N. raphe)—or those promoting sleep—GABA (Ventrolateral preoptic nucleus), adenosine, galanin, melatonin—implicate a great deal of interconnection of delirium and sleep. Apparently, delirium could be considered as an example of a "twilight" condition (along with sleep and hypnotic or dissociative trance) that is characterized by disturbance in consciousness that, in turn, should be interpreted as reduced clarity of awareness of the environment and self with reduced ability to focus, sustain, or shift attention and altered level of arousal (in a continuum from coma and stupor to normal alertness and even hyper-arousal state). Needless to say, the etiology and intricate mechanisms of aforementioned "twilight" conditions are different.

DSM-5 uses specifiers to identify the etiologic factors of delirium (drug intoxication/withdrawal, another medical condition, or multiple etiologies). *DSM-5* has included "medication-induced delirium" to specify iatrogenic delirium, which is frequently observed in recovery from general anesthesia, Propofol sedation, or treatment with some antibiotics, anticonvulsants, anticholinergic and other prescription medications (in contrast to recreational use of medications). In addition, *DSM-5* introduces the terms "acute" and "persistent" to specify the length of delirious conditions, which may range from a few hours or days to weeks and months, respectively. To specify another clinically important characteristic of delirium—psychomotor activity—*DSM-5* uses the terms "hypoactive," "hyperactive," and "mixed level of activity."

DSM-5 introduces a new category "other specified delirium" to be used in situations in which "the presentation does not meet the criteria for delirium or any specific neurocognitive disorder." As an example, *DSM-5* uses a category of "attenuated delirium syndrome"—delirium in which some, but not all, diagnostic criteria for delirium are met (e.g., lack of significant cognitive impairment). "Unspecified delirium" is another new category in *DSM-5* that is intended to be a provisional diagnosis of delirium (e.g., in emergency room settings).

Differential Diagnosis

Delirium is included in the differential diagnosis of many mental conditions such as dementia, amnesia, catatonia, insomnia, nightmares, mania, depression, anxiety, and psychosis.

Dementia and Amnesia

The differential diagnosis of delirium and other neurocognitive disorders—dementia and amnesia—is the most challenging task because dementia itself is a risk factor for the development of delirium, and these two conditions may coexist. Nevertheless, thorough evaluation of the course and main features of the clinical presentation provide clues necessary to distinguish these conditions (see Table 10.3).

Some patients with amnesia (post-traumatic or substance-induced) may confabulate, which means that they recite imaginary events to fill in gaps in their memory. These may be perceived by an observer as confusion or even psychosis. *Attention, level of consciousness, thought processes, and perception* as well as overall cognitive functioning in amnestic patients are usually preserved.

Catatonia

Catatonia can present with odd behaviors, confusion, impairments in speech and communication, and fluctuation during the course of the day.

Table 10.3 Clinical Presentation and Symptoms of Dementia and Delirium

	Dementia	Delirium
Onset	Insidious	Acute (hours/days)
Course	Slowly progressing	Fluctuating
Level of consciousness	Normal	Waxing/waning
Attention	Normal	Inattention
Memory	Impaired	Impaired
Thinking	Word-finding difficulties, Impoverished	Disorganized
Orientation	Intact (in early dementia)	Disoriented
Reversibility	Progressive	Reversible
Sleep disturbance	Insomnia	Sleep/wake cycle disturbance

Distinct features of catatonia such as *mutism, echolalia, echopraxia, and waxy flexibility* may complicate the testing of thought process, attention, and orientation, but, on the other hand, may provide important clues to distinguish these two conditions. According to catatonic patients (reported after recovery), their level of consciousness is preserved (and they *do* remember the doctors who applied painful stimuli to elicit their reaction).

Insomnia and Nightmares

Delirium is characterized by sleep-wake cycle disturbances. Therefore, patients with sleep-wake disorders such as insomnia, hypersomnolence, and parasomnias may present in medical settings with features resembling those in delirious patients. However, these conditions usually last for months or years, in contrast to delirium precipitated by acute medical illness. Insomniacs may suffer from attention compromise. Critical for delirium, fluctuation of *consciousness* is not observed in patients with insomnia or nightmares.

Depression and Mania

It is not rare that a psychiatrist is called to see a patient for depression or mania and encounters a patient either in hypoactive or hyperactive delirium, respectively. A differential diagnosis of hypoactive delirium and severe melancholic depression is easy to establish because of clear differences in *onset and course* of the disease. Depression has a more insidious onset and is chronic in course. Mania can have an abrupt onset, particularly if triggered by medications and sleep disturbance in the hospital. Attention and memory may be compromised in depression and mania. However, awareness and arousal are usually preserved, as well as perception and thought process. However, in psychotic depression and mania, delusional thinking (usually mood congruent) may be present.

Psychosis

For a psychiatrist, the differential diagnosis of delirium and psychotic disorders is usually not difficult since no impairment of *consciousness* occurs in psychosis. *Speech and attention* are also preserved in psychosis. Psychotic features such as *hallucinations* are usually visual in delirium and auditory in schizophrenia spectrum disorders.

Anxiety

Delirious patients may sometimes appear anxious or restless, which makes it difficult to distinguish between delirium and anxiety. Evaluating the history and current presentation helps with the diagnosis—anxiety disorders usually have a protracted *course* and lack altered *consciousness*.

The Treatment and Management of Patients with Delirium

Treatment of delirium is a multitask endeavor that consists of the treatment of underlying etiologies, preventive measures, interventions directed to improve patient functioning and comfort, and assurance of safety. Treatment requires collaboration with other services: Toxicology (management of intoxication and withdrawal), Pain Management Service, Neurology (brain pathology, seizures), Internal Medicine, Cardiology, Infectious Diseases, Oncology, Social Work, Ethics, and Security. Psychosomatic physicians should be proactive in providing systematic education about delirium for colleagues from other medical specialties, as well as clinical administration, in relentless efforts to improve the hospital environment and patients' care that can prevent or minimize risks of delirium.

1. Acute interventions to avoid catastrophic decompensation of causative medical condition (usually in cooperation with Toxicology service, Neurology/Neurosurgery service, ICU team):
   - Wernicke's encephalopathy (IV administration of thiamine, 500 mg three times a day, monitoring cognitive improvement, then tapering to 100 mg and switching to PO);
   - Withdrawal from alcohol/GABA agonist (administration of benzodiazepines using a taper, front-loaded, symptom-triggered approach, adding barbiturates or other anticonvulsants);
   - Hypoglycemia (glucose repletion as clinically indicated);
   - Hypoxemia/hypoperfusion (blood transfusion, aggressive treatment of CHF);*
   - Hypertensive encephalopathy (e.g., hydralazine IV);
   - Intoxication with alcohol, cocaine, hallucinogens (quiet protective environment, constant observation, use of sedatives);
   - Meningitis/encephalitis (specific antibiotic/antiviral therapy);
   - Poisoning/drug overdose (Acetylcysteine, Naloxone, Fomepizole, Flumazenil);
   - Seizures (loading doses of anticonvulsant);
   - Stroke (anticoagulation when indicated).
     * Delirium may be the main clinical feature of acute brain hypoxia and indication for blood transfusion (Note: hypoxia may occur in severely anemic patients with pulse oximetry readings of 92%–99%).

2. Multimodal therapy targeting the underlying medical condition (in cooperation with primary medical/surgical team):
   - Correct abnormal electrolytes, Mg, Ca, Phos, BUN, creatinine, LFT/NH3, blood glucose, blood gases, B_{12}, folate, TSH, abnormal medication levels;
   - Treat infections while monitoring CBC with differential count, UA, blood cultures;
   - Consider additional medical workup when clinically indicated: blood cultures, blood gases, urine (comprehensive) toxicology screen, LP (with HIV, RPR, PCR tests), heavy metal screen, brain

imaging, EEG studies. (Sometimes lack of an identifiable medical condition, especially in elderly patients, should raise a concern for initial presentation of another neurocognitive disorder, particularly dementia with Lewy bodies);

- Optimize pain management (pain control in opioid dependent patient using opioid and non-opioid modalities), change of opioid medication.

3. Preventive/ameliorating measures (including environmental interventions):
   - Implement safety measures—electronic alarm devices, low bed, mats, bed rails, placement near nursing station (fall and wandering precautions), judicial use of soft restraints, safety sitters to prevent unintentional self-harm (e.g., disconnection of life lines);
   - Minimize polypharmacy, reconsider or avoid use of anticholinergic medications (including eye drops), opioids (or change the pain medication), benzodiazepines/hypnotics (including zolpidem). It may be appropriate to hold some non-essential medications in acute phase of delirium to avoid drug-drug interactions;
   - Provide strong environmental cues to maintain normal sleep-wake cycle. During the day, nursing staff should be instructed to engage in frequent verbal interactions with patients, to promote visual, auditory, tactile stimulation, and exposure to daylight in the room. At night, all efforts should be directed to protect night-time sleep by reducing light, noise, avoiding non-essential procedures between midnight and 6 a.m.; consider normalizing sleep cycle with melatonin (3 mg) or melatonin agonists PO HS;
   - Encourage family to visit and bring from home personal items, patient's eyeglasses and hearing aids, CPAP machine;
   - Provide the patient with emotional support directed to reduce anxiety, uncertainty by frequent inquiries about level of pain, needs for assistance, environmental comfort;
   - Activate HELP—Hospital Elderly Life Program (where available), which is designed to assess patients at risk of delirium (70+ years old), provide daily follow-up visits monitoring for incident delirium, education for patients, families, and nursing staff—it uses volunteers in direct bedside interaction (orientation, socialization, mental stimulation, mealtime assistance).

4. Pharmacological interventions:
   - Antipsychotics. There is evidence that small doses of haloperidol (< 3.5 mg/24 h) decrease intensity and duration, but not incidence of delirium. Second-generation antipsychotics at average clinical doses appear to have no advantage over haloperidol. More research is required to assess the efficacy of the antipsychotic medications (e.g., Olanzapine 10 mg) to prevent post-surgical delirium. Use of antipsychotics in hypoactive delirium is still controversial, despite the fact that patients with hypoactive delirium are just as distressed as patients with hyperactive delirium. Use of antipsychotics in an elderly patient could increase mortality and requires thorough risk/benefit evaluation and discussion with patient's family.

- Benzodiazepines are known to be efficient medications for treatment of alcohol/sedative/hypnotic delirium. Flumazenil (benzodiazepine antagonist, 0.2–0.5 mg IV push q min, up to 5 mg) has shown its efficacy to briefly improve mental status in delirious patients with hepatic failure (helpful for consent purposes). The medicine should be used with great caution in patients with GABA agonist intoxication/withdrawal as it may result in seizures.
- No advantage of acetylcholine esterase inhibitors (Donepezil, Rivastigmine) was found in ameliorating the course of delirium (as anticholinergic hypothesis of delirium could suggest). On the other hand, physostigmine remains a standard treatment of propofol-induced delirium (watch for seizures).

5. Evaluation and treatment of comorbid psychiatric illness (mania/hypomania, psychosis, PTSD, OCD, panic disorder, personality disorders, etc.):
   - Assess and monitor mental status (including cognitive function)
   - Optimize psychopharmacological treatment
   - Bedside supportive psychotherapy
   - Disposition planning

6. Family/patient/team education: Delirium is a highly distressing experience for spouses, caregivers, and nurses who are caring for delirious patients. Prompt recognition and treatment of delirium is critically important to reduce suffering and distress. More than half (53.5%) of patients recall their delirium experience. Short-term memory impairment, delirium severity, and the presence of delusions and perceptual disturbances were significant predictors of delirium recall and of spouse/caregiver distress. Delirium severity and the presence of perceptual disturbances were the most significant predictors of nurse distress.
   - Educate the nursing staff on how to diagnose delirium and monitor mental status of delirious patients;
   - Educate the patient and family regarding the illness (early recognition, reassurance of reversibility, variability of time course—delirium may last weeks after the diagnosis);
   - Establish and maintain alliances with family and other healthcare providers;
   - Assess individual and family psychological and social characteristics (dealing with anxiety).

7. Management of behavioral disturbance (see more details in Chapter 7):
   - Use verbal redirection/de-escalation in order to engage the patient in discussion and search for a mutually acceptable solution of the problem. Ask, "What usually helps you to feel better when you are frustrated (angry, anxious, etc.)?"
   - Use restraining devices to prevent physical harm (e.g., discontinuation of life-preserving medical treatment such as oxygen or lines). Need for restraints should be re-evaluated frequently as the course of delirium fluctuates.

- Use sedative medications for severe agitation (patient is violent, does not cooperate, and physical restraints are not sufficient to maintain safety).

8. Decision-making capacity: Patients in delirium do not usually have capacity to make healthcare decisions, including the decision to discontinue treatment and leave against medical advice (AMA). If they lack capacity to leave AMA, this should be noted clearly in the record and should be reassessed at times that the patient requests to leave. The patient does not need to be committed for involuntary psychiatric evaluation to be held in the medical hospital against his or her will (remember, the patient's consciousness is clouded). On the other hand, with protracted and waxing/waning course of delirium, patients may have periods of lucidity when their capacity to communicate their choice of care may be consistent and valid.

9. Disposition: Patients who have experienced delirium frequently have residual symptoms at the time of discharge. They are likely to require significant support either at home or in a structured environment such as a skilled nursing facility or personal care home.

Key Points

- Delirium is the most frequent condition that requires a psychiatrist's expertise in medical settings because it can mimic a wide range of mental disorders.
- Delirium should be considered as acute brain failure, which requires immediate clinical attention and aggressive multimodal therapy targeting the underlying medical condition.
- Delirium may occur in verbal and nonverbal patients and is a highly distressing experience for patients, families, caregivers, and medical personnel.
- Systematic education provided by psychosomatic physicians, as well as relentless efforts to improve the hospital environment and patients' care, can prevent or minimize risks of delirium.

Disclosures

Dr. Gushchin has no conflicts of interest to disclose.

Further Reading

Ely EW, Inouye SK, et al. (2001). Delirium in mechanically ventilated pateints: Validity and reliability of the Confusion Assessment Method for the intensive care unit (CAM-ICU). *JAMA*, *286*(21), 2703–2710.

Inouye SK, Westendorp RJ, et al. (2014). Delirium in elderly people. *Lancet*, *383*(9920), 911–922.

Lipowski ZJ. (1990). *Delirium: Acute Confusional States.* New York: Oxford University Press.

Marcantonio ER (2011). In the clinic: Delirium. *Ann Intern Med.*, *154*, ITC6 1–16.

Maldonado JR (2013). Neuropathogenesis of delirium: Review of current etiologic theories and common pathways. *Am J Geriatr Psychiat.*, *21*, 1190–1222.

Meagher DJ, Moran M, et al. (2007). Phenomenology of delirium: Assessment of 100 adult cases using standardized measures. *Br J Psychiat.*, *190*, 135–141.

Trzepacz PT, Mittal D, et al. (2001). Validation of the Delirium Rating Scale-Revised-98: Comparison with the Delirium Rating Scale and the Cognitive Test for Delirium. *J Neuropsych Clin N.*, *13*, 229–242.

Wise MG, Rundell JR (2005). *Clinical Manual of Psychosomatic Medicine: A Guide to Consultation-Liaison Psychiatry.* Washington, DC: American Psychiatric Publishing.

Exercises

1. A 50-year-old patient with alcohol dependence is admitted to the emergency department for confusion, oculomotor disturbances, ataxia, and dysarthria. The first step in acute management of this patient's condition would be to administer which of the following medications?
   a. Haloperidol
   b. Thiamine
   c. Glucose
   d. Lorazepam
   e. Phenytoin

2. Which of the following better describes delirium?
   a. Motor agitation, delusion, auditory hallucinations
   b. Motor agitation, lability of affect, thought process abnormalities
   c. Poor attention, sleep-wake cycle disturbance, disorientation
   d. Poor attention, poor memory, language disturbances

3. A 64-year-old woman with metastatic breast cancer is hospitalized for the third cycle in a series of 10 cycles of chemotherapy. She also is receiving sulfasalazine treatment for a urinary tract infection. During her hospitalization, she confides to a nurse that a catlike creature sleeps on her bed at night. Although she likes animals, she believes that certain individuals send the cat to her room to monitor her. The woman has no prior history of psychotic illness. What is the most likely diagnosis?
   a. Depressive disorder
   b. Schizophrenia
   c. Dementia
   d. Delirium

4. A 69-year-old man is brought to the emergency department after being found walking down the middle of a highway. During the psychiatric interview, the patient refuses to cooperate, and no collateral systems are available. The patient's hospital records reveal no history of psychiatric admissions. His last visit was two months ago for a transurethral prostatectomy, at which time the patient was oriented and able to give informed consent. Differential diagnosis should include which of the following?
   a. Delirium
   b. Major depression
   c. Dementia
   d. Dissociative amnesia
   e. All are correct

Answers: (1) b (2) c (3) d (4) e

Neurocognitive Disorders in the General Medical Setting

Ghennady V. Gushchin

Introduction

"Dementia" (from the Latin for "out of mind") is a term long used to describe the deterioration of intellectual/cognitive function (with relatively spared consciousness and perception), accompanied by behavioral abnormalities and changes in personality. Historically, dementia was associated with a neurodegenerative (dementing, senile) illness and connotes a condition of the elderly (compare with Kraepelin's "Dementia praecox" for schizophrenia). The term "neurocognitive disorder" (NCD), which was introduced in the fifth edition of the *Diagnostic and Statistical Manual of Mental Disorders* (*DSM-5*), is more inclusive and is applicable to conditions that may affect young individuals (e.g., traumatic brain injury or HIV infection). Nevertheless, the term "dementia" is most frequently used in medical settings, where it has long been the accepted term. It will be used in this chapter to designate the most severe end of the NCD spectrum. This chapter will help consultation-liaison (C-L) clinicians to meet the diagnostic challenges of NCDs and to educate patients and families about the diagnosis and management of NCDs. We will focus initially on the cross-sectional epidemiology, assessment, and initial workup for cognitive impairment in the medical setting. Core features of major and mild NCD and specific features of each of the primary neurocognitive disorders will then be reviewed. The chapter will conclude with a review of differential diagnosis and illness, and symptom-management for patients with NCDs in a medical setting.

Epidemiology

Dementia is a major public health problem, causing disability for patients and anguish for families. It is estimated that 2%–10% of individuals at age 65 have mild NCD, and 1%–2% have major NCD. Furthermore, by age 85, about 30% of individuals will develop major NCD (dementia).

A number of recent studies have refined the epidemiology of dementia. Nevertheless, the most prevalent subtype of dementia remains Alzheimer's disease (60%–90% of all dementia cases), followed by vascular dementia (8%–35%), with a significant portion of demented patients showing features of both types on autopsy (2%–46%). In recent years, the contribution of other subtypes of NCD to the overall disease burden of dementias has been increasingly recognized; NCD with Lewy bodies has been identified in a significant proportion of cases (2%–30%), and frontotemporal NCD and normal pressure hydrocephalus currently account for 5% and 2.5% cases of NCDs, respectively. Other NCDs, including those that occur as a result of traumatic brain injury, substance/medication use, Parkinson's disease, Huntington's disease, progressive supranuclear palsy, multiple sclerosis, HIV infection, progressive paralysis, and prion disease, likely represent < 2.5% of cases.

Assessment of Patients with Cognitive Impairment

Thorough history-taking is by far the most efficient element of clinical assessment of patients with cognitive impairment. Initial evaluation of high-risk patients should include questions about their memory and independent functioning at home: how are they getting meals, who is doing finances and medication management, and so on. It is also important to obtain collateral information from previous medical records, family, and outpatient caregivers corroborating the gradual decline in functioning, because patients may be not aware of or may hide their cognitive impairment.

Screening Tools (Psychometrics)

A psychosomatic physician begins the assessment of the patient with suspected cognitive impairment using available screening tools specifically designed for bedside cognitive examination (see Chapter 2). The Montreal Cognitive Assessment (MoCA) appears more versatile in covering all neurocognitive domains described for NCDs in *DSM-5* (e.g., complex attention, executive function, learning and memory, language, perceptual and motor function, and social cognition), with the exception of social cognition. This shortfall could be supplemented with the story card test (e.g., NIH Stroke Scale—Picture Description; http://www.ninds.nih.gov/doctors/NIH_Stroke_Scale.pdf) which can reveal the inability to identify the emotional state of persons depicted on the test card or to recognize their intentions or possible thoughts.

Sometimes it is prudent to repeat the bedside cognitive testing while the patient is in the hospital. Evidence of variability in cognitive tests and even a reversal of previously detected deficiencies may be critical for differential diagnosis, especially of superimposed delirium.

Initial Medical Workup

Cognitive deficits revealed by psychometric screening should prompt a vigorous search for reversible causes of cognitive impairment. Given the high probability of delirium in medically ill patients, psychosomatic physicians should begin an assessment by reviewing available clinical data, including medical records, labs, and brain imaging, to identify medical conditions that convey a high risk of delirium (see Chapter 10 for discussion of delirium risk factors).

As a first step, it is important to check:

• Vital signs and pulse oximetry
• Blood level of electrolytes (with Ca and Phos), BUN/Creatinine, LFTs, ammonia, CBC with differential
• Urine analysis.

If necessary, a C-L psychiatrist could recommend additional medical workup to determine whether the cognitive impairment is a feature of delirium or an NCD due to another medical condition (see the relevant section later in this chapter). This may include the following:

- Blood: B_{12}, folate, TSH/T3/T4, blood gases/glucose, specific drug levels
- Urine drug screen
- Brain imaging (CT, MRI): evidence of bleeding/ischemia or hydrocephalus, space-occupying tumors, etc.
- EEG: epileptic spikes, generalized slowing.

Evidence of metabolic, infectious, hematological, and/or toxic etiologies of the cognitive impairment should trigger aggressive treatment of the underlying medical condition.

In addition, PT/OT evaluation of activities of daily living (ADLs) could help gauge the patient's level of independence in everyday activities, which may be important for aftercare/disposition planning.

Diagnosis of Neurocognitive Disorders

Currently, the NCDs are viewed in a continuum of "normal aging—mild NCD—major NCD (dementia)," characterized by progressive decline in cognition and impairment in functioning due to acquired cognitive deficits. *DSM-5* emphasizes a quantitative approach to diagnosis of NCD. Performance in quantitative neuropsychological tests two or more standard deviations below the appropriate norms (based on age, educational attainment, and cultural background) signifies the presence of major NCD. Mild NCD is defined by performance between one and two standard deviations below norms. Interference of these cognitive deficits with independence of daily living and need for assistance to complete routine tasks (or their abandonment) are characteristics of major NCD, whereas patients with mild NCD are typically able to maintain independence (although compensation strategies may be required).

DSM-5 uses two sets of diagnostic criteria for NCDs:

1. Generic criteria (common for all NCDs, regardless of etiology)
2. Disorder-specific criteria (including definitions of probable and possible disorder).

DSM-5 identifies 11 subtypes of NCDs depending on their etiology: Alzheimer's disease (AD), vascular disease, Lewy body disease (LBD), frontotemporal lobar degeneration (FTLD), trauma, substance/medication use, Parkinson's disease, Huntington's disease, HIV or prion infections, and another identifiable medical condition (e.g., hydrocephalus, multiple sclerosis, endocrinopathy, syphilis, etc.).

DSM-5 provides clinically important specifying criteria of NCD such as "probable or possible disease" and "with or without behavioral disturbance."

Generic diagnostic criteria of major and mild NCD are almost identical, with only some quantitative differences. Criteria of major NCD are listed below, with distinction of mild NCD criteria indicated in parentheses.

1. Evidence of significant (modest) decline of performance in one or more neurocognitive domains as revealed by:
   - History, that is, patient's complaints; concerns of relatives, friends, and the observant clinician; AND
   - Mental Status Exam, that is, decreased performance in cognitive tests below two (between one and two) standard deviations;
2. Interference of these cognitive deficits with independence in everyday activities (requirement of greater efforts to preserve independence in routine complex activities);
3. Lack of clinical evidence that another mental illness, such as schizophrenia or major depression, can account for the symptoms above.

Disorder-Specific Diagnostic Criteria

This section discusses clinical features, labs, and imaging data important for diagnostic considerations. It also aids psychosomatic physicians with educating patients and families when the diagnosis of an NCD is suspected or was recently established. Not all sophisticated laboratory tests and instrumental studies are available for routine clinical use, and their ordering should be deferred to specialized clinics/services.

Alzheimer's Disease

In 1906, Alois Alzheimer, a German psychiatrist, presented a case report of a 51-year-old woman with short-term memory loss and strange behavior, and, using Nissl's silver staining, demonstrated morphological abnormalities in the brain, which later were identified as amyloid-predominant neuritic plaques and Tau-predominant neurofibrillary tangles, and cerebral amyloid (congophilic) angiopathy. Genetic mutations in presenilin 1 (PSEN1), presenilin 2 (PSEN2), or autosomal dominant mutation of amyloid precursor protein (APP) can be found collectively in 2% of Alzheimer's disease (AD) patients. There is an increased risk of illness in ApoE4 homozygous patients (7%–15%) and patients with Chromosome 21 trisomy (Down syndrome).

Age of onset: before age 65 (5%), after age 65 (95%).

Clinical Presentation and Natural Course

Alzheimer's disease is characterized by a gradual onset and a continuous slow but steady decline in prior intellectual and functional capacities, especially memory. In the early stages, the most common symptoms are difficulty remembering recent events, anomia, paraphasic errors, and perseveration, while maintaining a "good façade." Often, AD begins with an accentuation of the patient's premorbid character traits. Depression may also be present when the patient is aware of the cognitive deficits. The progression of the disease with further memory decline is accompanied by impairment in orientation, judgment, ability to cope in the community and at home, and personal care and attention, as well as personality changes, loss of flexibility, and lability of affect. In advanced dementia, individuals may become totally oblivious to their surroundings and require constant care. Patients with AD live an average of 10 years following diagnosis. The degree to which patients with NCDs have premature death is difficult to measure, as elderly patients with NCDs typically die of other medical disorders.

Brain Imaging

- Head CT/MRI: hippocampal and temporoparietal atrophy, ventriculomegaly (hydrocephalus *ex vacuo*); MRI: punctate hemosiderin residue in cortical/subcortical locations;
- PET (if available) with Pittsburgh compound B (PiB), Amyvid F18 (Florbetapir), Vizamyl (flutemetamol): positive for amyloid deposition (helps to differentiate AD and FTLD);
- FDG-PET (if available): hypometabolism in hippocampal and temporoparietal brain regions.

Diagnosis

Probable NCD due to AD:

- There is evidence of a causative genetic mutation from family history or genetic testing, OR
- All three of the following features are present:
  a. Decline in memory and learning plus one or more other neuro-cognitive domains
  b. Steadily progressive, gradual decline in cognition without plateaus
  c. No evidence of mixed etiology.

Possible NCD due to AD:

- No evidence of a causative genetic mutation from family history or genetic testing, AND
- All three features of probable NCD due to AD are not present.

Vascular Dementia

Vascular dementia (VD) is the second most frequent NCD in the elderly. Risk factors of VD include hypertension, diabetes, smoking, obesity, hypercholesterolemia, high homocysteine level, and atrial fibrillation and other conditions with high risks of cerebral emboli.

For many years, cognitive impairment due to cerebral vascular disease or multi-infarct dementia was associated primarily with cerebrovascular accidents (CVA) or strokes. Only with the advent of modern neuroimaging techniques (brain CT/MRI) did it become possible to link impairment of cognitive function with "silent" cases of cerebrovascular diseases affecting primarily small-size vessels and known as "small vessel disease" and "lacunar infarcts." In 1894, Swiss psychiatrist Otto Binswanger was the first to describe a slowly progressing dementia and subcortical white matter atrophy that he attributed to "vascular insufficiency."

In addition, there is a hereditary disorder, cerebral autosomal dominant arteriopathy with subcortical infarcts and leukoencephalopathy (CADASIL), that is characterized by Notch 3 gene mutation in chromosome 19 and 28%–48% penetration at age 60. It presents with migraine attacks (with aura) and/or subcortical TIAs and frequently progresses to subcortical dementia associated with pseudobulbar palsy.

Age of onset: any age (35–55 for CADASIL), but increases exponentially after age 65.

Clinic Presentation and Natural Course

Vascular dementia in many CVA patients presents with an acute onset of cognitive deficits (with motor and behavioral signs, and affective symptoms), followed by a stepwise decline or fluctuating course with intervening periods of stability and even some improvement. No direct correlation between the magnitude of the affected area of the brain and the degree of cognitive impairment was established. Sometimes, a single small infarct located in a "strategic" area (e.g., thalamus, basal forebrain, angular gyrus) may be sufficient to cause dementia. If the frontal lobe is affected, the patient may present with abulia, apathy, poor attention, gait apraxia, and urinary incontinence.

VD may also present with more insidious onset of cognitive deficits and with predominant features of subcortical dementia: intellectual slowing, motor impairment, and executive function deficiencies. At times, sudden worsening of cognitive function in patients with a "silent" course of cerebrovascular disease may be triggered by non-neurologic illness or elective surgery, such as open heart surgery, when transient brain hypoxia and hypoperfusion can exhaust all compensatory mechanisms of the brain. Given the lack of premorbid history of strokes and minimal brain imaging findings, such as "small vessel disease" on head CT/MRI scans, the patient and family may experience frustration and have difficulty accepting the diagnosis of vascular neurocognitive disorder.

Patients with VD commonly survive for an average of four to eight years after onset of dementia, and death usually results from cardiovascular disease or stroke.

Brain Imaging

- Head CT/MRI: blood deposits in brain tissue, lesions and atrophy of cortical and/or subcortical structures corresponding to CVA (especially in thalamus, basal forebrain, angular gyrus), cerebral white matter changes ("small vessel disease" or leukoaraiosis) and/or subcortical lacunar infarcts;
- MRI: punctate hemosiderin residue in cortical/subcortical locations (microhemorrhages).

Diagnosis

Probable Vascular NCD:

- Neurocognitive syndrome is temporally related to one or more CVAs
- Significant decline in frontal/executive function, complex attention/processing speed
- Neuroimaging evidence of significant parenchymal injury
- Both clinical (history, physical exam) evidence and genetic (CADASIL) evidence of cerebrovascular disease are present
- Not better explained by another brain or systemic disease.

Possible vascular NCD could be established if generic criteria for major (or mild) NCD are met, but other criteria for probable diagnosis are not fully met.

Lewy Body Disease

Lewy Body Disease (LBD) is named after Friedrich H. Lewy, a German-American neurologist, who worked with Alzheimer in the 1910s and discovered rounded eosinophilic, intraneuronal inclusions (Lewy bodies) in dementia. These inclusions represent the accumulation of abnormal protein aggregates containing alpha-synucleins and ubiquitin, also found in Parkinson's disease (see discussion later in this chapter). LBD is usually associated with diffuse cortical location of Lewy bodies, whereas Parkinson's disease and dementia that develops in course of Parkinson's disease are characterized by the presence of Lewy bodies primarily in the basal ganglia: cholinergic neurons of Nucleus basalis of Meynert and dopaminergic neurons of Substantia nigra. No family history is usually identified for LBD.

Age of onset: age 65–75.

Clinical Presentation and Natural Course

LBD is a gradually progressive disorder with insidious onset. Often patients have a history of acute confusion (delirium), precipitated by illness or surgery, when no adequate underlying cause can be found. This should alert clinicians to consider LBD. The core features of LBD include the following:

- Fluctuating cognition with pronounced variations in attention and alertness
- Recurrent visual hallucinations (animals, humans) and misperceptions/misinterpretation (in 75% of cases)
- Spontaneous parkinsonism (tremor, rigidity, gait problems/falls), which must begin after the onset of cognitive decline (at least one year delay) (see NCD due to Parkinson's disease below).

Several features such as episodes of unexplained loss of consciousness, orthostatic hypotension, and urinary incontinence are suggestive of LBD. Two suggestive features are included in *DSM-5* diagnostic criteria:

- Presence of REM sleep behavior disorder
- Severe sensitivity to neuroleptics and antiemetics (patients may develop catatonia, loss of cognitive function, and life-threatening muscle rigidity, NMS).

The course of LBD may have occasional plateaus. It eventually progresses through severe dementia to death faster than AD, with average duration of five to seven years.

Brain Imaging
- Head CT/MRI: no brain atrophy
- SPECT/PET (if available): reduced striatal dopamine transporter ligand uptake.

Diagnosis
Probable NCD with Lewy bodies:

- Insidious onset and gradual progression
- Presence of two or more core features, or one suggestive feature with one or more core features
- No evidence of other neurological or neurocognitive disorders.

Possible NCD with Lewy bodies could be established if generic criteria for major (or mild) NCD are met, but other criteria for probable diagnosis are not fully met.

Frontotemporal Lobar Degeneration

In case reports from 1892 to 1906, Czech psychiatrist Arnold Pick described a group of patients with circumscribed brain pathology (atrophy of frontal and temporal lobes and spared parietal and occipital lobes), unusually severe aphasia (he introduced the term "agrammatism"), and apraxia. In 1994, Pick's disease was relabeled as a variant of Frontotemporal Lobar Degeneration (FTLD), a group of neurodegenerative disorders characterized by neuronal cellular inclusions containing tau-protein (Pick's disease, corticobasal degeneration, progressive supranuclear palsy, and amyotrophic lateral sclerosis) and/or other specific proteins and different degrees of cognitive impairment. Frontotemporal NCD (FTD) has strong genetic predisposition: 40%–50% of patients have a family history of early dementia, and collectively 10%–20% of patients have mutations of microtubule-associated protein-tau (MART), granulin (GRN), or C9orf72 genes with autosomal dominant inheritance pattern linked to Chromosome 17 (Tau gene) and Chromosome 3.

Age of onset: before age 65 (75%–80%), after age 65 (20%–25%)

Clinical Presentation and Natural Course

FTD may present as one of two syndromic variants occurring in almost equal proportion and featuring either progressive development of behavioral/personality changes (behavioral variant FTD) or language impairment (language variant FTD, additionally distinguished by semantic, agrammatic/nonfluent, and logopenic subtypes). Both major variants demonstrate relative sparing in learning, memory, and perceptual-motor domains. The progression is more rapid than AD, with death typically in three to eight years (11 years for the language variant). There is male preponderance of the behavioral variant FTD, and female preponderance of the agrammatic/nonfluent subtype of language variant FTD.

Patients with behavioral variant FTD present with prominent decline in the social cognition domain: **behavioral disinhibition**, aggression, substance addiction, **compulsions** (sometimes creative ones), odd affiliations, **perseverative/stereotyped behavior, hyperorality, or apathy/ inertia. Loss of empathy** in behavioral variant FTD can be evident in the lack of concern for a loved one's illness, cruelty, rudeness, not respecting interpersonal space, and a diminished response to pain. It is usually attributed to right temporal lobe degeneration. In early stages, cognitive decline is not prominent, and formal testing may show relatively few deficits. Fifty percent of patients with behavioral variant FTD in the early stages are misdiagnosed with other psychiatric disorders. In the course of the illness, the patient's personal care rapidly deteriorates, with increased apathy, stereotypy, and loss of expressive speech with late mutism and amimia. Temporal and spatial orientation is usually preserved for a long time, in contrast to Alzheimer's.

The language variant of FTD presents with gradual onset of language problems and primarily progressive aphasia. Behavioral and personality changes similar to those in behavioral variant FTD may appear later. The semantic (fluent) subtype presents with "difficulties in remembering the names of people, places, and things" during questioning of word meaning in conversation, and prominent impairment of single-word comprehension. The agrammatic (nonfluent) subtype presents with severe distortion of speech output: hesitant effortful speech, stutter, anomia, phonemic paraphasia, agrammatism (using the wrong tense or word order) with preserved single-word comprehension (some similarity with Broca's aphasia). As the disease progresses, speech quantity decreases, and patients become mute. The logopenic subtype presents as anomic aphasia with a slowly progressing and debilitating impairment of reading, writing, and comprehension, with a mixed pattern of semantic and agrammatic subtypes.

Brain Imaging

- Head CT/MRI: atrophy of medial frontal/anterior temporal lobes (behavioral variant), bilateral asymmetric atrophy of temporal lobes (semantic variant), predominantly left posterior fronto-insular (nonfluent), or left posterior perisylvian or parietal atrophy (logopenic) with sparing most of parietal and occipital lobes;

- F-MRI (if available): hypoperfusion and cortical hypometabolism in corresponding brain regions (present in the early stages);
- PET (if available) with Pittsburgh compound B (PiB), Amyvid F18 (Florbetapir), Vizamyl (flutemetamol): Negative for Amyloid deposition.

Diagnosis

Probable frontotemporal NCD:

- Insidious onset and gradual progression
- Presence of three or more behavioral symptoms (highlighted above) OR prominent decline in language
- Relative sparing of memory, perceptual, and motor functions
- Causative genetic mutation (from family history or genetic testing), OR
- Evidence of disproportionate frontal and/or temporal lobe atrophy on neuroimaging.

Possible frontotemporal NCD could be established if generic criteria for major (or mild) NCD are met, clinical history is consistent with FTD, but other criteria for probable diagnosis are not fully met (no genetic evidence, no neuroimaging data).

Substance/Medication-Induced Neurocognitive Disorder

Since the classical description of amnestic-confabulatory syndrome in his thesis "Alcoholic paralysis" by Russian neuropsychiatrist Sergei S. Korsakoff in 1887, alcohol is by far the most known substance that can cause persistent cognitive impairment. Besides alcohol, recreational use of intoxicative chemical products (inhalants) or sedative-hypnotic-anxiolytic medications can result in persistent cognitive impairment. Growing literature suggests that a substantial group of patients who receive aggressive chemotherapy for breast, ovarian, and prostate cancer may experience significant difficulties with memory, attention, fluency, and motor coordination ("chemo brain").

Age of onset: any age (depending on substance), increased prevalence after age 50.

Clinical Presentation and Natural Course

Initial manifestation could be a slower recovery of brain functions from a period of prolonged substance use with cognitive improvements seen over many months. However, with continuous use after certain age (for alcohol, age 50), the neurocognitive deficits may become persistent. Korsakoff's dementia presents with memory deficits (anterograde amnesia, retrograde amnesia with confabulations) and impairment of executive function. Barbiturates/benzodiazepines can cause impairment in several neurocognitive domains, including attention, memory, and learning.

Brain Imaging

- Head CT/MRI: cortical thinning, white matter loss, enlargement of sulci and ventricles, mammillary body/medial thalamus atrophy (alcohol), microhemorrhages or infarcts (methamphetamines)
- FDG-PET (if available): decreased metabolism in frontal, parietal, and cingulate areas.

Diagnosis
Substance/medication-induced NCD:
- Criteria for major (or mild) NCD are present
- Impairment persists beyond the duration of intoxication/withdrawal
- Not exclusively in the course of delirium
- Duration, extent of use, and substance involved are capable of producing impairment
- Symptoms don't worsen without continued use and may improve after abstinence.

Traumatic Brain Injury

Traumatic brain injury (TBI) is defined as brain trauma caused by a bump, blow, or jolt to the head or a penetrating head injury that disrupts the normal function of the brain, including cognition. However, the degree of cognitive impairment does not necessary correspond to severity of the TBI. The most common etiologies of TBI in the United States are falls (35%), motor vehicle/traffic accidents (17%), being struck on the head (17%), assaults (10%), and others (21%). Currently, neurocognitive impairment resulting from brain surgery is considered in this category.

Age of onset: any age (highest prevalence before age 4, in late teens, and after age 65).

Clinical Presentation and Natural Course
Neurocognitive deficits must be present immediately after injury occurs or immediately after the individual recovers consciousness. Impairments in complex attention, executive function, learning and memory, social cognition, and slowing of processing speed are common features of TBI. More severe TBI patients may present with aphasia, neglect, and constructional dyspraxia. NCD due to TBI may be accompanied by disturbances in emotional function, personality changes, somatic disturbances (e.g., HA, fatigue, sleep disorder, vertigo, dizziness, tinnitus, hyperacusis, photosensitivity, anosmia, reduced tolerance to psychotropic medications, seizures, visual deficits, neurological deficits such as hemiparesis, and cranial nerve palsy).

NCD due to mild TBI tends to resolve within days to weeks after the injury, with complete resolution typically by three months. However, repeated mild TBIs may result in persistent post-traumatic dementia, for example, dementia pugilistica (boxer's syndrome), featuring a clinical picture of dementia and parkinsonism (non-progressing).

Brain Imaging
- Head CT/MRI: petechial, subarachnoid hemorrhages, signs of brain contusion.

Diagnosis
NCD due to traumatic brain injury:
- Impact to the head causing one or more of the following:
  - Loss of consciousness
  - Disorientation and confusion
  - Post-traumatic amnesia

- Neurological signs and symptoms (neuroimaging evidence of injury, new-onset seizures, visual field cuts, anosmia, hemiparesis).
- Deficits present immediately after brain injury or immediately after the individual recovers consciousness and persist past the acute post-injury period.

Neurocognitive Disorder Due to Another Medical Condition

This etiologic subtype requires the prioritized attention of psycho-somatic and primary medical clinicians, pursuing a vigorous search for reversible causes of cognitive impairment and suggesting appropriate treatment for the causative condition.

Impairment of cognitive function can be found in numerous medical conditions with different etiologies:

- Intracranial lesions (primary and secondary brain tumors, SDH, NPH)
- Endocrine diseases (hypothyroidism, hypercalcemia, hypoglycemia)
- Nutritional deficiency (thiamine, niacin, B_{12})
- Hypoxia (CHF/hypoperfusion)
- CNS infections, for example, neurosyphilis, Cryptococci infection (see section on NCD due to HIV and prion infection below)
- Autoimmune diseases (SLE, temporal arteritis, multiple sclerosis)
- Hepatic and renal failure
- Epilepsy
- Status post-ECT and brain irradiation.

In addition, rare genetic metabolic disorders are characterized by enzymatic deficiency and the accumulation of abnormal byproducts in the CNS with damage of brain tissues, "storage diseases" (e.g., neuronal ceroid-lipofuscinosis, Lafora's disease, adrenoleukodystrophy, multiple system atrophy (parkinsonian symptoms that do not respond to dopamine [DA] agonists), Gaucher's disease, metachromatic leukodystrophy, Niemann-Pick disease, familial British and Danish dementia, and Wilson's disease (hepatolenticular degeneration)).

Age of onset: varies (childhood, adolescence, adulthood).

Clinical Presentation and Natural Course

Ordinarily, these diseases manifest themselves with features that are primarily the focus of other medical specialties. Some NCDs present with typical symptoms that assist with the diagnosis and treatment of the underlying medical condition, for example, normal pressure hydrocephalus (urinary incontinence, and gait apraxia/"magnetic floor") or hypothyroidism (cold intolerance, slow deep reflexes, low body temperature, weight gain). Progression of cognitive impairment is commensurate with progression of the underlying medical condition, and usually will improve or stabilize in response to appropriate treatment.

Labs

Depending on the specific etiology of the medical condition, these may include:

- Histopathology: biopsy reveals accumulation of the byproducts in skin, arterial walls, and so on;

- Blood: abnormal TSH/T3/T4, electrolytes, creatinine/BUN, LFT/NH3, blood gases/glucose, thiamine, B_6, B_{12}, folate, positive RPR, ANA, ESR, CPK, toxic screen, low ceruloplasmin;
- CSF: Positive for cryptococcal antigen, fluorescein treponemal antibody absorption/treponema immobilization test, oligoclonal IgG bands, increased protein, pleocytosis;
- EEG: epileptic spikes.

Brain Imaging (When Indicated)
- CT/MRI: lesions of the brain, enlargement of ventricle system.

Diagnosis
- Criteria for major (or mild) NCD are present
- Evidence that NCD is the pathophysiological consequence of the medical condition in question.

Neurocognitive Disorder Due to Parkinson's Disease

A psychosomatic physician can be called to see a patient with an established diagnosis of Parkinson's disease who appears depressed. Remember the high prevalence of NCDs in patients with this condition.

Age of onset: age 60–80 (at least one year after the onset of motor symptoms).

Clinical Presentation and Natural Course
Gradual cognitive decline develops relatively early in the disease course. Approximately 27% of patients with Parkinson's have mild NCD. With further progression of Parkinson's, up to 75% of patients will develop major NCD.

Diagnosis
Probable NCD due to Parkinson's disease:
- Insidious onset and gradual progression
- Diagnosis of Parkinson's is established, and Parkinson's clearly precedes the onset of cognitive impairment
- Not better explained by other neurological or neurocognitive disorders.

Possible NCD due to Parkinson's disease could be established if generic criteria for major (or mild) NCD are met, but other criteria for probable diagnosis are not fully met.

Differential diagnosis of NCD due to Parkinson's and NCD with LBD (see above) is conventionally based on the time frame of cognitive and Parkinsonian symptoms presentation: in NCD with LBD, cognitive symptoms begin shortly before, or concurrently with, motor symptoms; in NCD due to Parkinson's, motor symptoms begin at least a year before the onset of cognitive symptoms.

Neurocognitive Disorder Due to Huntington's Disease

The disease carries the name of George Huntington, an American physician, who published in 1872 a thorough description of the disease he called chorea and identified the inheritance pattern as an autosomal dominant disease. The illness equally affects men and women, and has variable geographic and ethnic prevalence (e.g., the incidence is higher in people with Western European descent, at 7 per 100,000). A psychosomatic physician should be vigilant because cognitive impairment and psychiatric symptoms can predate the motor abnormality by at least 15 years.

Age of onset: age 35–45.

Clinical Presentation and Natural Course

The illness presents with changes in the patient's character: annoying, impulsive, suspicious, eccentric, with poor self-control, accompanied by excessive unintentional movements in any part of the body. Cognitive impairment and psychiatric symptoms can predate the motor abnormality and can further progress with the disease, with early changes in executive function (processing speed, organization, and planning) and attention, followed by a decline in communication, social withdrawal, and other signs of subcortical dementia. Life expectancy is 20 years from onset of visible symptoms.

Labs (if Available)

- Genetics: 100% penetration, 40 or more CAG repeat expansion in the Huntington Disease Gene (Chromosome 4).

Brain Imaging

- CT/MRI: volume loss of the caudate nucleus and putamen.

Diagnostic Criteria

- Insidious onset and gradual progression
- Diagnosis of Huntington's is established, or risk for Huntington's based on family history or genetic testing
- Not better explained by another medical condition.

Neurocogntive Disorder Due to HIV Infection

It is estimated that from one-third to over one-half of patients with HIV infection have neurocognitive impairment as a result of viral infection/opportunistic infection and/or medication treatment. Three populations of individuals are at highest risk of contracting HIV infection: adults with risky behaviors (unprotected sex, drug use with sharing needles), children of HIV infected mothers (perinatal transmission), and recipients of blood transfusions or organ transplantation. According to the United States Centers for Disease Control and Prevention (CDC), recipients of infected blood/organs have the highest risk of contracting the infection after an exposure (90%), followed by perinatal transmission (25%), unprotected intercourse with HIV+ partners (0.01–3%) and drug use with sharing of needles (0.3–0.67%).

Age of onset: any age.

Clinical Presentation and Natural Course

Impaired cognitive functioning in HIV-infected patients has an insidious onset, and a slow, fluctuating course with periods of worsening and improvement. An estimated 25% will develop mild NCD and 5% major NCD. Clinical presentation is typical subcortical dementia with motor slowing and social withdrawal. "If an AIDS patient seems to have depression, he probably has dementia" (Kaufmann, 2001).

Brain Imaging
- Head CT/MRI: white matter atrophy (leukoencephalopathy).

Diagnosis
NCD due to HIV infection:
- Documented HIV infection
- Not better explained by secondary brain disease (progressive multifocal leukoencephalopathy or cryptococcal meningitis)
- Not attributable to another medical condition.

Neurocognitive Disorder Due to Prion Disease

These NCDs include subacute spongiform encephalopathies (Creutzfeldt-Jakob disease and its variants, kuru, Gerstmann-Sträussler-Scheinker syndrome, fatal familial insomnia) caused by transmissible agents known as prions (from PRotein infectION; Prusiner, 1982).

Age of onset: age 20–60.

Clinical Presentation and Natural Course
The disease begins with prodromal symptoms: fatigue, anxiety, difficulties with concentration, and appetite and sleep disturbance. A few weeks later, incoordination, altered vision, abnormal gait, and myoclonic, choreoathetoid, or ballistic movements appear, with rapidly progressive dementia. The disease typically progresses to major impairment over several months. The onset of Gerstmann-Sträussler-Scheinker syndrome involves slowly, developing dysarthria/ataxia/dementia and affects 1–10 per 100 million. Fatal familial insomnia onset is age 18–60 with complete loss of sleep (hypnotics are not helpful and paradoxically worsen the course). The disease lasts 7–18 months until death (40 known families in the world).

Labs (if Available)
- CSF: elevated 14-3-3 protein, Tau protein testing of cerebrospinal fluid;
- Real-time quaking-induced conversion (RT-QuIC) (in vitro PrP^{CJD} amplification);
- EEG: periodic sharp, triphasic discharges;
- Genetics: autosomal dominant prion disease Chromosome 20.

Brain Imaging
- MRI (DWI or FLAIR): multifocal grey matter hyperintensities in subcortical and cortical regions.

Diagnosis
NCD due to prion disease:
- Insidious onset and rapid progression
- Myoclonus or ataxia, or biomarker evidence.

Differential Diagnosis of NCDs

Unless the direct cause of cognitive impairment is readily identifiable, making a diagnosis of a particular subtype of NCD can be challenging, especially in early stages. Thorough history-taking and attention to specific clinical details can be critical.

Multiple NCDs

It may be more difficult to make a diagnosis of NCD if the features of two conditions coexist (e.g., Alzheimer's disease and vascular dementia), whereas diagnosis of NCD due to multiple etiologies may be appropriate. For psychosomatic clinicians, evaluating cognitive impairment when dementia and delirium are superimposed can be extremely challenging. Close watch and serial bedside cognitive testing (using standard cognitive rating scales) may reveal waxing/waning changes in behavior and cognitive function, making a case for delirium (although patients with NCD often struggle in new environments and may have intermittent worsening due to unidentified triggers). Sometimes EEG evidence of "generalized slowing" adds to the argument for delirium. Collateral information is often indispensable in determining the patient's baseline level of functioning.

Major Depressive Disorder

Cognitive deficits may be present in other mental disorders such as schizophrenia, anxiety, and ADHD, but these deficits appear subtle compared to the main clinical symptoms. However, aging presents additional diagnostic and treatment challenges when chronic mental illness and neurocognitive illness co-occur. Of particular interest is major depressive disorder (MDD) that can present with significant cognitive impairment, for years referred to as "pseudodementia" (Kiloh, 1961). In contrast to dementia, "pseudodementia" could have a more variable length of onset, history of prior affective illness, presence of neuro-vegetative signs, and marked variability in cognitive performance with inconsistent efforts. Patients with major depression usually do not conceal cognitive deficits, as patients with dementia do. Recent and remote memories are equally poor in patients with "pseudodementia." They rarely have "sundowning," and they respond to standard treatment for depression with improvement of cognition. Recent studies, however, suggest that despite the beneficial effect of antidepressants, some cognitive deficits may persist, indicating a prodromal stage of NCD.

Amnesia

NCDs of different etiologies (e.g., post-traumatic NCD, substance-induced NCD) may present with impairment of memory as the main clinical feature. However, memory disturbance may occur in the absence of NCD (e.g., transient global amnesia, dissociative amnesia, pseudologia fantastica, and Ganser syndrome).

Treatment of Cognitively Impaired Patients in Medical Settings

Early diagnosis and specific therapy of reversible causes of cognitive impairment are the main priorities in the treatment of NCDs. However, due to the insidious onset and slow progression of most conditions, NCDs may remain undiagnosed and untreated until an unrelated medical crisis triggers an exacerbation of the clinical features of NCD and requires the assistance of a psychosomatic physician.

Therapeutic options for NCDs can be divided into three categories: specific treatments (when etiology of the condition is known), illness-modifying therapies (directed to modify the disease course), and symptom-modifying treatment (targeting the prominent and disturbing features).

A psychosomatic physician should promote the implementation of specific and symptom-modifying treatment options whenever possible. Regarding illness-modifying modalities, no universal recommendation exists; psychosomatic physicians have the option to defer the decision to Neurology/Geriatric services, or to discuss the risks/benefits of a particular treatment with family and patient, start the treatment, and make arrangement for appropriate follow-up.

Specific Therapies

Currently available for a small proportion of NCDs, mainly those due to another medical condition, treatments of causative medical conditions, such as infections, brain tumors, autoimmune disease, renal or liver failures, circulatory abnormalities, endocrinopathies, vitamin deficiencies, substance use disorders, seizures, and hydrocephalus, can slow and possibly reverse the progression of the NCD. Progression of vascular dementia can be modified by addressing the cause of strokes (e.g., HTN, dyslipidemia, coagulopathies, etc.).

Illness-Modifying Therapies

For the great majority of NCDs with neurodegenerative features, including Alzheimer's disease, FTD, and LBD, etiology remains uncertain, and for some neurodegenerative NCDs with known etiology, including Huntington's and prion diseases, curative treatment options are not yet available. Here therapeutic efforts are directed to slowing the course of presumed pathological processes and/or compensating for the consequences of neural damage to prevent further cognitive decline.

- Cholinesterase inhibitors were the first group of medications that the US Food and Drug Administration (FDA) approved for the treatment of Alzheimer's (1997). These medications were designed to compensate for the deficiency/loss of cholinergic neurons by increasing acetylcholine neurotransmission. The clinical efficacy of these medications (e.g., donepezil [Aricept], galantamine [Razadyne], and rivastigmine [Exelon]) is considered very modest, although some patients may have more robust responses. There is no evidence that one inhibitor is more effective than the others. Some data suggest that donepezil has a modest effect, improving cognition, global functioning, and ADLs in patients with dementia associated with Parkinson's and LBD. Galantamine can provide benefit in Parkinson's and vascular dementia. Rivastigmine is available as pills, oral solution, and patch. Transdermal application of rivastigmine has fewer gastrointestinal side effects than the oral formulation and is useful for patients with limited GI access. It is also used for treating Parkinson's disease–related NCD.

- Memantine (Namenda), an N-methyl-D-aspartate (NMDA) receptor antagonist, was introduced in 2003 to treat moderate-severe Alzheimer's, and can be administered alone or in combination with acetylcholinesterase inhibitors. Its effect is likely mediated through non-competitive antagonism with glutamatergic neurotransmission and prevention of neuronal excitotoxicity. Namenda usually starts at 5 mg (pill or oral solution) daily with slow titration up to 10 mg twice daily. Sustained released formulation of memantine seems more convenient. The medication is usually well-tolerated. Some data indicate that memantine may be used as an effective alternative to antipsychotics in management of behavioral abnormalities in Alzheimer's patients.

- The dopamine precursor (L-DOPA) has been used since the 1960s for treatment of Parkinson's to compensate for progressive loss of dopaminergic neurons in the substantia nigra. Although no evidence exists that treatment with Sinemet affects the progression of NCD due to Parkinson's, some medications used for treatment of Parkinson's are known to have beneficial effects on cognition. A dopamine agonist Amantadine helps to restore cognitive function in TBI patients. The MAOI-B inhibitor Selegiline in the short term can improve cognition and ADLs in demented patients.

- A miscellaneous group of pharmacological agents and food supplements have beneficial effects on cognitive function in patients with NCDs: Cytidine 5'-diphosphocholine (CTD-choline, citicoline), Piracetam (Nootropil), and Axona. Drugs that target production, deposition or clearance of β amyloid or phosphorylation/assembly of tau-proteins in the CNS are currently under different stages of development. The future of this new approach of illness-modifying therapy for Alzheimer's relies on the validity of the assumption that deposition of these byproducts is a core mechanism of neurodegeneration and cognitive impairment, rather than a "tombstone" of the neural death. Gene therapy with nerve growth factor hyperexpression and stem cell transplantation in the brain—promising approaches in the treatment of neurodegenerative diseases—are in their nascent state.

Symptom-Modifying Therapies

Independent of disease-specific therapies, clinical attention is focused on managing the most disturbing symptoms and/or behaviors of patients with dementia, including agitation, psychosis, "sundowning," impulsivity, apathy, and urinary incontinence. Symptom-modifying therapy uses both pharmacological and non-pharmacologic modalities, relying heavily on preventive measures, behavioral modifications, and environmental interventions.

- **Agitation**: Patients with cognitive impairment feel vulnerable and experience significant stress in the foreign environment of a medical floor. In addition, for the person with dementia who has impaired problem-solving ability or deficits in receptive and expressive language, agitation or odd behaviors may be a form of communication. Exploration of the behavior's cause, such as pain, illness, urges for excretion, or overstimulation or deficit of sensory input, is of paramount importance before jumping to pharmacological "pacifiers." Observant clinicians can evaluate what preceded the behavior, the behavior itself, and its consequences in an attempt to identify patterns. At times, room placement that provides adequate sensory stimulation can make a difference. Normal day/night light cycle maintenance, presence of family members/familiar items from home, and hearing aids and glasses are helpful for orientation and prevention of agitation and, its extreme form, aggression. The latter requires a prompt reaction that may include restraints and therapeutic sedation (see Chapter 7).
- **Psychosis**: Delusions and hallucinations are significant problems in managing demented patients. Recent findings of the high death rate in patients with dementia treated with neuroleptics, reflected in the 2005 FDA black box warning, suggest that antipsychotics be used judiciously in patients with dementia complicated by psychosis or agitation, with open discussion of risks/benefits with patients and families. Completely avoiding the use of antipsychotics is not feasible in many patients with dementia and severe psychosis who require urgent treatment, and when preventive measures or behavioral interventions alone are insufficient to alleviate suffering. The recommended strategy is to start the antipsychotic at a low dosage and to raise the dosage slowly, constantly reviewing the response and side effects. Due to fewer extrapyramidal effects, second-generation antipsychotics have some advantage and are used more frequently: olanzapine (Zyprexa), risperidone, or aripiprazole (Abilify).
  - Use of antipsychotics in patients with LBD should be avoided due to the severe sensitivity of the patients to these medications. Treatment of psychosis in patients with NCD due to Parkinson's may be challenging due to the obvious dilemma: treat psychosis with dopamine (DA) antagonists or treat stiffness/tremor of Parkinson's with DA precursors/agonists, which may be a cause of psychosis. The best results of psychosis treatment in this case can be achieved with clozapine (Clozaril); however, an initial trial of low doses of quetiapine (Seroquel) may be warranted.
- **"Sundowning"**: This is a characteristic exacerbation of behavioral symptomatology such as confusion, agitation/restlessness, anxiety, mood swings and irritability, suspiciousness, and aggressiveness in patients with dementia, usually occurring in the late afternoon, evening (6–7 p.m.), or night (nocturnal wandering). Many features of sundowning, such as diurnal waxing/waning changes of consciousness (orientation, arousal), agitation, and perceptual abnormalities, are similar to those observed in delirium, and some clinicians consider this phenomenon a variant of delirium. One hypothesis associates sundowning with the malfunction/degeneration of the

suprachiasmatic nucleus in the hypothalamus, which plays a key role in the body's circadian rhythms, including the sleep-wake cycle. Interventions aimed to maintain proper circadian rhythms and sleep, such as bright light therapy, good sleep hygiene, and treatment with melatonin agonists, have shown some beneficial effects. However, behavioral disturbance from sundowning can be very challenging for caregivers at home and are likely a common cause of institutionalizing patients with dementia. When behavioral approaches are not effective, low doses of sedatives, such as trazodone, olanzapine (Zyprexa), quetiapine (Seroquel), or risperidone in the evening (5–6 p.m.), can help manage behavioral disturbance.

- **Impulsivity**: Patients with cognitive impairment can present with disinhibited behavior, impulsiveness, and, at times, unprovoked acts of violence. The primary treatment approach is to examine the behavior (triggers, patterns, consequences) and to use both behavioral modifications and medications to help patients maintain control. Among the drugs used are SSRIs (citalopram, sertraline), anticonvulsants (valproate, carbamazepine, topiramate), and antipsychotics (see Chapter 7 on agitation).

- **Falls and wandering**: Precautions for these are an integrative part of managing patients with dementia and should be implemented according to the safety policy on the floor (low bed, safety mattress, hospital gown, safety attendant, etc.).

- **Incontinence**: Toilet assistance, including timed voiding, in combination with additional interventions, and prompted voiding are established evidence-based interventions for incontinent persons with dementia that can help to reduce anxiety and prevent agitation. Indwelling catheters should be avoided.

- **Apathy**: Decreased motivation in patients with dementia can be associated with frontal and subcortical pathology. Supportive psychotherapy and psychostimulants (modafinil, methylphenidate) have beneficial effects in treating apathy.

Psychotherapeutic Interventions

Psychotherapeutic interventions can be used separately or as part of a comprehensive behavioral plan combined with psychopharmacology. Several therapies, such as reality orientation and stimulation-oriented therapy that utilizes art, music, pets, exercise, recreational activities and aromatherapy, have beneficial effects in dementia.

Caregiving

With 80% of patients with dementia residing at home, caregiving remains the primary management approach. It is important to educate patients and caregivers about the challenges in managing NCDs, to set expectations, to encourage close monitoring, to refer to online resources, and to coordinate a referral for appropriate follow-up. Interaction with family may be a sensitive task; family members may be in denial of the cognitive deficits of their loved ones and may feel embarrassed if the cognitive exam of the patient occurs in their presence.

Evaluation of Decision-Making Ability

Patients with cognitive impairment do not necessarily lack the capacity to make decisions regarding their care. The relationship between intellectual capacity and decisional capacity is always case-specific and should be evaluated on a continuum of importance of the decision, risk/benefit ratio, and impact on the patient and others (see Chapter 9). Patients may lack the capacity to make complex medical decisions, but retain the capacity to choose a surrogate decision-maker and should be encouraged early on to consider living wills, and so on. A psychosomatic physician should consider whether driving privileges should be suspended for significantly impaired patients. Procedures vary based on state and local statutes.

The main treatment goal for patients with NCDs is to help maintain the highest quality of life for patients and family.

Conclusion

NCDs are becoming a substantial portion of psychosomatic medical practice due to demographic changes and an aging population. It is not rare, especially in community hospitals, for elderly individuals to be admitted from home after falls, odd behaviors, or a failure to thrive. Evaluation may suggest that the primary issue is progression of an NCD. Psychosomatic physicians should be vigilant and proactive in efforts to detect NCDs as early as possible, should educate patients and families about etiology and treatment options, and should provide appropriate referrals for further evaluation and management.

Disclosures

Dr. Gushchin has no conflicts of interest to disclose.

Key Points

- Neurocognitive disorders (NCDs) are becoming a substantial portion of psychosomatic medical practice due to an aging population.
- Psychosomatic physicians should be cognizant of NCDs, as we are frequently the initial clinicians to diagnose NCD and have a responsibility to educate patients and families about clinical features and treatment.
- Evaluating patients with features of more than one NCD, such as dementia and delirium, can be extremely challenging.
- For the NCDs with unknown etiology or unavailable curative treatment options, therapeutic efforts are directed to slowing the course of presumed pathological processes (illness-modifying therapies), and to targeting the prominent and disturbing features (symptom-modifying treatment).

Further Reading

American Psychiatric Association (2013). *Diagnostic and Statistical Manual of Mental Disorders*, 5th ed. Arlington, VA: American Psychiatric Association.

Kaufman DM (2001). *Clinical Neurology for Psychiatrists*, 5th ed. Philadelphia: W.vB. Saunders.

Jellinger, KA (2008). Morphologic diagnosis of 'vascular dementia": A critical update. *J Neurol Sci.*, *270*, 1–12.

Kiloh LG (1961). Pseudo-dementia. *Acta Psychiat Scand.*, *37*(4), 336–351.

Lippa CF, Duda JE, et al. (2007). DLB and PDD boundary issues: Diagnosis, treatment, molecular pathology, and biomarkers. *Neurology*, *68*, 812–819.

McKhann GM, Knopman DS, et al. (2011). The diagnosis of dementia due to Alzheimer's disease: Recommendations from the National Institute on Aging—Alzheimer's Association workgroups on diagnostic guidelines for Alzheimer's disease. *Alzheimer's Dement.*, 7, 263–269.

Nasreddine ZS, Phillips NA, et al. (2005). The Montreal Cognitive Assessment, MoCA: A brief screening tool for mild cognitive impairment. *J Am Geriatr Soc.*, *53*(4), 695–699.

Rabinovici GD, Miller BL (2010). Frontotemporal lobar degeneration. *CNS Drugs*, *24*(5), 375–398.

National Institute of Neurological disorders and Stroke. NIH Stroke Scale. Rev. 10/1/2003. Retrived from http://www.ninds.nih.gov/doctors/NIH_Stroke_Scale.pdf

Exercises

1. Dementia characterized by personality changes, attention deficits, impulsivity, affective lability, indifference, perseveration, and inability to plan and organize is most commonly associated with dysfunction in which brain region?
   a. Frontal lobe
   b. Arcuate gyrus
   c. Hypothalamus
   d. Corpus callosum
   e. Medial temporal lobe

2. A 75-year-old patient presents with mild forgetfulness and intermittent episodes of hallucinations, paranoid delusions, and confusion. His wife reports frequent falls, and he complains of frequent episodes of dizziness when getting out of bed. His blood pressure lying down is 135/90, standing is 100/55. On examination, he has bilateral limb and axial rigidity without tremor. This presentation is most consistent with:
   a. Alzheimer's disease
   b. Creutzfeldt-Jacob disease
   c. Pick's disease
   d. Lewy body disease
   e. Progressive supranuclear palsy

3. Which of the following MRI findings is the most consistent characteristic of Alzheimer's disease?
   a. Frontal lobe atrophy
   b. Occipital lobe atrophy
   c. Caudate nucleus atrophy
   d. Reduced hippocampal volumes
   e. Periventricular white matter lesions

4. The MRI of a 68-year-old woman with slowly progressive dementia shows multiple areas of increased signal intensity on the T2-weighted images in the periventricular white matter. This finding is most consistent with:
   a. Pick's disease
   b. Pseudotumor cerebri
   c. Vascular dementia
   d. Neurocognitive disorder due to Parkinson's disease
   e. Normal pressure hydrocephalus

5. Caudate head atrophy on CT and MRI scans and a reduction in basal ganglia glucose metabolism on PET scan most strongly support a diagnosis of:
   a. Huntington's disease
   b. Binswanger's disease
   c. Alzheimer's disease
   d. Neurocognitive disorder due to HIV infection
   e. Progressive supranuclear palsy

Answers: (1) a (2) d (3) d (4) c (5) a

Psychiatric Presentations Associated with Neurologic Illness

Ellen M. Whyte

Introduction

This chapter contains two sections. The first section, "General Neuropsychiatric Syndromes," describes common neuropsychiatric manifestations and treatment of central nervous system (CNS) disorders that involve the brain without regard to the specific underlying disease. The neuropsychiatric presentation of CNS disorders is more closely related to which brain regions are involved and, to some extent, how much of the brain is involved, than to the etiology of the underlying neurological disease. Hence, neuropsychiatric manifestations present similarly and are managed similarly across an array of CNS disorders. The second section of this chapter, "Disease-Specific Features," highlights the neuropsychiatric manifestations of specific CNS disorders that affect the brain (Table 12.1), including acquired brain injury (i.e., stroke and traumatic brain injury [TBI]), seizure disorders, neurodegenerative diseases, inflammatory diseases, and infectious diseases. The reader is encouraged to consult both sections.

Cognitive Impairment

The behavioral manifestations of neurological disorders are frequently inseparable from its cognitive consequences. For example, a patient with impaired executive functions but with intact language and memory abilities may primarily be viewed as apathetic, impulsive, anxious, or agitated, but not cognitively impaired. In this example, apathy reflects the patient's inability to initiate and maintain activity, whereas impulsivity reflects an inability to inhibit behavior in a socially appropriate way; both reflect the underlying executive impairment. Depression, anxiety and agitation may emerge from frustration over the cognitive inability to navigate day-to-day life. Clarifying the patient's cognitive status is an important role of the consulting psychiatrist. Knowledge of the patient's cognitive profile (1) informs treatment planning, (2) helps the treatment team and family understand the patient's behavior, and (3) circumvents the patient being blamed for his or her behavior (e.g., the apathetic patient being labeled as "lazy"). A careful history obtained from family regarding cognitive function prior to the acute illness can be informative.

Table 12.1 Relative Incidence of Various Neuropsychiatric Symptoms in Common Neurological Disorders

	Depression	Mania	Pseudo-bulbar Affect	Apathy	Anxiety	Fatigue	Agitation and Aggression	Psychosis	Significant Cognitive Impairment
Stroke	+++	rare	+++	+++	+++	+++	variable	rare	+++
TBI	++++	+	+++	+++	+++	+++++	variable	rare	variable
MS	++	rare	++	++	+++	+++	variable	+	++
Parkinson's Disease	++++	+[e]	+	++	+++	+++	---[c]	+++++[a,e]	+++
Huntington's Disease	+++	++	---	+++++	++++	---	++++	++[a]	+++++[d]
HIV/AIDS	+++	+	---[b]	++	++	+++	---[c]	++[a]	+++
Epilepsy	+++	rare	---	---	+++	---	---	variable	variable

Key: Plus signs reflect relative prevalence of neuropsychiatric symptoms; the greater number of + signs indicate that the symptom is more common.
+++++ indicates that maximum reports of incidence are > 75%; ++++ (> 50%); +++ (> 25%); ++ (> 10%); + (1–9%)
[a] More common in later stage disease
[b] Reported in progressive multifocal leukoencephalopathy, a complication of AIDS
[c] Agitation/aggression can be seen during delirium or when dementia is present
[d] Dementia is a common manifestation of late disease
[e] Likely induced by dopamine replacement therapy

General Neuropsychiatric Syndromes

Depression

Etiology

Mood disturbance is very common in CNS disorders and primarily presents as depression. Depression can be both a psychological reaction to a devastating neurological illness and a basic biological outcome of the illness. Evidence supporting the latter etiology includes studies demonstrating that the prevalence of depression in CNS disorders is greater than that in similarly disabling non-CNS disorders. In addition, damage to key brain regions, especially basal ganglia, have been consistently implicated in depression; for example, depression is commonly seen in Parkinson's disease (PD) and after basal ganglia stroke. Yet, one of the strongest risk factors for developing depression is a personal pre-morbid history of depressive illness, suggesting that personal genetic and psychological makeup plays a strong role in mental health, even in the setting of CNS disorders. Depression in neurological disorders can also be induced by medications used to treat the illness. For example, interferon beta-1a, a first-line medication in relapsing-remitting multiple sclerosis (MS), is associated with an 18%–25% incidence of depressive symptoms.

Illness Course

The onset of depression is variable and is influenced by the specific underlying disorder. For example, in stroke, the peak incidence appears to be three to six months post-injury, whereas in Parkinson's disease, depression can appear at any time and, in some cases, can be one of the presenting symptoms of the neurological disease.

Although the peak incidence of depression will vary for different neurologic disorders, in most cases the point prevalence of depression remains elevated throughout the illness course—while some patients will improve after an index episode of depression, others will suffer from chronic depressive symptoms.

Diagnosis

The *DSM-5* diagnostic code typically used is "Depressive Disorder Due to Another Medical Condition," with the further specifiers of *with depressive features, with major depressive-like episode,* or *with mixed features.* This diagnosis is used when the mood disturbance is the direct pathophysiological consequence of the neurological disorder and the symptoms are not better accounted for by another psychiatric disorder. However, making this diagnosis presumes reliable knowledge of etiology of the depressive episode for the unique patient, which is seldom the case. The clinician needs to use his or her best judgment when making a diagnosis. The differential diagnosis includes major depressive disorder, substance/medication-induced depressive disorder, other specified depressive disorder, and unspecified depressive disorder. Adjustment disorder, where the neurological illness is the stressor, should also be considered.

We favor an inclusive approach that counts all symptoms toward the syndromal diagnosis of depression, even if there may be another possible etiology for that symptom (e.g., fatigue, which is common in MS, would "count" toward a diagnosis of depression). The rationale for this approach is that if the depression is successfully treated, any depressive symptoms, even if caused by multiple etiologies, should improve. Of course, only patients with either depressed mood and/or anhedonia would be considered for a depression diagnosis.

Impairments in language ability or other cognitive domains can make assessment challenging. See Table 12.2 for techniques to overcome language/cognitive barriers. A "quick and dirty" method for assessment of verbal comprehension is to ask the patient a series of yes/no questions in which you provide them the opportunity to truthfully answer yes or no. For example, ask the patient to verify personal information, such as confirming her middle name or the year that she was born, and provide the patient with the opportunity to truthfully answer "no" by purposefully providing her with false information. Once confirmed that the patient can correctly answer yes/no questions, then questions such as "Are you feeling sad?" are appropriate.

Differential Diagnosis

Depressed patients can demonstrate lack of motivation or goal-directed behavior, which may be better attributed to primary apathy or

Table 12.2 Techniques to Overcome Barriers to Assessment

Barrier to Assessment	Potential Solutions
Expressive Aphasia (e.g., can comprehend simple spoken language)	• Utilize yes/no questions (e.g., Yessevage Geriatric Depression Scale or simple questions) • Use Picture Board • Use Visual Analog Scale
Receptive Aphasia	• If mild, restate question in different words and/or use Picture Board
Memory Impairment	• Gather collateral information from family, friends, hospital/nursing home staff. Front line staff, e.g., personal care aides, physical therapists, etc., who spend significant amounts of time with the patient, are an excellent source of information. • Request log of the person's sleep and appetite.

pathological fatigue. Crying can be seen both in depression and in pseudobulbar affect (i.e., emotional lability, emotional incontinence). Agitation can be seen in depression, anxiety, psychosis, and impulse control disorders. While a single patient may have more than one neuropsychiatric disorder concurrently, the absence of low mood and anhedonia rules out a depressive diagnosis.

Patients with CNS disorders are typically burdened by significant medical comorbidity in addition to the multiple complications of their neurological illness. These factors can contribute to depression, and need to be identified and modified (if possible) as part of a holistic approach to disease management. A select subset of these factors is listed in Table 12.3. The reader should also consult Chapter 3.

Treatment/Management
Studies suggest that standard antidepressants can be effective. Side-effect profile is an important consideration in selecting an antidepressant. For example, medications with anticholinergic properties

Table 12.3 Common Factors Contributing to Depression, Fatigue, and Apathy in the Context of Neurological Illness

Cardiovascular	Ischemic heart disease
	Congestive heart failure
	Endocarditis
	Hypotension/orthostatic hypotension
Impaired Sleep	Sleep apnea (a risk factor for stroke; a common sequelae of acquired brain injury)
	Chronic sleep impairment due to pain, motor symptoms, loss of bladder/bowel control
	Excessive daytime sleepiness in Parkinson's disease
Metabolic/Nutritional	Poorly controlled diabetes mellitus
	Severe B_{12} deficiency
	Chronic renal inefficiency
Rheumatological	Fibromyalgia
	Lupus
	Vasculitis
Medication-Induced	Glucocorticoids
	Interferon
Other	Severe deconditioning
	Grief/stress/anxiety
	Chronic pain

(e.g., TCAs) should be avoided, as they can impair cognitive functioning and worsen the urinary retention commonly seen in stroke. Bupropion's risk of seizure would make it a poor choice in patients with a known seizure disorder. Non-pharmacological interventions are useful, including psychotherapy to address life changes caused by the neurological illness and cognitive retraining to reduce frustration related to cognitive impairment.

There are no studies exploring how long a patient needs to remain on antidepressants after remission of symptoms. Given that the risk of depression remains elevated throughout the illness course, lifelong maintenance use of an antidepressant should be considered.

Suicide

As with all patients with depression, a thoughtful suicide assessment is indicated. Patients demonstrating impulsivity may be at heightened risk, for example, patients with Huntington's disease. Survivors of TBI have particularly elevated rates of hopelessness and suicidal ideation. One survey of TBI survivors reported that 18% of TBI survivors have had a suicide attempt (Simpson & Tate, 2002). The risk of suicidality post-injury appears to be independent of gender, age, race, income, education, injury severity, or length of time since injury (Tsaousides et al., 2011).

Clinical Pearl

Disability and depression have a reciprocal and reinforcing relationship. While persons with functional limitations due to physical disability are more likely to become depressed, those with depression will demonstrate increased functional limitations due to diminished effort, decreased engagement in rehabilitation, or the motor effects (typically slowing) of depression. Treatment of depression can thereby improve a person's ability to function.

Clinical Pearl

Selective serotonin reuptake inhibitors (SSRIs) and serotonin norepinephrine reuptake inhibitors (SNRIs) are first-line treatments of depression in Parkinson's disease, even though some case reports suggest that SSRI/SNRI antidepressants can worsen the motor symptoms. Sertraline may be the SSRI least likely to worsen motor symptoms. In addition, the use of antidepressants in combination with monoamine oxidase B inhibitors (e.g., selegiline and reasagiline) has the potential to cause serotonin syndrome. However, this is unlikely when both classes of drugs are used within the recommended dose ranges. Finally, use of high-dose monamine oxidase inhibitor MAOi-B also results in inhibition of MAO-A; under this condition, concomitant use of an antidepressant may result in a hypertensive crisis.

Pseudobulbar Affect

Pseudobulbar affect (PBA), also known as emotional lability, emotional incontinence, or pathological laughing and crying, is abnormal emotional expression characterized by sudden onset of crying (or laughing), which the patient does not feel is under his control and which occurs in situations that would not previously have provoked such behavior. In addition, the crying is not simply an expression of depression or grief. The content of the provoking situation can be congruent, neutral, or incongruent with the expressed affect. PBA is frequently misdiagnosed as depression.

> *Case Vignette:* Mr. J is a 68-year-old white male admitted for rehabilitation after suffering a right middle cerebral artery stroke that has resulted in dense left hemiparesis. This is his second stroke. A psychiatry consult is requested, as the patient cries throughout the day. On interview, the patient denies feeling sad and denies anhedonia. He is optimistic, but realistic, about his future. While he admits that there will be challenges, he is determined to be the "best husband, father, brother and grandfather possible despite the stroke." He is tearful at several points during the interview. He denies feeling sad when tearful. He reports that since the stroke, he will cry whenever he feels a moderately strong emotion. For example, he cried when his grandchildren came to see him. He is embarrassed by this crying and does not feel that he can control it.

Etiology
The etiology of PBA is unkown. However, PBA is more common when the underlying disease process affects multiple brain regions, for example, in later stages of MS and in persons who have suffered multiple strokes. Glatiramer acetate, used in relapsing-remitting MS, is associated with a 1% incidence of PBA.

Diagnosis
PBA is not included as its own diagnosis in *DSM-5*, although it appears as "emotional lability" in both *ICD-9* and *ICD-10*. When occurring in the setting of cognitive impairment, PBA may be subsumed under the "behavioral disturbance" specifier of neurocognitive disorders.

Illness Course
Pathological crying is the most common variant. Pathological laughing and mixed crying/laughing are less common. The natural history of PBA is unclear. In stroke patients, some evidence suggests that the prevalence decreases over time (a 20%–25% prevlance within first six months after stroke vs. a 10%–15% prevalence at 12 months).

Treatment
Patient and family education are important, as pathological crying can be misinterpreted as depression and pathological laughing is viewed as rude and socially inappropriate. Nudexa (dextromethorphan hydrobromide 20 mg with quinidine sulfate 10 mg) is the only FDA-approved treatment. However, older studies indicate that both SSRIs and TCAs are effective in controlling the symptoms of PBA in stroke and MS. Onset of response is usually within 24–48 hours of starting a low-dose antidepressant.

Clinical Pearl

While PBA is a distinct syndrome that is separate from depression, the two commonly coexist. In addition, the presence of PBA in the absence of depression after stroke is associated with a 50% risk of developing depression subsequently.

Apathy

Definition

Apathy is a lack of motivation that is not attributable to intellectual impairment, emotional distress, psychiatric disorder, or diminished level of consciousness. While not formally part of *DSM-5*, criteria for apathy have been proposed by Roberts and colleagues (2009). The key features of the proposed criteria include that the patient needs to demonstrate (1) a reduction in motivation compared to his or her prior level of function that is inconsistent with the patient's age/culture, and (2) a decrease in goal-directed behavior, cognitive activity, and/or emotion over a least a four-week period. In addition, apathy symptoms must cause significant impairment in functioning and cannot be better explained by decreased level of consciousness or other physical disability and cannot be substance induced.

Etiology

Evidence suggests that disruption of the prefrontal cortex-basal ganglia circuits is common in patients with apathy. The prevalence of apathy has been reported to exceed 20% in a variety of disorders, including Alzheimer's disease, Huntington's disease, MS, and stroke.

Diagnosis

Apathy is not included as its own diagnosis within *DSM-5*, although it appears as "demoralization and apathy" in both *ICD-9* and *ICD-10*. Diagnostic criteria for apathy have been proposed and should be based on both informant reports of the patient's behavior and the patient interview. The diagnosis can only be established once other disorders, such as depression or hypothyroidism, are ruled out.

Treatment

There is no definitive treatment for apathy. However, the general approach to minimize apathy and increase function across CNS disorders is similar:

1. Undertake a thorough workup to diagnosis any psychiatric and medical conditions associated with diminished motivation, for example, identify and treat obstructive sleep apnea.
2. Educate the patient, family, and caregivers regarding the nature of apathy and the goals of treatment (i.e., often remediation, not cure).
3. Consider an empirical trial of an antidepressant to exclude the possibility of an anhedonic major depression without insight.
4. Consider other medication trials. There is little empirical evidence supporting any pharmacological interventions due to paucity of studies. Agents to consider include antidepressants, stimulants (e.g., methylphenidate starting at 5–10 mg/d, amphetamine mixed salts starting at 10 mg/d) and, in the setting of cognitive

impairment, acetylcholinesterase inhibitors (e.g., donepezil starting at 5 mg/d).
5. Utilize non-pharmacological treatments, which are a mainstay of treatment. Behavioral strategies include providing the patient with structured daily activities, a more rewarding and stimulating environment, and increased socialization. Consideration can be given to a token economy in which the patient earns desired rewards for participating in specified behaviors. However, a token economy can only be set up with the full consent of the patient, in consultation with his or her family, and conducted in a manner that is not punitive.

Fatigue

Chronic pathological fatigue may be best described as a pathological feeling of tiredness that is disproportionate to the person's level of actual physical or mental exertion and is poorly relieved by rest. Chronic pathological fatigue differs from everyday fatigue that is experienced by healthy individuals in that "everyday" fatigue can be linked to an identifiable cause such as exertion or stress, and is relieved by rest. Chronic pathological fatigue negatively influences social, physical, and cognitive functioning and leads to decreased quality of life. When present, patients often label chronic pathological fatigue as their most disabling symptom. Fatigue is often comorbid with depression, but is an independent syndrome.

Etiology

The etiology is unknown. Factors such as age, gender, race, and, for traumatic brain injury patients, injury severity and time since injury are not associated with fatigue.

Illness Course

Fatigue is a chronic syndrome whose overall prevalence appears to remain constant over time. While commonly comorbid with depression, it can also be present (and disabling) in the absence of depression.

Diagnosis

Fatigue is not included as its own diagnosis within *DSM-5*, although it appears in *ICD-9* as "other malaise and fatigue" and in *ICD-10* as "other fatigue." Diagnosis is based on the patient's subjective report of fatigue that is not relieved by rest and that is out of proportion to the amount of physical or mental activity. It is a diagnosis of exclusion and is made only after other causes of fatigue, including any comorbid depressive and medical illnesses, are addressed. In contrast to apathy and some cases of depression, motivation is intact in chronic pathological fatigue.

Treatment/Management

There is no definitive treatment for chronic pathological fatigue. However, a general approach to minimize fatigue would include the following:
1. Normalize the fatigue experience for the patient and their family so that it is accepted as a common consequence of neurological illness and not as a moral failure.

2. Treat other illnesses potentially contributing to fatigue (see Table 12.3).
3. Treat any underlying sleep disturbance.
4. Address acquired physical deconditioning, which can develop as a person increasingly limits his or her activity due to fatigue, which then compounds fatigue.
5. Encourage patients to set realistic goals, and to modify how they work toward goals in order to conserve energy. Occupational therapists can help teach patients energy conversation strategies.
6. Consider pharmacological interventions. Suggested pharmacological management of fatigue is based on limited trials. The most commonly used agents include stimulants (e.g., methylphenidate starting at 5–10 mg/d, amphetamine mixed salts starting at 10 mg/d), wakefulness-promoting agents (e.g., modafinil 200 mg/d), dopaminergic agents (e.g., amantadine 100 mg qd or bid), and non-sedating antidepressants (especially bupropion starting at 100 mg/d or an SNRI (e.g., venlafaxine XR starting at 37.5 mg/d)).

Psychosis

Definition
Psychosis can include delusions and/or hallucinations, although the latter are more common in neurological disorders.

Etiology
While the exact etiology of psychosis is unknown, lesions of the occipital lobes are closely associated with visual hallucinations, whereas lesions of the temporal lobes are associated with auditory hallucinations.

Diagnosis
The *DSM-5* diagnostic code typically used is "Psychotic Disorder Due to Another Medical Condition" with the further specifiers of *with delusions* or *with hallucinations*. This diagnosis is used when the psychosis is thought to be the direct pathophysiological consequence of the neurological disorder and is not better accounted for by another psychiatric disorder. When occurring in the setting of cognitive impairment, psychosis may be subsumed under the *behavioral disturbance* specifier of neurocognitive disorder.

Treatment/Management
The emergence of psychosis should trigger an assessment for a possible delirium. Patients with brain damage (e.g., due to stroke or MS) are at increased risk of developing delirium while simultaneously being the patients least likely to be able to report the symptoms of intervening medical illnesses. If no delirium is identified, the use of low-dose antipsychotic medication can be initiated. However, based on evidence in the treatment of psychosis in Alzheimer's disease, a trial of an SSRI antidepressant (e.g., citalopram 10–20 mg/d) is reasonable before turning to an antipsychotic medication. Second-generation antipsychotics are preferred due to the increased risk of adverse effects of antipsychotics in this population (e.g., increased risk of tardive dyskinesia and extrapyramidal symptoms).

Clinical Pearl

The most common form of psychosis in epilepsy is postictal psychosis, which affects 6%–10% of patients with epilepsy and typically occurs one to three days post-seizure. Less common are ictal psychosis, seen in non-convulsive seizures, and interictal psychosis, which emerges between episodes of seizures, has no association with the timing of seizures, and is mostly associated with partial epilepsy. In all forms of epilepsy-associated psychosis, treatment is primarily the control of the seizure disorder and, if needed, use of antipsychotic medications.

Clinical Pearl

Psychosis affects up to 40% of Parkinson's patients who receive drug treatment and typically presents as visual hallucinations or paranoia. Psychosis in PD can be due to the underlying Lewy body disease or a side effect of antiparkinsonian medication. The management of psychosis in PD involves a stepwise algorithm:

1. Assess for and treat any delirium due to another medical illness.
2. Attempt to minimize the amount of antiparkinsonian medications being used to control the motor symptoms. A suggested order of dose reduction or discontinuation is anticholinergic drugs first, followed by amantadine, then catechol-O-methyl transferase inhibitors, and then dopamine agonists (e.g., pramipexole, ropinirole), followed by an attempt at reducing Levodopa/Carbidopa.
3. Treat with a low dose of either quetiapine or clozapine if psychosis persists despite medication reduction, or if medication reduction is not possible due to the worsening of motor symptoms. Due to the risk of agranulocytosis and the need for regular blood tests with clozapine, quetiapine is generally used as first line.

Aggressive Behaviors

Readers are referred to Chapter 7 for a discussion of the management of agitation and aggression.

Disease-Specific Features

Stroke

- Depression, pseudobulbar affect, apathy, and fatigue are all common after stroke, frequently co-occur, and are associated with increased disability.
- Depression affects approximately 34% within the first year of stroke. The risk of depression remains elevated for years after a stroke. Depression with onset soon after stroke is associated with left frontal lobe lesions.
- Pseudobulbar affect (i.e., emotional lability, emotional incontinence) occurs in 20%–25% of stroke survivors within the first six months after stroke and is a risk factor for subsequently developing depression.
- Apathy affects approximately one-third of stroke patients, both in the acute post-stroke phase and in the long term.

Traumatic Brain Injury

- Depression is common and can be chronic.
- Up to 18% of TBI survivors have had a suicide attempt.
- Fatigue is commonly labeled as the most disabling post-injury symptom among community-dwelling TBI survivors.
- Use of antipsychotics should be avoided, as blockade of the dopamine-2 receptor may interfere with brain recovery.
- New onset temporal lobe epilepsy should be considered as a potential cause of agitation/aggression.

Multiple Sclerosis

- Depression is common. Interferon beta-1a, used to treat relapsing forms of MS, may induce depression.
- Pseudobulbar affect afflicts 10% of MS patients.
- Apathy afflicts approximately 20% of MS patients.
- Fatigue affects > 75% of MS patients and significantly impacts daily function.

Parkinson's Disease

- Depression is common and can be the earliest presenting symptom. SSRI or SNRI are first-line medication treatments but potentially can worsen motor symptoms.
- Fatigue is a common problem.
- Psychosis affects 40% of patients and is typically due to medications used to manage motor symptoms. Initial treatment includes reducing/eliminating offending medications; then, if needed, low-dose quetiapine or clozapine can be used.

Huntington's Disease

- Neuropsychiatric symptoms can develop at any point in the disease course.
  - Agitation and depression can present years before onset of motor symptoms.

- Agitation/aggression can stem from loss of ability to inhibit behaviors as the striatum and orbitofrontal-subcortical circuits degenerate.
- Atypical antipsychotics may improve both psychotic and motor symptoms.
- Anxiety, including symptoms of obsessive-compulsive disorder, are common.
- HD patients have an elevated suicide risk, as do non-symptomatic HD mutation carriers.

HIV/AIDS

- Major depression is seen in 15%–40% of patients.
- AIDS mania is seen in late-stage HIV infection and can respond to antipsychotic monotherapy. Anticonvulsants can be used, but carbamazepine and valproate should be used cautiously due to risk of agranulocytosis and thrombocytopenia, respectively.
- The non-nucleoside reverse transcriptase inhibitor (NNRTI) efavirenz and rilpivirine plus other medications used to treat HIV can induce significant changes in mood and behavior and may be associated with increased risk of suicide attempts.
- HIV-related neurocognitive disorder typically includes deficits in executive functions, processing speed, complex attention, and acquisition of new information.
- Psychotic symptoms are more common in later stage disease, especially if cognitive impairment is present.

Epilepsy

- Depression is the most common neuropsychiatric symptom in epilepsy and is more common in patients with partial seizure disorders of temporal and frontal lobe origin. Some anticonvulsant medications (e.g., phenobarbital, primidone, vigabatrin, levetiracetam, felbamate, topiramate) can contribute to depressed mood.
- The clinical presentation of depression may not be consistent with *DSM-5* criteria and may be described relative to the symptoms' temporal relationship to the seizure:
  - Pre-ictal affective symptoms are seen in 10%–20% of patients.
  - Ictal affective symptoms are part of a simple partial seizure.
  - Postictal affective symptoms can last for one hour to three days post-seizure.
  - Interictal affective symptoms tend to follow a waxing and waning course.
- Depression treatment should include improving the control of underlying seizure disorder. Judicious use of antidepressants is appropriate. Bupropion and tricyclic antidepressants should be avoided due to an elevated risk of seizures.
- Psychosis is more common in the postictal setting and may not require use of an antipsychotic agent. Interictal psychosis is less common and typically requires use of an antipsychotic. All antipsychotic medications can lower seizure threshold. Clozapine should be avoided because of the high risk of seizures.

Key Points

- Psychiatric symptoms are common in neurological disorders affecting the brain. These symptoms contribute greatly to patient suffering and disability.
- Depression, pseudobulbar affect, apathy, and fatigue are all common in neurological disorders and frequently co-occur.
- Pharmacotherapy, behavioral interventions, and education can have a positive impact on symptom burden.
- While suicidality can occur with depression in the setting of any neurological illness, patients with Huntington's disease or traumatic brain injury have an especially high risk of suicide.
- Psychosis affects 40% of patients with Parkinson's disease and is typically due to medications used to manage motor symptoms. First-line management is to reduce or eliminate offending medications.
- Antipsychotic medication should be used only when absolutely necessary. This is especially true for traumatic brain injury patients, as research suggests that D_2 blockade interferes with brain recovery.

Disclosures

Dr. Whyte receives grant support from the USPHS NICHD/NCMRR (R01 067710) and NIMH (5U01MH062565). Study medication has been provided for the later study by Eli Lilly Company and Pfizer Pharmaceutical Inc.

Further Reading

De Groot MH, Phillips SJ, et al. (2003). Fatigue associated with stroke and other neurologic conditions: Implications for stroke rehabilitation. *Arch Phys Med Rehabil.*, *84*(11), 1714–1720.

Draper K, Ponsford J, et al. (2007). Psychosocial and emotional outcomes 10 years following traumatic brain injury. *J Head Trauma Rehabil.*, *22*(5), 278–287.

Gallego L, Barreiro P, et al. (2011). Diagnosis and clinical features of major neuropsychiatric disorders in HIV infection. *AIDS Rev.*, *13*(3), 171–179.

Hackett ML, Köhler S, et al. (2014). Neuropsychiatric outcomes of stroke. *Lancet Neurol.*, *13*(5), 525–534.

Haussleiter IS, Brüne M, et al. (2009). Psychopathology in multiple sclerosis: Diagnosis, prevalence and treatment. *Ther Adv Neurol Disord.*, *2*(1), 13–29.

Hubers AA, Reedeker N, et al. (2012). Suicidality in Huntington's disease. *J Affect Disord.*, *136*(3), 550–557.

Reekum R, Stuss DT, et al. (2005). Apathy: Why care? *J Neuropsychiat Clin Neurosci.*, *17*(1), 7–19.

Robert P, Onyike CU, et al. (2009). Proposed diagnostic criteria for apathy in Alzheimer's disease and other neuropsychiatric disorders. *Eur Psychiat.*, *24*(2), 98–104.

Schwarzbold M, Diaz A, et al. (2008). Psychiatric disorders and traumatic brain injury. *Neuropsychiatr Dis Treat.*, *4*(4), 797–816.

Simpson G, Tate R (2002). Suicidality after traumatic brain injury: Demographic, injury and clinical correlates. *Psychol Med.*, *32*(4), 87–97.

Tsaousides T, Cantor JB, et al (2011). Suicidal ideation following traumatic brain injury: Prevalence rates and correlates in adults living in the community. *J Head Trauma Rehabil.*, *26*(4), 265–275.

Whyte EM, Mulsant BH (2002). Post stroke depression: Epidemiology, pathophysiology, and biological treatment (Review). *Biol Psychiat.*, *52*(3), 253–264.

Exercises

1. Which of the following is true regarding neuropsychiatric complications of neurological disorders?
   a. These disorders are only responsive to medication interventions.
   b. Neuropsychiatric complications are highly specific to the underlying neurological disorder.
   c. The disorders of depression, apathy, and fatigue are distinct clinical syndromes.
   d. The presence of depression does not exacerbate disability.

2. In pseudobulbar affect, patients typically report low mood during episodes of crying.
   a. True
   b. False

3. Management options for chronic pathologic fatigue would include all of the following except:
   a. Education for the patient and family regarding fatigue as a consequence of neurologic illness.
   b. A recommendation to rest and to limit all physical activity in order to conserve energy.
   c. A trial of a stimulant, such as methylphenidate starting at 5–10 mg/d.
   d. Workup to identify other potential causes of fatigue.

4. In Parkinson's disease, strategies for treating hallucinations would include all except:
   a. Start quetiapine 12.5–25 mg po qd
   b. Assess for another medical illness inducing a delirium
   c. Reduce anticholinergic drugs
   d. Start risperidone 0.25–0.5 mg po qhs.

5. The following statements about suicidality in traumatic brain injury are true, except:
   a. Poor impulse control may be associated with a higher risk of suicide.
   b. The presence of suicidal thoughts decreases as the time since the injury increases.
   c. Men and women seem to have an equal risk of suicidality.

Answers: (1) c (2) b (3) b (4) d (5) b

Psychiatric Presentations Associated with Organ Failure and Systemic Illness

Pierre N. Azzam, Priya Gopalan, Abhishek Jain, Francis E. Lotrich, and Kevin R. Patterson

Introduction

The complex interplay between systemic or peripheral organ pathology and that of the brain lies at the heart of psychosomatic medicine. In the clinical setting, an appreciation for the breadth of psychiatric presentations associated with metabolic, end-organ, rheumatologic, endocrine, and infectious pathology prepares the psychiatrist to predict and identify that which is seen at the bedside. Attempts to understand the underpinnings of this brain-body connection drive the academic and research endeavors that guide qualified provision of patient care. This chapter will focus on various systemic diseases and end-organ dysfunction, and the relationship of each to affective, behavioral, and neurocognitive presentations.

Cardiovascular Disease

In this section, the following topics are reviewed:
- Cardiac contributions to psychiatric conditions
- Psychiatric contributions to cardiac disease
- Psychotropic medication use in the setting of cardiovascular disease.

Cardiac Contributions to Psychiatric Conditions

Coronary Artery Disease and Congestive Heart Failure

Coronary artery disease (CAD) is the most prevalent cardiac illness and accounts for one in six US deaths (Murphy et al., 2013); congestive heart failure (CHF) contributes to one in nine US deaths (Go et al., 2013). Among individuals with CAD, an estimated 15%–20% meet criteria for a depressive disorder, and 5%–10% for an anxiety disorder (Lichtman et al., 2008). Among individuals with CHF, an estimated 10%–60% meet criteria for a depressive disorder, and 11%–45% for an anxiety disorder (Yohannes et al., 2010); the wider range of estimates in CHF may be related to a broader array of CHF severity. Psychological stressors, such as facing mortality, caretaker dependence, and adapting to new routines, often contribute to low mood, fear, and anxiety. Decreased physical functioning may worsen psychiatric symptoms, such as poor sleep, energy, and concentration.

Effects of Cardiac Medications

Several medications that are commonly prescribed for cardiovascular disease have been implicated in precipitating or exacerbating psychiatric syndromes. For example, depression may be a side effect of alpha-blockers or methyldopa; ACE inhibitors may induce mood elevations; and digoxin toxicity may present with hallucinations. Though statins and beta-blockers were previously thought to cause depression, meta-analyses do not support direct causation; nevertheless, beta-blockers may contribute to fatigue in depressed patients (Young-Xu et al., 2003; Ko et al., 2002). From clinical experience, we do not recommend reflexive discontinuation or avoidance of necessary cardiovascular medications save for debilitating associated psychiatric symptoms.

Psychiatric Contributions to Cardiac Disease

Psychiatric Conditions Associated with Heart Disease

Patients with major depressive disorder, bipolar disorder, and schizophrenia generally have increased rates of CAD and myocardial infarction (MI) when compared to the general population. Depression has been consistently associated with at least a twofold increased mortality in both post-myocardial infarction (MI; Meijer et al., 2011) and CHF patients (Jiang et al., 2001). Data regarding associations between anxiety, CAD, and CAD-related mortality are mixed. Scientific evidence does suggest an elevated risk for fatal coronary heart disease and sudden cardiac death among patients with phobic anxiety (Albert et al., 2005), and that moderate use of anti-anxiety medications (e.g., benzodiazepines) following an MI is associated with decreased mortality and hospitalization (Wu et al., 2014).

Sedentary lifestyle, smoking, and medication non-adherence (Gehi et al., 2005) among patients with mental illness often contribute to increased heart disease. Psychological factors and personality traits, such as low frustration tolerance, may also predict coronary artery disease (Williams et al., 2013). Emotional stress has been well documented to trigger acute coronary events (Zupancic, 2009), whereas positive adaptive functioning may reduce the risk of chronic heart disease (Williams et al., 2013).

Potential Links Between Cardiac and Psychiatric Pathology

Among depressed patients, biological factors may mediate the relationship between psychiatric illness and heart disease; these include lower heart rate variability, greater platelet adhesion, higher cortisol levels, elevation of inflammatory cytokines (e.g., IL-1, IL-6, TNF-α), and activated hypothalamic-pituitary-adrenocortical and sympathetic adrenal medullary systems (Pozuelo et al., 2009). Metabolic factors, such as obesity, diabetes, and hypertension, are highly prevalent in patients with serious and persisting mental illness, particularly schizophrenia; this may be exacerbated by antipsychotic medication use.

Emerging research has identified mechanisms that may be linked independently to both heart disease and psychiatric illness. For example, an increased risk for comorbid depression and myocardial infarction may be associated with variations in the serotonin transport promoter region gene (5-HTTLPR). Previously, panic disorder and mitral valve prolapse were thought to have a bidirectional association; recent studies suggest the cluster of mitral valve prolapse, interstitial cystitis, migraines, thyroid disease, and panic disorder may have a common linkage through chromosome 13 (Talati et al., 2007).

Psychotropic Medication Use in the Setting of Cardiovascular Disease

Increased collaboration among cardiologists and mental health providers has become critical in improving cardiac and psychiatric outcomes. The American Heart Association has published screening and treatment recommendations for patients with depression and heart disease (Lichtman et al., 2008). For example, a positive response on one item of the Patient Health Questionnaire (PHQ-2) has up to 90% sensitivity in screening for depression in the medically ill (Kroenke et al., 2003; Pozuelo et al., 2009), and should prompt further evaluation. Studies have demonstrated that SSRIs, particularly sertraline, are safe after myocardial infarction and are effective in treating associated depression (Glassman et al., 2002). Non-pharmacologic interventions, such as cognitive behavioral therapy and cardiac rehabilitation, can be invaluable in improving depression and cardiac outcomes. Despite strong associations between depression and poor cardiac outcomes, and between depression recovery and improved cardiac outcomes, to date studies have not definitively shown that treating depression directly improves cardiac outcomes. However, studies and clinical experience do suggest that treating depression in cardiac patients improves quality of life and medication adherence (Rieckmann et al., 2006).

Cardiac complications may develop with psychotropic medication use through various mechanisms (see Chapter 6):

- **Direct cardiac effects of the medication** (e.g., tricyclic antidepressants have a quinidine-like effect and may cause ventricular arrhythmias, cardiac conduction delays, and prolonged QRS and QT intervals)
- **Side effects** (e.g., increased blood pressure with venlafaxine or bupropion)
- **Drug-drug interactions** (e.g., fluoxetine raises serum beta-blocker levels via cytochrome 2D6 metabolism).

Of potential direct cardiac effects of psychotropic medications, prolongation of the corrected QT interval (QTc) on EKG and Torsade de Pointes (TdP) represents a growing concern, particularly with antipsychotic medications. Owing to the relatively low incidence of drug-induced TdP and the inherent challenges associated with studying cases of transient dysrhythmia, most research has focused on QTc prolongation as a marker for TdP risk. Among antipsychotic medications, aripiprazole has consistently demonstrated the lowest tendency to prolong the QTc interval, whereas high-dose or parenteral administrations of thioridazine and haloperidol have been more strongly implicated in QT prolongation, and rarely in cases of dysrhythmia. Other atypical antipsychotics, particularly ziprasidone and quetiapine, have been implicated in QT-prolongation; nevertheless, their potential to unilaterally induce cardiac dysrhythmia appears to be low. In a recent review of 61 publications, including 18 clinical trials, the balance of evidence suggests that antidepressants, particularly SSRIs, are generally safe in cardiac patients (Mavrides & Nemeroff, 2013). Among SSRIs, the US Food and Drug Administration (FDA) issued a warning in 2011 for citalopram, citing a dose-dependent association with prolonged QTc; in May 2012 the FDA revised the recommendations, including a maximum dose of 20 mg daily for patients older than 60 years of age or with cardiac disease.

Overall, important clinical considerations regarding the risk of QTc prolongation and TdP with psychotropic medications include:

- **Reviewing medical, cardiac, and family histories** (e.g., for history of congenital long QT syndrome, familial history of sudden cardiac death)
- **Reviewing recent medication use** (e.g., for medications that may prolong QT or inhibit metabolism of QT-prolonging agents)
- **Checking and correcting electrolytes** (e.g., hypomagnesemia, hypokalemia)
- **Obtaining baseline and serial EKGs, when indicated** (e.g., patients with high cardiac risk, who are routinely taking QT prolonging agents)
- **Obtaining informed consent from patients and/or families** (i.e., with review of cardiac risk).

A helpful online resource for QTc-prolonging medications is through the Arizona Center for Education and Research on Therapeutics (www.crediblemeds.org).

Pulmonary Disease

In this section, the following topics are reviewed:
- Pulmonary contributions to psychiatric conditions
- Psychiatric contributions to pulmonary disease
- Psychotropic medication use in the setting of pulmonary disease.

Pulmonary Contributions to Psychiatric Conditions

Chronic Obstructive Pulmonary Disease

Among patients with chronic COPD, the prevalence of depression has ranged from 10% to 71%, depending on the screening instrument, sampling method, and breathing impairment (Jain & Lolak, 2009). Generalized anxiety disorder has been estimated to be up to five times as common among COPD patients as compared to the general population (Brenes, 2003), with a prevalence range of 6%–33% (Willgoss & Yohannes, 2013). The prevalence of panic disorder among patients with severe COPD can be as high as 44% (Potoczek et al., 2008).

Asthma, Interstitial Lung Disease, Cystic Fibrosis

Varying rates of depression and anxiety have been reported in asthma patients; these have typically been at least double that of the general population (Lavoie et al., 2006), with anxiety correlating most strongly to asthma (Roy-Byrne et al., 2008). Among patients with interstitial lung disease (ILD; e.g., idiopathic pulmonary fibrosis), limited data are available to describe the nature of psychiatric presentations, though lower quality of life and impaired functioning associated with ILD mirror the impact of COPD (Tomioka et al., 2007). About 30,000 Americans have cystic fibrosis (CFF, 2010) with patients and parents both at increased risk for depression and anxiety (Tluczek et al., 2013).

Psychiatric Contributions to Pulmonary Disease

Psychiatric and respiratory symptoms share a complex bidirectional relationship. Depression, anxiety, low motivation, low energy, and hopelessness may contribute to poor treatment adherence and poor respiratory outcomes. Respiratory symptoms may also worsen psychiatric symptoms, such as shortness of breath leading to panic, fear, and distress, and decreased physical functioning leading to poorer quality of life. More subtle mechanisms, such as chronic hypoxemia leading to disruptions in neurotransmitter synthesis and poor oxygenation in vulnerable brain regions, may also contribute to depression and anxiety (Norwood, 2006). Medications that are used to treat respiratory conditions, such as albuterol, prednisone, and theophylline, may contribute to symptoms of mood, anxiety, psychosis, and impaired cognition. Physiological changes, such as increased inflammatory markers interleukin (IL)-4, IL-5, and interferon-gamma (IFN-γ) in asthma patients have also been identified, but with unclear clinical significance.

Psychotropic Medication Use in the Setting of Pulmonary Disease

Practical considerations for patients with primary psychiatric conditions, especially those who smoke, include promoting routine primary care and monitoring of respiratory symptoms. Among patients with primary respiratory conditions, routine screening for anxiety and depression can prove useful. For example, the PHQ-9 can help in detecting a depressive disorder with a score of 5 or more (sensitivity 100%; specificity 72%) (Lamers et al., 2008).

In the management of depression and anxiety, SSRI agents such as sertraline and paroxetine are generally well tolerated and provide symptomatic relief, often within weeks. Buspirone can help as a non-benzodiazepine alternative for anxiety treatment, and is generally well tolerated; however, similar to SSRIs, it may take weeks for effectiveness, and study results have been mixed regarding its efficacy (Putman-Casdorph & McCrone, 2009). Bupropion was shown to improve depression symptoms in asthma patients who did not respond to SSRI therapy with citalopram (Brown et al., 2007), and may assist with smoking cessation. Tricyclic antidepressants can reduce symptoms of anxiety, depression, and pain; at the same time, cardiac side effects, such as ventricular arrhythmias and conduction delays, must be considered before use (Putnam-Casdorph & McCrone, 2009).

Benzodiazepines are frequently prescribed for patients with respiratory conditions such as COPD; 31.7% of elderly COPD patients received a new benzodiazepine in the prior year in one Ontario-based study (Vozoris et al., 2013). At the same time, caution must be used due to the potential for respiratory depression, especially in high doses or in combination with medications such as opiates. Benzodiazepines are best prescribed on a short-term basis only, particularly with comorbid respiratory disease.

Non-pharmacologic treatments of anxiety include cognitive behavioral therapy (CBT), pulmonary rehabilitation, progressive muscle relaxation, and biofeedback. Although studies show mixed results in respiratory patients—ranging from improvement in both psychiatric and physical symptoms to no improvement in either—non-pharmacologic interventions possess several advantages: they may be cost-effective, have no pharmacological side effects, present an opportunity for collaboration between mental health providers and pulmonary teams, and can serve as an adjunctive treatment during medication titration.

Renal Disease

In this section, the following topics are reviewed:
- Renal contributions to psychiatric conditions
- Psychiatric contributions to renal disease
- Psychotropic medication use in the setting of renal impairment.

Renal Contributions to Psychiatric Conditions

Uremia and Dialysis-Related Encephalopathy

Renal injury and uremia can induce various neuropsychiatric conditions, often based on the severity of kidney impairment, as shown in Table 13.1.

Serum labs typically reveal elevations in BUN and creatinine, along with electrolyte disturbances such as hyponatremia and hyperkalemia. While head imaging may be undertaken to evaluate for other potential contributors to encephalopathy, it rarely confirms uremic contributions to delirium. Uremia-related encephalopathy is frequently associated with generalized slowing on EEG, with triphasic wave patterns in some cases. Encephalopathy may complicate the period during and shortly after dialysis (typically hours), likely related to rapid osmolar and electrolyte shifts and neuronal swelling. This syndrome may be prevented by slowing the course of dialysis and monitoring electrolyte shifts.

Sodium Regulation: Hyponatremia and Hypernatremia

Clinically significant decline in serum sodium (normal range: 135–145 mEq/L), or rapid shifts in plasma sodium levels, can precipitate various neuropsychiatric and physical changes, as shown in Table 13.2.

Medical complications of hyponatremia are typically driven by the severity and speed of decline in serum sodium. Seizures, coma, and death are severe complications associated with extremes of hyponatremia (e.g., Na < 120 mEq/L) or sudden osmolar shifts.

Hyponatremia can be precipitated by a number of conditions (e.g., burns, gastrointestinal fluid losses); the consultation psychiatrist is most frequently presented with questions around two conditions: the syndrome of

Table 13.1 Neuropsychiatric Presentations of Mild, Moderate, and Severe Uremia

Mild	Moderate	Severe (typically, limited to GFR < 30 mL/min)
Fatigue	Lethargy	Coma
Poor concentration	Encephalopathy	Myoclonic jerks, hiccups
Mild cognitive changes	Sleep/mood disturbances	Seizures
		Peripheral neuropathy, cramps

Adapted from Harrison & Kopelman (2009).

Table 13.2 Clinical Features of Hyponatremia

Mild-Moderate	Severe
Fatigue	Delirium
Poor food intake, nausea	Seizures
Headache, blurred vision	Coma
Insomnia	Death

inappropriate antidiuretic hormone (SIADH), discussed below, and primary polydipsia, discussed in the following subsection "Psychiatric Contributions to Renal Disease." Excessive ADH release from the posterior pituitary may be precipitated by a multitude of conditions (see Table 13.3).

Management of hyponatremia involves slow, steady correction of sodium; with SIADH, this is most frequently achieved by fluid restriction.

Table 13.3 Causes and Risk Factors for the Syndrome of Inappropriate Antidiuretic Hormone

Causes of SIADH	
Medical Conditions	Head injury
	Hypothyroidism
	Intracranial hemorrhage
	Lung cancer (particularly, small-cell variants)
	Pneumonia
	Stroke
Medications	Selective serotonin reuptake inhibitors (SSRIs)
	Serotonin norepinephrine reuptake inhibitors (SNRIs)
	Antipsychotic medications
	Anticonvulsant medications (e.g., carbamazepine, oxcarbazepine)

Risk Factors for Iatrogenic Development of SIADH	
	Advanced age
	Female sex
	Prior episodes of hyponatremia
	Concurrent illness of the respiratory or central nervous system
	Smoking

Less frequently utilized, administration of intravenous saline or medications that interfere with action or binding of ADH (e.g., demeclocycline, conivaptan) must be undertaken carefully, not to exceed correction of sodium by greater than 10 mmol/L in 24 hours. For more detail about psychotropic medication-induced hyponatremia, please refer to the following subsection, "Psychiatric Contributions to Renal Disease."

As with hyponatremia, elevations in serum sodium are most often symptomatic when they occur abruptly or severely (e.g., Na > 155 mEq/L). Neuropsychiatric symptoms of hypernatremia are included in Table 13.4.

Hypernatremia may result from excessive sodium intake (e.g., excess hypertonic saline hydration) or dehydration without compensatory water intake. Hypernatremia may also occur in the context of pathologic processes that interfere with ADH production, release, or effect at the kidneys. Long-term use of lithium, for example, can decrease sensitivity of the renal collecting ducts to the activity of ADH, thereby precipitating nephrogenic diabetes insipidus (DI). Correction of hypernatremia typically hinges on treating the precipitating pathology and the slow, steady reduction of sodium with IV hydration, at no greater than 10 mmol/L per day. Nephrogenic DI may be treated with thiazide diuretics; if the decision is made to continue lithium use, the addition of a thiazide will often require a reduction in lithium dosing to compensate for the diuretic's interference with lithium clearance. Central DI may prompt administration of synthetic ADH, in the form of desmopressin (DDAVP).

Psychiatric Complications of Chronic Kidney Disease and Dialysis Requirement

As with other potentially debilitating conditions, chronic kidney disease—particularly when dialysis is necessary—is commonly complicated by depression and anxiety. The process of hemodialysis, itself, may trigger significant anxiety with recurrent hospital visits, phlebotomy, and rapid electrolyte changes that can induce physical discomfort. Existential fears over the reliance of technology to maintain vitality may manifest with helplessness. In this context, dialysis-dependent patients may question their desire to continue this degree of care, and therefore struggle with adherence. Clinicians must

Table 13.4 Neuropsychiatric Symptoms of Hypernatremia

Mild-Moderate	Severe
Acute confusion	Seizures
Somnolence	Coma
Myalgia	Death
Myoclonus	

weigh these considerations when assessing medical decision-making capacity for patients with kidney disease who request to terminate treatment. Maximizing quality of life, facilitating future planning, and promoting an individual's sense of control prove to be vital in this process.

Psychiatric Contributions to Renal Disease

Psychotropic Medication-Induced Hyponatremia

The relation of psychotropic medications to sodium abnormalities is often independent of dose or treatment duration. Complicating matters further, many medications that are associated with sodium dysregulation are used to treat serious and persisting mental illnesses. The consultation psychiatrist is often at the forefront of the decision to continue or to withhold an often-necessary and long-standing medication.

Of psychotropic medications, SSRIs are among the most heavily studied contributors to hyponatremia by SIADH, though precise epidemiology of this complication is unclear. Advanced age is a particularly notable risk factor; 10%–25% of patients over the age of 65 experience some degree of hyponatremia after starting an SSRI, often within two weeks of initiation (Jacob & Spinler, 2006), and the condition is believed to be dose-independent. Detection hinges on obtaining a serum sodium level before starting a potentially offending agent and repeating in the first weeks of use. SIADH can be diagnosed by comparing osmolality and sodium concentrations in the serum and urine; typically, with SIADH, urine osmolality (U_{osm} > 100 mOsm/kg) and sodium (U_{Na} > 40 mEq/L) are elevated in spite of low serum sodium and osmolality (P_{osm} < 275 mOsm/kg). The concurrent presence of polydipsia or other conditions that interfere with free water or sodium excretion may complicate the definitive diagnosis of SIADH based on lab studies.

Management

- When patients develop hyponatremia during psychiatric medication use, providers should pursue further medical workup to clarify the underlying mechanism. If SIADH is suspected, the provider should engage the patient in a risk-benefit discussion of medication continuation versus cessation.
- If a potentially offending psychotropic agent is discontinued, an alternate medication with lower risk for SIADH should be considered (e.g., mirtazapine, bupropion for depression).
- If a potentially offending psychotropic agent is continued, the following steps are prudent: frequent monitoring of serum sodium (e.g., weekly in the first month and monthly for the next three months), ongoing education of the warning signs/symptoms and risks of hyponatremia, and guidance for fluid restriction, when appropriate.

Primary Polydipsia

Primary polydipsia, pathologic excess in fluid consumption, impacts 6%–20% of individuals with psychiatric conditions, most notably psychotic disorders (Dundas, 2007). Hyponatremia is commonly observed, and is typically marked by low urine and serum osmolality. The etiology of primary polydipsia is likely multifactorial, including changes to central thirst regulation or the hypothalamic-pituitary response to osmoreceptors, and is exacerbated by medications that cause dry mouth. Treatment includes avoidance of anticholinergic agents and careful fluid restriction. As with correction of hyponatremia of other etiologies, care must be taken to avoid sudden elevations in serum sodium for individuals with long-standing polydipsia.

Psychotropic Medication Use in the Setting of Renal Impairment

In general, psychiatric medications are extensively metabolized through the liver; as such, few adjustments are required for mild to moderate renal disease. In severe or end-stage kidney disease, direct effects of impaired medication and metabolite excretion are complicated by other pharmacokinetic factors, such as shifts in protein binding from circulating urea and gastric alkalization. Common considerations for psychiatric medication use in kidney impairments are as follows (see Chapter 6 for details):

- As a class, SSRIs are not affected significantly by kidney disease, and dose adjustment is often not required. In cases of moderate-severe renal impairment, clearance of mirtazapine and venlafaxine may be reduced by 30%–50%, and duloxetine is not recommended for use in individuals with creatinine clearance under 30 mL/min.
- Of the antipsychotic medications, few require dose adjustment in renal impairment. First-generation antipsychotics are generally used without significant adjustment. Metabolites of risperidone are excreted renally, and slow titration of dosing is recommended when this agent is used in moderate-severe renal disease. Likewise, paliperidone is not recommended for severe renal impairments, and mild-moderate kidney disease typically requires dose reduction by 50%–75%.
- Various anticonvulsant medications require dose adjustment based on renal function, including gabapentin (25%–75% reduction based on creatinine clearance), oxcarbazepine (50% reduction in severe renal impairment), and topiramate (50% reduction in mid-moderate renal impairment, avoidance in severe cases).
- Lithium use may result in renal impairment from acute toxicity or chronic exposure. In addition to excessive lithium intake, acute toxicity may be precipitated by impaired lithium clearance from the renal tubules, specifically by concurrent medication use (e.g., thiazides, non-steroidal anti-inflammatory medications). Potential effects include hyponatremia and acute renal failure, in severe cases requiring emergent hemodialysis (e.g., serum lithium level > 4.0 mEq/L). Chronic, high-dose lithium use may precipitate nephrogenic diabetes insipidus (DI), resulting in polyuria and requiring close scrutiny of the risk-benefit ratio of continuing or suspending lithium use. In cases for which mood stability is reliant on lithium, amiloride may be used to correct the effects of lithium on vasopressin.

Hepatic Disease

In this section, the following topics are reviewed:
- Hepatic contributions to psychiatric conditions
- Hepatotoxicity related to psychiatric medications
- Special topic: Psychiatric clearance for interferon-alpha (IFN-α) therapy.

Hepatic Contributions to Psychiatric Conditions

Hepatic Encephalopathy

In the context of liver failure, hepatic encephalopathy (HE) may induce symptoms ranging from mild behavioral dysregulation to confusion, somnolence, and coma; these may be mediated by the toxic effects of ammonia (NH3) to astrocytes and resultant cerebral edema. Serum NH3 is often used as a marker for the severity of HE. However, the association between hyperammonemia and severity of neuropsychiatric effects is less clearly correlated. Regardless, the diagnosis of HE is based principally on clinical findings. Physical examination may reveal tremor, asterixis, and jaundice. Brain MRI may show T1 hyperintensities in the basal ganglia, and EEG may reveal generalized slowing with triphasic morphology; these too are not unilaterally diagnostic of HE.

In addition to the effects of ammonia, hepatic encephalopathy has been linked to endogenous benzodiazepine and neurosteroid production. SPECT has revealed decreased regional blood flow in the fronto-temporal areas of the brain, as well as the basal ganglia in individuals with HE. Treatment of HE includes supportive care; treatment of the underlying cause of HE, when possible; reduction of serum ammonia levels with lactulose; and empiric antibiotics.

Wilson's Disease (Hepatolenticular Degeneration)

Wilson's disease is a genetic disorder with autosomal recessive inheritance that typically presents in the second or third decade of life, with a prevalence of approximately 1:25,000. The Chromosome 13 mutation results in altered coding of the ceruloplasmin protein, which is responsible for copper transport, metabolism, and excretion. The result is excess copper deposition in various organs, including the liver and brain, with predilection for the basal ganglia. Associated clinical features include those listed in Table 13.5.

Management of Wilson's disease includes the administration of copper chelating agents, such as zinc, penicillamine, and tetrathiomolybdate; this is principally in an effort to minimize liver damage. Unfortunately, even when chelation is undertaken successfully, the complications associated with established intracranial copper deposition tend to reverse minimally, if at all. As such, early diagnosis is critical. Management of psychiatric features is typically symptom-based, with little evidence to guide unique treatment considerations.

Pharmacologic Considerations in Hepatic Disease

Though the incidence of liver toxicity from psychiatric medications is lower than 0.1%, certain circumstances require selection of medications

Table 13.5 Neuropsychiatric Features Associated with Wilson's Disease

Personality chang es
Mood disturbances
Impulsivity and disinhibition
Psychosis
Tremor
Asterixis
Dystonia

with lower tendency for hepatotoxicity. A guiding principle is to opt for less hepatotoxic medications when possible in patients with liver disease, while remembering that even somewhat hepatotoxic medications can be used safely, when necessary.

Most antidepressants have minimal evidence for hepatotoxicity, though some may cause elevations in hepatic enzymes:

- With exceptions noted below, **SSRIs** and **SNRIs** are associated with very low incidence (i.e., < 0.5%) of hepatic enzyme elevation.
- **Fluoxetine** and **sertraline** are associated with an approximately 0.5% and 0.8% incidence, respectively, of minor liver enzyme elevations.
- **Duloxetine** has been associated with tripling the rate of enzyme elevations with long-term use, and liver damage has been reported in 2:100,000 case exposures.
- Liver damage related to **TCAs** and **MAOIs** is greater than that seen in newer antidepressants.
- In clinical trials, under 1% of subjects developed an adverse hepatic event while taking **atomoxetine**, with none developing liver failure.
- Whereas only six cases of chronic liver damage have been described in patients taking **trazodone**, **nefazodone** carries an FDA black box warning for hepatotoxicity risk; literature suggests this is three to four times greater than that of other antidepressants.

Antipsychotic medications are more strongly associated with potential for hepatotoxicity:

- **Phenothiazines** increase liver enzymes in approximately 20% of patients, though the incidence of overt hepatotoxicity is lower than 1%.
- Half of patients receiving **haloperidol** develop minor enzyme elevations; about 17% experience a twofold elevation; 2.4%, a threefold elevation.
- **Clozapine** similarly causes hepatic enzyme elevations in 30%–50% of patients, though fulminant hepatitis only occurs in 1:100,000.
- **Risperidone** may be associated with mild transient enzyme elevation in up to half of cases.

- **Olanzapine** is associated with transient enzyme elevations in about 9% of cases.
- **Quetiapine** has only sporadically been associated with liver damage.
- **Ziprasodone, paliperidone,** and **aripiprazole** have limited evidence for hepatoxicity.

Of anti-epileptic agents with mood stabilizing properties, **carbamazepine** and **valproate** are well known for associated liver damage and should be avoided in patients with underlying hepatic disease, or those who are taking other hepatotoxic medications. Typically, this is independent of dose and serum level and can be reversed by stopping the medication. **Lamotrigine** is associated with hepatic inflammation in approximately 0.1% of cases, and can occasionally cause liver failure.

In treating drug and alcohol use disorders, approximately 25% of patients develop elevated hepatic enzymes during the first few months of **disulfiram** treatment. Significant liver injury is rare, and often the effects of chronic alcohol use cannot be differentiated from those of the medication itself. **Naltrexone** carries an FDA black box warning for hepatotoxicity, particularly when used at high doses. Reports of **methadone**- and **buprenorphine**-induced hepatitis are uncommon.

Special Topic: Psychiatric Clearance for Interferon-alpha Therapy

Interferon-alpha (IFN-α) is an immune modulator used to treat chronic hepatitis C viral (HCV) infection, typically for a course of 24–48 weeks. In its influence on neuronal function, IFN-α can precipitate depression, anger, and fatigue that may lead to treatment discontinuation and, in severe cases, suicide. HCV-infected individuals may have a pre-existing unrecognized psychiatric illness; current recommendations therefore dictate that all patients with HCV should be screened for psychiatric conditions before starting IFN-α.

If basic screening raises suspicion for a psychiatric condition, then further assessment (a "psychiatric clearance") is indicated. This process often includes the steps described in Table 13.6.

Management of Psychiatric Conditions Associated with Interferon Treatment

- **Depression** may present in 15%–40% of patients during treatment with IFN-α and is often managed effectively with SSRIs. Ensuring appropriate management of any pre-existing depressive disorder is particularly prudent.
- **Fatigue** is less responsive to antidepressants, and case reports support use of exercise or, in some scenarios, a psychostimulant or modafinil for apathy syndromes.
- **Insomnia** may respond well to cognitive behavioral therapies that target sleep hygiene. When necessary, sedating antidepressants such as mirtazapine and trazodone may be effective, though trazodone has rarely been associated with liver toxicity.
- **Mania** less frequently complicates IFN-α use. Regardless of the indication, it is most prudent to avoid potentially hepatotoxic medications.
- **Alcohol use**, which may affect depression risk, treatment efficacy, and adherence, should be strongly discouraged.

Table 13.6 Psychiatric Evaluation Associated with "Clearance" for Interferon-alpha Use

Assessment of psychiatric follow-up and symptom stability

Survey of available psychosocial supports and barriers to adherence

Consideration of risks-benefits for prophylactically treating subsyndromal features of depression

Education about potential psychiatric symptoms and associated treatments

Establishment of regular mental health monitoring

Anticipation of potential medication interactions

Laying groundwork for regular communication with the hepatologist

Human Immunodeficiency Virus Infection

In this section, the following topics are reviewed:
- Contributions of HIV to psychiatric conditions
- Pharmacologic considerations in HIV
- Special topic: Substance use and HIV.

Contributions of HIV to Psychiatric Conditions

In the recent past, HIV (human immunodeficiency virus) infection and acquired immune deficiency syndrome (AIDS) represented the leading killers of people aged 18–45 in the United States; they continue to hold this distinction in Africa. Today, as a result of increasingly effective medications, HIV infection is often experienced as a chronic condition rather than an acute threat, presenting similar challenges to other longitudinal, multisystem illnesses.

Approximately half of HIV-seropositive adults experience a diagnosable psychiatric condition (Bing et al., 2001), and may be most vulnerable to adjustment, mood, and anxiety disorders at particular stages of the disease process: diagnosis, progress of physical symptoms, start of antiretroviral therapy, and first AIDS-defining condition. Adults with HIV may ruminate about external perceptions of being diseased or dangerous, or become suspicious of others' abilities to detect HIV status. These anxieties are often manageable with psychosocial and educational interventions. Comorbid psychiatric conditions and substance use (often dubbed "dual diagnosis") are so prevalent in the HIV+ population (see Table 13.7) that the term "triple diagnosis" has become popularized (Samet et al., 2004).

HIV is also associated with direct neuropsychiatric effects. Marked by confusion, impaired balance and movement, and psychotic experiences, HIV encephalopathy may present at any stage of infection, but is most prevalent in periods of high viral load. Late in the course of infection, HIV may be associated with mild or major neurocognitive disorders. Dementia affects 18%–30% of otherwise asymptomatic adults with HIV-1 infection in the United States and Europe, and presents with chronic, insidious decline in cognition (Heaton et al., 2004). Infectious

Table 13.7 Rates of Psychiatric Diagnosis in HIV+ Individuals

Anxiety Disorders	25%–36%	Jayarajan & Chandra, 2010
Depressive Disorders	20%–30%	Bing et al., 2001
Severe Mental Illness	1%–24%	DeHert et al., 2011
Substance Use Disorder	32%	Whetten et al., 2005

CNS lesions (e.g., cryptococcal meningitis) may result in a variety of clinical presentations, often based on the lesion site.

Pharmacologic Considerations in HIV

Psychiatric Complications of HIV Treatment

Treatments for HIV can induce neurovegetative symptoms, in addition to having direct effects on mood and motivation. In particular, agents of highly active antiretroviral therapy (HAART) protocols are known to have the psychiatric side effects, as outlined in Table 13.8.

In considering the impact of HAART on major depression, evidence is conflicting; the medications themselves may induce neurovegetative symptoms, whereas the associated decrease in viral load may result in offsetting improvements (Turjanski & Lloyd, 2005). Current guidelines encourage treatment for depression before implementing HAART, so as to improve adherence to HIV management; at the same time, HIV management should not be delayed in patients who choose not to engage in mental health care.

Psychiatric distress should be treated symptomatically, considering patient function and HAART adherence, even when diagnostic criteria for mood and anxiety disorders are not met strictly. Psychiatric consultants can play a key role in identifying the link between cognitive and

Table 13.8 Adverse Psychiatric Effects Associated with Antiretroviral Medications

Protease Inhibitors	
Amprenavir	Mood changes
Indinavir	Mood changes
Lopinavir	Agitation, anxiety
Ritonavir	Anxiety
Nucleoside Reverse Transcriptase Inhibitors	
Didanosine	Lethargy, anxiety, sleep disturbance, mood disorder, psychosis
Lamivudine	Insomnia, mood disorder
Zalcitabine	Somnolence, mood disorder, delirium
Zidovudine	Sleep disturbance, agitation, mania and depression, psychotic symptoms, delirium
Non-Nucleoside Reverse Transcriptase Inhibitors	
Efavirenz	Agitation, depersonalization, hallucination, psychosis, catatonia, delirium

mood symptoms, decreased motivation, adherence to HAART protocols, and viral load. Minimizing this cycle can have a profound impact on
both the medical course and the patient's mental health.

Considerations for Psychiatric and HIV-Related Pharmacotherapies

Concerns about medication-based treatments in patients with HIV
include increased sensitivity to psychotropic medications, impaired
liver function as a result of comorbidities (e.g., HCV co-infection) and
HAART therapies, and drug-drug interactions. Most psychotropic
medications can be tolerated fairly well and do not impede HIV management. Nonetheless, given the complex nature of HIV protocols and
psychopharmacologic treatments, we recommend checking for medication interactions utilizing an electronic medication interaction database.
Optimizing the use of as few medications as possible—particularly when
multiple benefits can be obtained from one agent (e.g., mirtazapine
for depression and sleep)—is prudent. Table 13.9 summarizes several
nuances of psychiatric treatment in this setting.

Special Topic: Substance Use and HIV

Habitual substance use can pose serious barriers to the management
of HIV. Blank and Eisenberg (2013) found that alcohol use was a factor
in predicting non-adherence to HIV treatments. In addition to impact-
ing viral load, substance use may compete with general pursuits of
health: from missed HAART doses to a decreased perception of the benefits of treatment. Finally, substance use may alter end-organ function,
causing changes to absorption and metabolism of HAART medications,
and potentiating drug interactions and side effects.

Delay of HAART implementation until full recovery from substance
use was once advocated to prevent resistance to treatment, both for
the patient's sake and for public health. A harm-reduction model provides a pragmatic alternative; while full recovery from addiction certainly
improves HIV treatment outcomes, partial reduction in substance use is
also correlated with improved medication adherence. Medication-based
treatments for substance use disorders (e.g., methadone maintenance
therapy) tend to be as successful as behavioral approaches, and with
either option, ongoing intervention is prudent for sustained compliance.

Table 13.9 Psychiatric Treatment Consideration for Individuals with HIV

Medication Class	Preferred Agents	Cautions and Considerations
Antidepressants	Citalopram Mirtazapine Venlafaxine	• Fluoxetine and fluvoxamine may increase HAART drug levels • TCAs can have many useful side effects, but should be avoided with ritonavir
Antipsychotics	Olanzapine Risperidone	• Risk for neutropenia with clozapine warrants cautious use • Atypical agents preferred due to increased sensitivity to extrapyramidal effects
Anxiolytics	Clonazepam	• Short-acting benzodiazepines may carry fewer drug-drug interactions but higher likelihood for abuse.
Mood Stabilizers	Olanzapine Risperidone Valproate Lamotrigine Lithium (monitor levels closely)	• Anticonvulsants may influence levels of HAART agents • Avoid carbamazepine due to bone marrow suppression

Endocrine and Metabolic Diseases

In this section, psychiatric manifestations of the following conditions are reviewed:
- Diabetes mellitus
- Thyroid disease
- Hypercortisolemia
- Pheochromocytoma.

Diabetes Mellitus

Diabetes mellitus is the most commonly diagnosed endocrine condition and is complicated by depression in 14%–32% of cases. For the consulting psychiatrist, management of depression becomes imperative, as untreated depression may lead to poor adherence with insulin regimens and may interfere with adequate blood glucose control. Functional impairments related to chronic illness and reduction in quality of life may exacerbate depression. Mechanisms of depression related to inflammatory processes from the chronic illness require further study.

Psychotropic medications are associated with metabolic risks in patients with pre-existing or newly acquired diabetes. Second-generation antipsychotics (SGAs) are highly associated with the development of diabetes and warrant risk-benefit discussion with patients in advance of a medication trial, in addition to frequent monitoring of glucose, body mass index, and lipids. Alternate agents must be considered for patients who are already at risk for diabetes. Recent studies suggest a reduction in the development of diabetes with use of metformin alongside an SGA. The consulting psychiatrist may opt to discuss this option with the patient's primary physician in advance of starting an SGA.

Thyroid Disease

Dysfunction in the hypothalamic-pituitary-thyroid system can lead to hypothyroidism (elevated TSH, low T3 and T4) or hyperthyroidism (low TSH, high T3 and T4). Psychiatric symptoms can herald both conditions; an awareness of the common presentations associated with each is critical for the psychiatric consultant (see Table 13.10).

Treatment of thyroid dysfunction should help to ameliorate psychiatric symptoms, though effects may be delayed. Symptomatic management with SSRIs, antipsychotics, and benzodiazepines is recommended in the interim.

Hypercortisolemia

Cushing's syndrome is a state of hypercortisolemia caused by endogenous or iatrogenic processes. The most common precipitant is excessive intake of oral corticosteroids; other causes include disruptions to the hypothalamic-pituitary-adrenal (HPA) axis (e.g., pituitary adenoma), ACTH-secreting tumors, or excess release of corticotropin-releasing hormone (CRH) by a neuroendocrine tumor. Patients with hypercortisolemia may present with distinct physical features and an array of psychiatric ones, as listed in Table 13.11.

Table 13.10 Clinical Signs and Symptoms Associated with Thyroid Disease

Clinical Features of Hypothyroidism	
Causes	Hashimoto's thyroiditis
	Iron deficiency
	Postpartum/Postoperative thyroiditis
	Iatrogenic hypothyroidism
Physical Indicators	Cold intolerance
	Alopecia, Dry skin
	Non-pitting edema (myxedema)
	Delayed deep tendon reflexes
	Goiter (may also be present in hyperthyroidism)
Possible Psychiatric Complications	Fatigue
	Depression
	Psychosis
	Cognitive effects
Clinical Features of Hyperthyroidism	
Causes	Grave's disease
	Thyrotoxicosis
	Toxic multinodular goiter
	Thyroid nodules
	Iatrogenic hyperthyroidism
Physical Indicators	Heat intolerance
	Heart palpitations
	Warm, moist skin
	Diarrhea, polyuria
	Tremor, muscle weakness
	Goiter (may also present in hypothyroidism)
Possible Psychiatric Complications	Generalized anxiety, panic (classically)
	Apathy, cognitive disturbances
	Mania
	Psychosis

Table 13.11 Clinical Signs and Symptoms Associated with Cushing's Syndrome

Physical Features	Psychiatric Symptoms
Truncal obesity	Mood lability
Buffalo hump malformation	Irritability
Hirsutism	Depression
Moon facies	Encephalopathy
Striae and telangiectasia	Personality changes
	Psychosis

Pheochromocytoma

Pheochromocytomas are neuroendocrine tumors that originate in the adrenal medulla and secrete catecholamines, principally norepinephrine and epinephrine. As a result, associated physical signs and symptoms include diaphoresis, tachycardia, hypertension, palpitations, and weight loss. Pheochromocytomas may be acquired through familial heritance or may be part of a wider syndrome, such as neurofibromatosis. Pheochromocytomas are rare, with a prevalence rate of 1:100,000. Diagnosis is made via elevation of metanephrines in serum or a 24-hour urine collection.

Associated catecholamine excess frequently leads to anxiety, panic, and irritability; these may represent the patient's principal complaint. Clinicians must therefore maintain a broad range of differential diagnoses for new-onset panic with autonomic changes. Timely workup and diagnosis are vital to appropriate management of pheochromocytoma. For the psychiatric provider, subjective symptoms of anxiety should always be considered in the context of the patient's medical history and physical signs and symptoms. In patients with panic symptoms, the absence of anticipatory anxiety should serve as an indication for consideration of pheochromocytoma.

Autoimmune and Rheumatologic Illness

In this section, psychiatric manifestations of the following conditions are reviewed:

- Systemic lupus erythematosus
- Multiple sclerosis
- Rheumatoid arthritis.

Systemic Lupus Erythematosus

Systemic lupus erythematosus (SLE) is a systemic autoimmune disorder that affects the CNS. SLE presents with a female-to-male ratio of 9:1, and the course is episodic with flares and remissions. Primary treatment approaches include use of immune-modulating agents such as immunosuppressants and corticosteroids during syndrome exacerbations. Direct CNS effects of the disease include neuronal injury and microvasculopathy, along with greater permeability of the blood-brain barrier over the course of the illness.

Depression and psychosis have long been associated with SLE, and psychiatric symptoms may persist well after disease flares have remitted. Cognitive symptoms are common, affecting up to 80% of patients with SLE; these features appear to present independently of direct CNS pathology. Further complicating the clinical picture of SLE is the required use of corticosteroids for treatment of acute flares.

Multiple Sclerosis

Multiple sclerosis (MS) is a demyelinating neurologic condition that preferentially affects women and has a typical age onset in the twenties. The diagnosis is classically made after an acute neurologic insult, such as optic neuritis. The course of the syndrome is variable, with numerous subtypes including relapsing-remitting, primary progressive, and secondary progressive MS. A number of psychiatric conditions can complicate the course of MS, as listed in Table 13.12.

Interferon therapy, the primary treatment for MS, is also associated with depression and other neuropsychiatric symptoms. In individuals with MS, depression serves as a risk factor for suicide and is associated

Table 13.12 Neuropsychiatric Complications of Multiple Sclerosis, with Prevalence Rates

Fatigue: up to 80%, either accompanying depression or independently
Cognitive impairment: 70%, typically minor decline with subcortical predilection
Depression: lifetime prevalence 50% for MDD, often presenting in advance of MS diagnosis

with poor quality of life and poor functional status. Suicide rates among MS patients may be high, with rates as high as 15% in one study (Sadovnick et al., 1991).

Rheumatoid Arthritis

Rheumatoid arthritis (RA) is a chronic inflammatory condition of the synovial joints that affects less than 1% of the general population. Unlike SLE, direct CNS involvement is not common in RA. Regardless, up to one-fifth of patients with RA develop a mood or anxiety disorder. Whereas depression was once thought to be a risk factor for the development of RA, more recent studies support the onset of depression after the diagnosis of RA in most cases.

Key Points

- Cardiac, pulmonary, hepatic, and renal disorders, and their related treatments, are associated with neuropsychiatric disturbances that can influence outcomes of chronic disease.
- Infectious, endocrine, and metabolic disturbances can precipitate affective and behavioral presentations that mimic primary psychopathology. Maintaining an awareness of the physical and laboratory markers of these conditions can help to define etiologies, thereby guiding appropriate treatment.
- Through physiological and psychological mechanisms, psychiatric conditions and treatments may place individuals at risk for end-organ, metabolic, endocrine, and infectious diseases.
- Psychotropic medication use requires awareness of potential medical complications, along with common drug-drug interactions associated with general medical pharmacotherapies.
- Comprehensive patient care requires a nuanced appreciation for the relationships between physical and mental presentations, subjective experiences and objective evaluation, and neurophysiological and psychological contributors to psychiatric presentations.

Disclosures

Dr. Azzam has no conflicts of interest to disclose.

Dr. Gopalan has no conflicts of interest to disclose.

Dr. Jain has no conflicts of interest to disclose.

Dr. Lotrich has no conflicts of interest to disclose.

Dr. Patterson has no conflicts of interest to disclose.

Further Reading

Cardiovascular Disease

Albert CM, Chae CU, et al. (2005). Phobic anxiety and risk of coronary heart disease and sudden cardiac death among women. *Circulation*, 111(4), 480–487.

Arizona Center for Education and Research on Therapeutics. List of drugs categorized by their potential to cause QT prolongation and/or torsades de pointes (n.d.) Retrieved August 8, 2014, from www.crediblemeds.org.

Gehi A, Haas D, et al. (2005). Depression and medication adherence in outpatients with coronary heart disease: Findings from the Heart and Soul Study. *Arch Intern Med*, 165, 2508–2513.

Glassman AH, O'Connor, CM, et al. (2002). Sertraline treatment of major depression in patients with acute MI or unstable angina. *JAMA*, 288(6), 701–709.

Go AS, Mozaffarian D, et al. (2013). Heart disease and stroke statistics—2013 update: A report from the American Heart Association. *Circulation*, 127, e6–e245.

Jiang W, Alexander J, et al. (2001). Relationship of depression to increased risk of mortality and rehospitalization in patients with congestive heart failure. *Arch Intern Med.*, 161, 1849–1856.

Ko DT, Hebert PR, et al. (2002). Beta-blocker therapy and symptoms of depression, fatigue, and sexual dysfunction. *JAMA*, 288, 351–357.

Kroenke K, Spitzer RL, et al. (2003). The Patient Health Questionnaire-2: Validity of a two-item depression screener. *Med Care*, 41, 1284–1292.

Lichtman JH, Bigger JT, Jr, et al. (2008). Depression and coronary heart disease: Recommendations for screening, referral, and treatment. *Circulation*, 118(17), 1768–1775.

Mavrides N, Nemeroff C. (2013). Treatment of depression in cardiovascular disease. *Depress Anxiety*, 30(4), 328–341.

Meijer A, Conradi HJ, et al. (2011). Prognostic association of depression following myocardial infarction with mortality and cardiovascular events: A meta-analysis of 25 years of research. *Gen Hosp Psychiat.*, 33(3), 203–216.

Murphy SL, Xu J, et al. (2013). Deaths: Final data for 2010. *National Vital Statistics Report*, 61(4), 1–117.

Pozuelo L, Tesar G, et al. (2009). Depression and heart disease: What do we know, and where are we headed? *Cleve Clin J Med.*, 76(1), 59–70.

Rieckmann N, Gerin W, et al. (2006). Course of depressive symptoms and medication adherence after acute coronary syndromes: An electronic medication monitoring study. *J Am Coll Cardiol.*, 48, 2218–2222.

Talati A, Ponniah K, et al. (2008). Panic disorder, social anxiety disorder, and a possible medical syndrome previously linked to chromosome 13. *Biol Psychiat.*, 63(6), 594–601.

Williams W, Kunik ME, et al. (2013). Can personality traits predict the future development of heart disease in hospitalized psychiatric veterans? *J Psychiatr Pract.*, 19(6), 477–489.

Wu CK, Huang YT, et al. (2014). Anti-anxiety drugs use and cardiovascular outcomes in patients with myocardial infarction: A national wide assessment. *Atherosclerosis*, 235(2), 496–502.

Yohannes AM, Willgoss TG, et al. (2010). Depression and anxiety in chronic heart failure and chronic obstructive pulmonary disease: Prevalence, relevance, clinical implications and management principles. *Int J Geriatr Psychiat.*, 25(12), 1209–1221.

Young-Xu Y, Chan KA, et al. (2002). Long-term statin use and psychological well-being. *J Am Coll Cardiol.*, 42, 690–697.

Zupancic ML (2009). Acute psychological stress as a precipitant of acute coronary syndromes in patients with undiagnosed ischemic heart disease: A case report and literature review. *Prim Care Companion J Clin Psychiat.*, 11(1), 21–24.

Pulmonary Disease

Akinbami LJ, Moorman JE, et al. (2012). Trends in asthma prevalence, health care use, and mortality in the United States, 2001–2010. *NCHS Data Brief*, 94, 1–8.

Brenes GA (2003). Anxiety and chronic obstructive pulmonary disease: Prevalence, impact, and treatment. *Psychosom Med.*, 65(6), 963–970.

Brown ES, Vornik LA, et al. (2007). Bupropion in the treatment of outpatients with asthma and major depressive disorder. *Int J Psychiatry Med.*, 37, 23–28.

Jain A, Lolak S (2009). Psychiatric aspects of chronic lung disease. *Curr Psychiatry Rep.*, 11(3), 219–225.

Lamers F, Jonkers CC, et al. (2008). Summed score of the Patient Health Questionnaire-9 was a reliable and valid method for depression screening in chronically ill elderly patients. *J Clin Epidemiol.*, 61, 679–687.

Lavoie KL, Bacon SL, et al. (2006). What is worse for asthma control and quality of life: Depressive disorders, anxiety disorders, or both? *Chest*, 130(4), 1039–1047.

Norwood R. (2006). Prevalence and impact of depression in chronic obstructive pulmonary disease patients. *Curr Opin Pulm Med.*, 12, 113–117.

Potoczek A, Nizankowska-Mogilnicka E, et al. (2008). Links between panic disorder, depression, defence mechanisms, coherence and family functioning in patients suffering from severe COPD. *Psychiatr Pol.*, 42(5), 731–748.

Putman-Casdorph H, McCrone S (2009). Chronic obstructive pulmonary disease, anxiety, and depression: state of the science. *Heart Lung*, 38, 34–47.

Roy-Byrne PP, Davidson KW, et al. (2008). Anxiety disorders and comorbid medical illness. *Gen Hosp Psychiat.*, 30(3), 208–225.

Tluczek A, Becker T, et al. (2013). Health-related quality of life in children and adolescents with cystic fibrosis: Convergent validity with parent-reports and objective measures of pulmonary health. *J Dev Behav Pediatr.*, 34(4), 252–261.

Tomioka H, Imanaka K, et al. (2007). Health-related quality of life in patients with idiopathic pulmonary fibrosis: Cross-sectional and longitudinal study. *Intern Med.*, 46(18), 1533–1542.

Vozoris NT, Fischer HD, et al. (2013). Benzodiazepine use among older adults with chronic obstructive pulmonary disease: A population-based cohort study. *Drugs Aging*, 30(3),183–192.

Willgoss TG, Yohannes AM (2013). Anxiety disorders in patients with COPD: A systematic review. *Respir Care*, 58(5), 858–866.

Renal Disease

Dundas B, Harris M, et al. (2007). Psychogenic polydipsia review: Etiology, differential, and treatment. *Cur Psychiatry Rep.*, 9(3), 236–241.

Harrison NA, Kopelman MD (2009). Endocrine diseases and metabolic disorders. In David AS, Fleminger S, Kopelman MD, Lovestone S, Mellers JDC (Eds.), *Lishman's Organic Psychiatry*, 4th ed. Oxford: Wiley-Blackwell.

Jacob S, Spinler SA (2006). Hyponatremia associated with selective serotonin reuptake inhibitors in older adults. *Ann Pharmacother.*, 40, 1618–1622.

Hepatic Disease

Batista-Neves, SC, Quarantini LC, et al. (2008). High frequency of unrecognized mental disorders in HCV-infected patients. *Gen Hosp Psychiat.*, 27, 431–438.

Castera L, Constant A, et al. (2005). Psychiatric disorders during treatment of chronic hepatitis C. *Gastroenterol Clin Biol*, 29, 123–133.

Dan AA, Crone C, et al. (2007). Anger experiences among hepatitis C patients: Relationship to depressive symptoms and health-related quality of life. *Psychosomatics*, 48, 223–229.

DeSanty KP, Amabile CM (2007). Antidepressant-induced liver injury. *Ann Pharmacother.*, 41, 1201–1211.

Ho SB, Nguyen H, et al. (2001). Influence of psychiatric diagnoses on interferon-alpha treatment for chronic hepatitis C in a veteran population. *Am J Gastroenterol.*, 96, 157–164.

Hosoda S, Takimura H, et al. (2000). Psychiatric symptoms related to interferon therapy for chronic hepatitis C: Clinical features and prognosis. *Psychiatry Clin Neurosci.*, 54, 565–572.

Lauterbach EC, Cummings JL, et al. (1998). Neuropsychiatric correlates and treatment of lenticulostriatal diseases: A review of the literature and overview of research opportunities in Huntington's, Wilson's, and Fahr's diseases. *J Neuropsychiatr Clin Neurosci.*, 10(3), 249–266.

Malek-Ahmadi P, Hilsabeck RC (2007). Neuropsychiatric complications of interferons: Classification, neurochemical bases, and management. *Ann Clin Psychiat.*, 19, 113–123.

Marwick KF, Taylor M, et al. (2012). Antipsychotics and abnormal liver function tests: systematic review. *Clinical Neuropharmacol.*, 35(5), 244–253.

Voican CS, Corruble E, et al. (2014). Antidepressant-induced liver injury: A review for clinicians. *Am J Psychiat.*, 171(4), 404–415.

HIV

Bing EG, Burnam MA, et al. (2001). Psychiatric disorders and drug use among human immunodeficiency virus-infected adults in the United States. *Arch Gen Psychiat.*, 58, 721–728.

Blank MB, Eisenberg MM (2013). Tailored treatment for HIV+ persons with mental illness: The intervention cascade. *J Acquir Immune Defic Syndr., 63*(Suppl 1), S44–48.

Centers for Disease Control (CDC). (2011). *HIV Surveillance Report: Diagnosis: Diagnoses of HIV Infection in the United States and Dependent Areas.* Vol. 23.

DeHert M, Cohen D, et al. (2011). Physical illness in patients with severe mental disorders. II. Barriers to care, monitoring and treatment guidelines, plus recommendations at the system and individual level. *World Psychiat., 10,* 138–51.

Heaton RK, Marcotte TD, et al. (2004). Impact of HIV-1 associated neuropsychological impairment on everyday functioning. *J Int Neuropsychol Soc., 10,* 317–331.

Jayarajan N, Chandra PS (2010). HIV and mental health: An overview of research from India. *Indian J Psychiat., 52,* S269–S273.

Parsons J, Rosoff E, et al. (2007). Patient-related factors predicting HIV medication adherence among men and women with alcohol problems. *J Health Psychol., 12,* 357–370.

Samet JH, Phillips SJ, et al. (2004). Detecting alcohol problems in HIV-infected patients: Use of the CAGE questionnaire. *AIDS Res Hum Retroviruses, 20,* 151–155.

Turjanski N, Lloyd GG (2005). Psychiatric side-effects of medications: Recent development. *Adv in Psychiatr Treat., 11,* 58–70.

Whetten K, Reif S, et al. (2005). Substance abuse and symptoms of mental illness among HIV positive persons in the southeast. *Southern Med J., 98,* 9–14.

Endocrine and Autoimmune Diseases

Anderson RJ, Freedland KE, et al. (2001). The prevalence of comorbid depression in adults with diabetes, a meta-analysis. *Diabetes Care, 24*(6), 1069–1078.

Carbotte R, Denburg SD, et al. (1986). Prevalence of cognitive impairment in systemic lupus erythematosus. *J Nerv Ment Dis., 174*(6), 357–364.

David S, Fleminger MD, et al. (Eds.), *Lishman's Organic Psychiatry,* 4th ed. Oxford: Wiley-Blackwell.

Dickens C, McGowan L, et al. (2002). Depression in rheumatoid arthritis: A systematic review of the literature with meta-analysis. *Psychosom Med., 64,* 52–60.

Kelly WF, Kelly MJ, et al. (2003). A prospective study of psychiatric and psychological aspects of Cushing's syndrome. *Clinical Endocrinol., 45,* 715–720.

Sadovnick AD, Eisen K, et al. (1991) Cause of death in patients attending multiple sclerosis clinics. *Neurology, 41,* 1193–1196.

Schaeffer JJW, Gil KM, et al. (1999). Depression, disease severity, and sickle cell disease. *J Behav Med., 22,* 115–126.

Exercises

1. Based on the 2004 INTERHEART Study, which of the following is the strongest risk factor for acute myocardial infarction?
   a. Obesity
   b. Hypertension
   c. Psychosocial factors
   d. All of the above
   e. None of the above

2. Which of the following treatment options should be considered in patients with severe pulmonary disease and mild anxiety?
   a. CBT
   b. SSRIs
   c. High dose benzodiazepines
   d. A and B
   e. None of the above

3. Which of the following medications is not recommended for use in severe renal impairment?
   a. Fluoxetine
   b. Paliperidone
   c. Haloperidol
   d. Quetiapine
   e. Citalopram

4. Which of the following constellation of features is associated with hepatic encephalopathy?
   a. Incontinence, gait apraxia, confusion
   b. Ataxia, ocular findings, delirium
   c. Asterixis, confusion, and jaundice
   d. Mydriasis, autonomic instability, piloerection
   e. Severe rigidity, nystagmus, incontinence

5. Which of the following is/are psychiatric manifestations of hypothyroidism?
   a. Fatigue
   b. Depression
   c. Psychosis
   d. Cognitive effects
   e. All of the above

Answers: (1) c (2) d (3) b (4) c (5) e

Part IV

Emergent Complications of Medication and Substance Use

Catatonia, Neuroleptic Malignant Syndrome, and Serotonin Syndrome

Pierre N. Azzam and Priya Gopalan

Introduction

Catatonia, neuroleptic malignant syndrome (NMS), and serotonin syndrome represent heterogeneous conditions that share phenotypic, phenomenologic, and pathophysiologic features. The consultation psychiatrist who attempts to understand all three conditions in relation to one another can better appreciate the unique elements of each one. This chapter begins with a discussion of catatonia, the fluctuating psychomotor syndrome that is precipitated by general medical conditions, psychiatric disorders, and pharmacologic interventions. In relation, NMS is believed to represent a highly malignant and iatrogenic variant of catatonia, and serotonin syndrome rests on a spectrum of drug-induced toxicities alongside NMS. By recognizing these conditions promptly and managing them aggressively, the consultation psychiatrist can provide maximal support to primary medical services, and can facilitate potentially life-saving measures.

Catatonia

Overview and History

Catatonia is a polymorphic syndrome of motoric and behavioral disturbances that fluctuate temporally. Common features include mutism, negativism (purposeless resistance), immobility, posturing, rigidity, repetitive or unusual movements, excitement, echophenomena (repetition of speech or behavior), and ambitendency (the sensation of feeling stuck) (Bush et al., 1997). Conceptualized historically as a variant of schizophrenia, catatonia is, in fact, precipitated by numerous medical and psychiatric conditions. Given its frequently missed diagnosis, heterogeneous presentation, and potentially fatal complications, learning to recognize catatonia proves critical to psychiatric care in the general medical setting.

Understanding the history of catatonia helps to frame its modern diagnostic and therapeutic challenges. In the late nineteenth century, German psychiatrist Karl Ludwig Kahlbaum coined the term "catatonia" to describe a condition that presented in vacillating stages of melancholy, excitement, and stupor. Subsequently, the syndrome found itself in Emil Kraepelin's concept of "dementia praecox," and by the turn of the century, joined Eugen Bleuler's psychodynamic framework for the illness of schizophrenia.

Twentieth-century descriptions of catatonia began to challenge psychodynamic and schizophrenia-specific conceptualizations, expanding the breadth of observed symptomatology and potential etiologies. Not only was catatonia increasingly diagnosed in patients with general medical and neurologic conditions, but a malignant variant of the syndrome was identified, characterized by physiologic deterioration and often fatal outcomes. By mid-century, electroconvulsive therapy (ECT) and amobarbital were used to treat the syndrome of catatonia, and by the end of the twentieth century, benzodiazepines became the mainstay of therapy. But the dilemma over a diagnostic home for catatonia in the American Psychiatric Association's *Diagnostic and Statistical Manual of Mental Disorders* (DSM) has persisted. In its first three editions, the DSM described catatonia exclusively as a subtype of schizophrenia. Reflecting the tendencies for affective and general medical disorders to induce the catatonic syndrome, a specifier was added to major depressive, manic, and mixed mood episodes in DSM-IV, along with the diagnosis of catatonia due to a general medical condition.

Responding to the etiologic and phenomenologic breadth of catatonia, DSM-5 has eliminated the catatonic subtype of schizophrenia and has clarified catatonia as a specifier for affective or psychotic states, as a syndrome due to another medical condition, or as an unspecified catatonic syndrome.

Identification and Diagnosis

In the inpatient psychiatry setting, the prevalence of catatonia has been reported from 7% to 31%; most cases are diagnosed in the context of the following conditions (Daniels, 2009):

- Affective disorders (~30%)
- General medical conditions (20%–25%)
- Schizophrenia (10%–15%).

The epidemiology of catatonia in the general medical setting remains elusive, though the syndrome is believed to go undetected frequently. In 2005, a Dutch study suggested under-recognition of catatonia by clinicians who used *DSM*, as compared to researchers who followed the World Health Organization's *International Classification of Diseases* (*ICD*) criteria (van der Heijden et al., 2005). The frequency with which medical conditions either precipitate or complicate catatonia underscores the need for diagnostic vigilance when providing psychiatric consultation in the general hospital.

For a diagnosis of catatonia, *DSM-5* requires three or more of the following: stupor, catalepsy, waxy flexibility, mutism, negativism, spontaneous posturing, mannerisms, stereotypy, purposeless agitation, grimacing, echolalia, and echopraxia (APA, 2013). These and additional features of catatonia are outlined in Table 14.1.

Catatonia is often described in terms of subtypes and variants:

- Individuals who present with some combination of immobility, mutism, staring, catalepsy, and waxy flexibility are frequently described as having *retarded, stuporous,* or *hypokinetic* catatonia.
- *Excited* or *hyperkinetic* catatonia is characterized by excessive motor activity, agitation, peculiar behaviors and speech, and echophenomena. Perhaps owing to a lesser appreciation for hyperkinetic aspects of the syndrome, excited catatonia is frequently misidentified as hyperactive delirium, mania, or other syndromes with accompanying agitation.
- Catatonia is defined as *malignant* when it is accompanied by autonomic instability and hyperthermia, typically with sudden onset, rapid progression, and more pronounced fluctuations. Motoric and behavioral signs most frequently displayed in malignant catatonia include posturing, rigidity, confusion, and intermittent excitement. Mortality rates are high, up to 30%. Malignant catatonia is clinically indistinguishable from NMS, and shared theories of pathophysiology suggest that NMS is a highly malignant iatrogenic variant of catatonia.

Evaluation and Underpinnings

The evaluation for catatonia should include full mental status and neurological examinations across multiple points in time, with a focus on assessing motor tone, monitoring for automatisms and echophenomena, eliciting frontal release signs, and observing for indicators of ambitendence. A full examination for catatonia should be considered for patients with prominent psychomotor slowing, posturing, agitation with mannerisms and stereotypies, perseveration, and echophenomena during clinical encounters. Information from family members, medical records, and clinical providers can provide a history of relevant risk factors, recent changes to medications, and substance use, in addition to providing a more comprehensive timeline of the presenting course.

Abnormal vital signs, labs, and studies often accompany catatonia; they may also herald the progression of malignant catatonia or the onset of a

medical complication. Individuals with catatonia present frequently with the following signs and symptoms:
- Elevation of pulse, blood pressure, and respiration rate
- Autonomic instability that warrants aggressive management in the critical care setting.

Table 14.1 Clinical Features of Catatonia with Definitions

Feature of Catatonia	Definition
Stupor	Minimal responsiveness or spontaneous motor activity
Waxy flexibility	Initial resistance to passive movement followed by yielding to repositioning, often with *catalepsy*
Negativism	Purposeless resistance to directions or passive movement
Mannerisms	Unusual behaviors that may be purposeful and often repetitive
Purposeless agitation	Extreme restlessness or excitement, often purposeless
Echolalia	Repetition of others' speech
Verbigeration	Monotonous repetition of a phrase
Oppositional paratonia	Proportional resistance to passive movement, most often appreciated in the upper extremities (motor negativism)
Catalepsy	Maintenance of unusual postures after passive repositioning
Mutism	Decreased production or volume of speech, absent in extreme forms
Posturing	Spontaneous maintenance of an abnormal position
Stereotypy	Repetitive non-purposeful movements
Grimacing	Abnormal facial positioning
Echopraxia	Repetition of others' actions
Automatic obedience	Immediate following of directions without thought to content
Frontal release signs	Primitive reflexes, including grasp, rooting, and glabellar reflexes

Serum labs frequently reveal the following:
- Elevated creatine phosphokinase (CPK)
- Leukocytosis
- Hyponatremia
- Low serum iron.

Head imaging and electroencephalography (EEG) may be used to evaluate for primary neurologic contributors to the syndrome, though no consistent findings are specifically associated with catatonia.

The catatonia workup should include consideration of general medical and neurologic conditions, in addition to toxidromes and withdrawal states, which can precipitate the syndrome (see Box 14.1). Depending on the clinical presentation, the differential diagnosis for catatonia includes akinetic or elective mutism, delirium, locked-in syndrome, and apathy syndromes (e.g., medial frontal stroke). As management of these conditions varies considerably, using history, brain imaging studies, and physical examination to differentiate between them also helps to guide management.

A multitude of diffuse neural networks and neurotransmitters are believed to contribute to the pathophysiology of catatonia. In particular, dysfunction of basal ganglia circuits has been implicated in rigidity and waxy flexibility; orbitofrontal and medial frontal networks are believed to contribute to amotivation, perseveration, and echophenomena; involvement of limbic structures likely dictates the intense fear associated with catatonia; and hypothalamic disturbances may precipitate the temperature and autonomic dysregulation seen most commonly in the malignant variant. Neurotransmitter deficits implicated in catatonia include dopamine and GABA hypoactivity, alongside glutamate hyperactivity that indirectly contributes to loss of GABAergic tone.

Management

Management of catatonia requires close observation, either in the medical hospital with psychiatric consultation, or in milder cases, on

---

Box 14.1 Psychiatric, Neurologic, Medical, and Drug-Induced Conditions That May Precipitate Catatonia

- *Psychiatric*: affective disorders, autistic spectrum disorders, conversion disorder, obsessive-compulsive disorder, schizophrenia
- *Neurologic*: Creutzfeldt-Jakob disease, encephalitis, encephalopathy, epilepsy, infarcts (cingulate, temporal, parietal), meningitis, traumatic brain injury
- *General Medical Conditions*: acute intermittent porphyria, AIDS/HIV, Cushing's disease, hepatitis, hyperparathyroidism, systemic lupus erythematosus, uremia
- *Medications/Drugs*: corticosteroids, disulfiram, MDMA ("Ecstasy," "Molly"), metoclopramide, neuroleptics, withdrawal states (alcohol, benzodiazepines, dopaminergic medications)

a psychiatric inpatient unit with close medical monitoring. Alongside pharmacologic treatment, essentials of care include management of precipitating conditions, elimination of all potentially offending agents (particularly dopamine antagonists), and implementation of preventive measures. The list of potential medical complications is extensive, including aspiration, pressure ulcers, muscle contractures, dehydration, end-organ failure, venous thromboembolism, and gastrointestinal bleed. Preventive care, namely optimizing anticoagulation, aspiration precautions, hydration, mobilization, and nutrition, is therefore key to mitigating the morbidity and mortality associated with catatonia.

Benzodiazepines constitute the mainstay of treatment for catatonia. ECT, the gold standard of care owing to effectiveness in all catatonic variants, is typically reserved for cases in which benzodiazepines are contraindicated or minimally effective, and for malignant catatonia. Prescribed antipsychotics should be discontinued in the initial phase of treatment. Dopamine agonists (e.g., amantadine, bromocriptine) can be helpful adjunctively, whereas antipsychotics and other dopamine antagonists have been shown to worsen cases of catatonia acutely. Antipsychotics may precipitate NMS when administered to patients with catatonia, even if the catatonic symptoms present in the setting of an exacerbated psychosis. As such, antipsychotics are better left for careful introduction, only as necessary for active psychotic symptoms, once an acute episode of catatonia is sufficiently treated. Additional pharmacotherapies have been used to treat catatonia, either monotherapy or adjunctively with varying degrees of success (see Box 14.2); of those, the muscle relaxant dantrolene is almost exclusively reserved for severe cases of NMS and malignant catatonia, owing to its multitude of toxicities and medical contraindications.

The clinician who suspects a patient has catatonia should be prepared to administer a benzodiazepine challenge dose while keeping a close watch on the patient's response at the bedside. Most authors advise parenteral administration of 1–2 mg lorazepam (or 5–10 mg diazepam), with graduated administration up to 6 mg lorazepam-equivalent in severe cases, and based on clinical response. With a successful trial, bedside monitoring should reveal improvement in motoric and behavioral signs.

Box 14.2 Case-Reported Adjunctive or Second-Line Agents for Management of Catatonia

Antiepileptic drugs (e.g., carbamazepine, topiramate, valproic acid)
Aripiprazole
Barbiturates
Dantrolene (in limited cases of severe rigidity/hyperthermia)
Dopamine agonists (e.g., amantadine, bromocriptine)
Lithium
Memantine
Psychostimulants
Zolpidem

Thereafter, most patients will require continuation of benzodiazepine therapy, in maintenance dosing, to prevent the return of catatonic features. Response to a challenge dose typically predicts response to maintenance dosing, with an average initial maintenance dose of lorazepam 3–6 mg, typically divided three times daily.

Maintenance dosing requires further adjustment based on clinical response, within days or weeks after initiating treatment of catatonia. Unfortunately, no standardized guidelines are available to guide this process. In many cases of partial response, incremental increases in total daily dose by 2–3 mg lorazepam-equivalent are undertaken, often to a maximum of 18 mg lorazepam per day. Benzodiazepine response rates average 70%–80% for non-malignant cases of catatonia and 40% for malignant cases; rates of response to ECT are more promising, reaching as high as 80%–90% in both non-malignant and malignant variants (Daniels, 2009). If no or limited response is noted to maximal benzodiazepine dosing, or if the syndrome progresses to malignant status, ECT must be sought quickly (i.e., within several days of either circumstance) in order to optimize rates of survival.

Duration of treatment for catatonia must be personalized, based on the status of the contributing condition and the patient's response to treatment, though general prognostic indicators can be helpful. Those who respond quickly and robustly to benzodiazepines are less likely to relapse with discontinuation of the medication, as are those who experience catatonia episodically as opposed to chronically. Those with good premorbid functioning and patients with mood disorders (i.e., as opposed to those with chronic medical conditions or psychotic conditions) also tend to have a better response, with shorter requirement for maintenance treatment. Conversely, patients who experience catatonia due to neurologic illness and those who require high-dose benzodiazepines for response are more likely to relapse with discontinuation of maintenance treatment. The decision to maintain versus withdrawing benzodiazepine agents should be made after discussion with the patient, based on the likelihood of relapse. Factors may include the status of the precipitating psychiatric or general medical conditions, duration of current catatonic episode, and history of prior episodes.

Suggested Guidelines for Management

1. Lorazepam test dose (1–2 mg IV) at the bedside with monitoring for response;
2. Lorazepam standing dose 1–2 mg every 8 hours as starting dose if treatment response is observed;
3. Daily titration to maximum tolerated dose or until treatment response;
4. If treatment response plateaus or if no response within one week, initiate institution-specific process for ECT.

Neuroleptic Malignant Syndrome

Overview and History

Neuroleptic malignant syndrome is a rare disorder most commonly associated with the initiation of antipsychotic medications. Thought to be similar in mechanism to both catatonia and malignant hyperthermia, NMS is associated with prominent neuromuscular findings (e.g., "lead pipe" rigidity), altered mental status, hyperthermia, and autonomic instability.

French physicians first described the *syndrome malin des neuroleptiques* in 1960. Since then, with the growth in clinical use of dopamine antagonists, NMS has been the subject of a growing body of case reports and clinical research. While NMS is relatively rare, its associated mortality rates have been reported at 10%–20%, and as high as 40%. NMS is precipitated by the initiation of dopamine antagonists or the abrupt withdrawal of a dopamine agonist (e.g., levodopa). In addition to antipsychotics, dopamine-blocking medications that have been associated with NMS include antiemetic drugs (e.g., metoclopramide, prochlorperazine) and the heterocyclic antidepressants amoxapine and maprotiline.

Identification and Diagnosis

In the inpatient psychiatry setting, NMS affects less than 1% of patients who take neuroleptic agents (Strawn et al., 2007). Older studies cite higher prevalence for NMS; development of second-generation antipsychotics and increased education on the syndrome likely explain the decrease over time. Age, race, and sex have not been cited as significant risk factors for the development of NMS, with only a slight predominance of men over women and an average age of middle-adulthood among diagnosed patients.

Causes of and risk factors for NMS include the following:

- High dosing, rapid titration, and parenteral or depot administration of antipsychotics;
- Chronic use of oral antipsychotics or other dopamine antagonists at therapeutic doses (most common);
- Concurrent lithium or anticholinergic medication use may increase risk of NMS;
- Other factors associated with NMS: dehydration, organic brain disease, mental retardation, previous episodes of NMS, and a history of receiving ECT.

Typically, NMS develops within two weeks after initiation of a dopamine antagonist (interval may be longer with intramuscular depot formulations) or after an increase in the dose of an established agent. On occasion, NMS occurs idiosyncratically after long periods of neuroleptic use. Careful history-taking is critical to identifying NMS; this includes a thorough review of recent medication changes, including non-psychotropic medications with dopamine-blocking properties and agents that interfere with metabolism or clearance of a dopamine antagonist (e.g., cytochrome P450 inhibitors). Since altered sensorium may preclude the patient from providing an accurate history, obtaining information from families, primary care physicians, psychiatric providers, and pharmacies is vital. Compared to other toxidromes and idiosyncratic drug reactions (e.g., serotonin syndrome), the course of NMS is usually more insidious and variable. While the average duration of the syndrome is one week, few reported cases have persisted for up to two months after discontinuation of the offending medication.

DSM-5 classifies NMS under the section "Medication-Induced Movement Disorders and Other Adverse Effects of Medication" and does not list specific criteria for diagnosing the syndrome (APA, 2013). The differential diagnosis of NMS is broad and includes catatonia, malignant hyperthermia, serotonin syndrome, stroke, seizures, and Parkinson's disease.

Evaluation and Underpinnings

The primary constellation of features identified in NMS includes the following:

- Fever
- Autonomic instability
- Neuromuscular symptoms (usually lead-pipe rigidity)
- Altered mental status.

Limited data suggest that altered mental status and neuromuscular abnormalities precede fever and autonomic signs in more than 80% of cases. Elevation of body temperature is associated with progressively higher morbidity and mortality. As such, clinicians must be vigilant in recognizing the early signs of NMS, as early detection may allow for interventions prior to the development of fatal hyperthermia.

Other associated features include:

- Tremor
- Sialorrhea
- Akinesia
- Dystonia
- Trismus (jaw spasm)
- Myoclonus
- Dysarthria
- Dysphagia.

Serum labs frequently reveal leukocytosis and elevated CPK (which can be extreme). Additional lab findings that are associated commonly with NMS, but not specific to the syndrome, include low serum iron, myoglobinuria, and metabolic acidosis. Neuroimaging and EEG should be undertaken when concerns arise for acute intracranial pathology or seizure activity, and a lumbar puncture may be considered based on clinical findings (e.g., isolated nuchal rigidity).

The pathophysiology of NMS is believed to involve central dopamine blockade within basal ganglia and hypothalamic projections, and more specifically down-regulation of D2 receptors in the striatum. In the acute phase of the syndrome, cerebrospinal fluid (CSF) analysis from afflicted patients has revealed decreased levels of homovanillic acid, a dopamine metabolite (Nisijima & Ishiguro, 1995). Still, second-generation antipsychotics with less prominent D2 blockade have been implicated in cases of NMS, suggesting more complex pathophysiology (e.g., sympatho-adrenal dysfunction leading to temperature dysregulation).

Management

Because NMS can develop precipitously and lead to death in up to 40% of cases, successful management hinges on quick diagnosis, early intervention, and prevention of associated medical complications.

Potentially fatal conditions associated with NMS include the following:

- Rhabdomyolysis
- Renal failure
- Disseminated intravascular coagulation
- Respiratory failure
- Autonomic instability
- Seizures
- Cardiac dysrhythmias.

Pharmacologic management of NMS starts with discontinuation of all dopamine antagonists and reintroduction of any recently discontinued dopamine agonists. Supportive measures can prove life-saving in cases of NMS; these include aggressive management of central body temperature, hydration, and vital functions in the intensive care setting.

Dopamine agonists, specifically bromocriptine (starting dose: 2.5 mg twice or three times daily; target daily dose: 45 mg in split dosing) and amantadine (starting dose: 50–100 mg twice daily; target daily dose: 200–400 mg), may alleviate the symptoms and vital sign abnormalities associated with NMS. Dantrolene, a calmodulin inhibitor that works at the sarcoplasmic reticulum, prevents muscle breakdown and may reduce fevers. Owing to adverse effects and risk for end-organ damage, dantrolene is used infrequently and only in the setting of severe muscle rigidity. Benzodiazepines are frequently used to manage anxiety and agitation in the setting of NMS.

ECT is typically reserved for cases that are refractory to supportive and pharmacologic treatments. In the acute phase of the syndrome, medical clearance for ECT requires deliberation, particularly given that autonomic instability increases the risk of cardiac and pulmonary complications associated with anesthesia. For patients who previously required long-term antipsychotic use, or for whom chronic treatment for psychosis is anticipated, ECT may be a reasonable option for both acute and long-term management.

Guidelines for Management of NMS

1. Discontinue offending agent and maximize supportive care;
2. Adjunctive use of benzodiazepines if needed;
3. Dopamine agonist if symptoms persist: bromocriptine (starting dose: 2.5 mg twice or three times daily; target daily dose: 45 mg in split dosing) and amantadine (starting dose: 50–100 mg twice daily; target daily dose: 200–400 mg);
4. ECT for treatment-refractory cases.

Many patients who develop NMS require long-term antipsychotic treatment; at the same time, up to 30% of patients who have experienced NMS once will re-experience the syndrome after reintroduction of an antipsychotic agent. When an antipsychotic agent is required after NMS, second-generation antipsychotics or low-potency first-generation agents should be tried preferentially, and titration should start at low doses and should be done slowly with careful monitoring of symptoms.

Serotonin Syndrome

Overview and History

Serotonin syndrome is an idiosyncratic drug reaction associated with serotonergic hyperactivity across multiple organ systems. Characterized by the classic triad of altered mental status, neuromuscular findings, and autonomic dysregulation, serotonin syndrome may also present with gastrointestinal (GI) distress, cognitive and perceptual disturbances, and other nonspecific features. Since the first case of serotonin syndrome was cited in 1955, numerous case reports and studies have helped to elucidate the etiology and pathophysiology of this rare and potentially fatal condition.

Any substance that promotes serotonergic activity can precipitate serotonin syndrome, including the following:
- Selective serotonin reuptake inhibitors (SSRIs)
- Serotonin norepinephrine reuptake inhibitors (SNRIs)
- Tricyclic antidepressants (TCAs)
- Monoamine oxidase inhibitors (MAOIs)
- Other commonly prescribed psychiatric medications: buspirone, lithium, mirtazapine, psychostimulants, trazodone
- Non-psychiatric serotonergic offenders: bromocriptine, linezolid, meperidine, ondansetron, tramadol
- Over-the-counter and herbal drugs: dextromethorphan, St. John's wort
- Drugs of abuse: MDMA (e.g., "Ecstasy," "Molly"), LSD.

Despite evidence to support the association of these agents with serotonin syndrome, little data help to explain individual susceptibility to the syndrome. Clinicians generally accept that the combination of two or more serotonergic agents puts patients at higher risk for serotonin syndrome than a single agent.

Identification and Diagnosis

Precise estimates for the incidence of serotonin syndrome are limited by the broad number of serotonergic agents and limited recognition of the symptoms. Approximately 14% of individuals develop serotonin syndrome after SSRI overdose (Isbister et al., 2004). Rates of serotonin syndrome at therapeutic antidepressant dosing are unknown, as are specific demographic risk factors. Known risk factors for serotonin syndrome include the following:
- Recent initiation or titration of a serotonergic agent
- Co-administration of multiple serotonergic medications
- Drug abuse involving MDMA or LSD
- Cytochrome P450 polymorphisms or drug-drug interactions that interfere with metabolism of serotonergic agents to cause higher serum drug levels.

The onset, progression, and course of serotonin syndrome are typically rapid. An individual may present with serotonergic features within minutes to hours of initiating or titrating an offending agent. Likewise, with appropriate recognition and management, symptoms typically abate within 48 hours. Because serotonin syndrome remains a clinical diagnosis without pathognomonic lab or study findings, maintaining vigilance for its clinical features is vital. Careful history-taking should clarify all recent ingestions, whether prescribed, over-the-counter, or illicit. Because serotonin syndrome is often associated with altered mental status, contact with family members, outpatient providers, and pharmacies is often necessary to ensure an accurate history.

Recommended diagnostic criteria for serotonin syndrome include the Hunter Serotonin Toxicity Criteria (Dunkley et al., 2003) or the Sternbach Criteria (Sternbach, 1991), as described in Table 14.2.

Evaluation and Underpinnings

A comprehensive mental status and physical examination should identify absent and present features among the classic triad of serotonin syndrome:

- Altered mental status
- Neuromuscular findings
- Autonomic signs.

A careful physical examination is particularly important when a patient's mental status precludes accurate history-taking. The neurologic examination should assess for clonus, myoclonic movements, tremor, rigidity,

Table 14.2 Diagnostic Criteria for the Evaluation of Serotonin Syndrome

Hunter Serotonin Toxicity Criteria	Sternbach Criteria
Recent use of one or more serotonergic agent AND	Recent addition or titration of a serotonergic agent AND
At least one of the following: a) tremor AND hyperreflexia b) spontaneous clonus c) muscle rigidity, temperature > 38°C, and either ocular clonus or inducible clonus d) either inducible or ocular clonus plus either agitation or diaphoresis	Three or more of the following: a) alteration in mental status b) agitation c) myoclonus d) hyperreflexia e) sweating f) shivering g) tremor h) diarrhea i) incoordination j) fever
	Absence of other likely etiologies or recent addition/increase to another psychotropic agent

Adapted from Denkley et al. (2003) and Sternbach et al. (1991).

and hyperreflexia in concert with the evaluation for encephalopathy and autonomic changes. Spontaneous clonus alone can be diagnostic of serotonin syndrome, and ocular clonus (i.e., uncontrolled rapid and equal movement of the eyes) is seen in few other conditions. Hyperreflexia is typically most prominent in the lower extremities, and most notably sustained with the patellar deep tendon reflex.

Serotonin syndrome may be conceptualized as a hyper-serotonergic spectrum disorder, with severity correlating with observed signs and symptoms, as listed in Table 14.3.

Though a hyper-serotonergic state may impact upon any of the 14 serotonin receptor subtypes currently identified, serotonin syndrome

Table 14.3 Clinical Signs and Symptoms of Serotonin Syndrome Based on Severity

Severity of Serotonin Syndrome	Clinical Features
Mild	• Diaphoresis, hot/cold flashes • Gastrointestinal symptoms (e.g., nausea, GI upset) • Subtle neuromuscular findings (e.g., hyperreflexia, tremor) • Restlessness • Tachycardia
Moderate	*As above, plus:* • Hypertension • Hyperthermia • Mental status changes • Notable neuromuscular findings (e.g., hyperreflexia, clonus)
Severe	*As above, plus:* • Agitation • Delirium • Pupillary changes (e.g., mydriasis) • Severe neuromuscular findings (e.g., hyperreflexia, clonus, rigidity)
Life-Threatening	*As above, plus:* • Autonomic instability • Coma • Hyperthermia (temperatures above 41.1°C) • Shock

has been associated predominantly with central and peripheral effects at the 5-HT$_{1A}$ and 5-HT$_{2A}$ receptors.

Management

Prognosis is favorable when clinicians identify serotonin syndrome promptly, discontinue all potentially offending medications immediately, and manage supportively. In most cases, serotonin syndrome will resolve within days after discontinuing serotonergic agents. Supportive measures include close observation, typically in the critical care setting; fluid resuscitation; management of severe hyperthermia, tachycardia, and hypertension; maintenance of fall and aspiration precautions; and management of agitation with benzodiazepines, as needed.

Despite theoretical support for use of cyproheptadine, a 5-HT$_{1A}$ and 5-HT$_{2A}$ antagonist, as an antidote for serotonin toxicity, little evidence supports its practical effectiveness, aside from limited case reports and anecdotal data. Because serotonin syndrome often resolves spontaneously with discontinuation of serotonergic agents, cyproheptadine is generally reserved for cases in which symptoms are persistent or prolonged.

Though no guidelines have been standardized for medication reintroduction, providers should wait at least two weeks after the syndrome's resolution before challenging with a serotonergic agent. A frank patient-provider discussion of potential risks, benefits, and alternative therapies may guide consideration of an agent with lesser serotonergic properties than the offending medicine, or for milder cases of depression and anxiety, consideration of psychotherapy alone, with close monitoring for relapse of psychiatric symptoms.

Key Points

- Catatonia is frequently misdiagnosed and is caused by a general medical condition in up to one-quarter of cases.
- Catatonia is a heterogeneous syndrome, associated with numerous neurologic and behavioral symptoms, and requires careful examination and expeditious treatment with benzodiazepines or electroconvulsive therapy.
- Neuroleptic malignant syndrome is a rare and potentially fatal condition that is associated with dopamine antagonism and is characterized by fever, autonomic instability, lead-pipe rigidity, and altered mental status.
- Neuroleptic malignant syndrome is managed by removal of the offending agent, potential use of dopamine agonists, and supportive care.
- Serotonin syndrome is caused by excessive use of serotonergic agents and is associated with the classic triad of altered mental status, neuromuscular findings, and autonomic signs.
- Serotonin syndrome is a short-lived phenomenon that generally responds to supportive care when the offending agent is promptly removed.

Disclosures

Dr. Azzam has no conflicts of interest to disclose.

Dr. Gopalan has no conflicts of interest to disclose.

Further Reading

American Psychiatric Association (2013). *Diagnostic and Statistical Manual of Mental Disorders*, 5th ed. Arlington, VA: American Psychiatric Publishing.

Boyer EW, Shannon M (2005). The serotonin syndrome. *New Eng J Med.*, *352*(11), 1112–1120.

Bush G, Petrides G, et al. (1997). Catatonia and other motor syndromes in a chronically hospitalized psychiatric population. *Schizophrenia Res.*, *27*(1), 83–92.

Daniels J (2009). Catatonia: Clinical aspects and neurobiological correlates. *J Neuropsychiat Clin Neurosci.*, *21*(4), 371–380.

Dunkley EJ, Isbister GK, et al. (2003). The Hunter serotonin toxicity criteria: Simple and accurate diagnostic decision rules for serotonin toxicity. *Quar J Med.*, *96*(9), 635–642.

Isbister GK, Bowe SJ, et al. (2004). Relative toxicity of selective serotonin reuptake inhibitors in overdose. *J Toxicol Clin Toxicol.*, *42*(3), 277–285.

Nisijima K, Ishiguro T (1995). Cerebrospinal fluid levels of monoamine metabolites and gamma-aminobutyric acid in neuroleptic malignant syndrome. *J Psychiat Res.*, *29*(3), 233–244.

Sternbach H (1991). The serotonin syndrome. *Am J Psychiat.*, *148*(6), 705–713.

Strawn JR, Keck PE, et al. (2007). Neuroleptic malignant syndrome. *Am J Psychiat.*, *164*(6), 870–876.

van der Heijden FM, Tuinier S, et al. (2005). Catatonia: Disappeared or under-diagnosed. *Psychopathology*, *38*(1), 3–8.

Exercises

1. Catatonia is associated with all of the following symptoms EXCEPT:
   a. Echophenomena
   b. Catalepsy
   c. Cataplexy
   d. Mutism
   e. Verbigeration

2. The most frequent cause of catatonia is:
   a. Schizophrenia
   b. Mood disorders
   c. General medical conditions
   d. Substance use disorders
   e. None of the above

3. Neuroleptic malignant syndrome may be caused by:
   a. Lithium
   b. Clonidine
   c. Haloperidol decanoate
   d. Fluoxetine
   e. Bromocriptine

4. Which of the following agents may cause serotonin syndrome?
   a. Linezolid
   b. Meperidine
   c. St. John's wort
   d. Tramadol
   e. All of these may induce serotonin syndrome

5. Differentiating between catatonia, neuroleptic malignant syndrome, and serotonin syndrome requires the clinician to:
   a. Obtain an MRI to look for differences in brain findings between the syndromes
   b. Obtain a comprehensive serum blood test to see what medications the patient has taken
   c. Obtain a thorough history, including a medication review, and conduct a careful physical examination for signs and symptoms of the different syndromes
   d. Perform benzodiazepine challenges on anyone with rigidity and altered mental status

Answers: (1) c (2) b (3) c (4) e (5) c

Toxidromes

Toxicology and the Psychiatric Patient

Michael G. Abesamis

Introduction

Patients with psychiatric disorders are uniquely susceptible to toxicologic issues. They have access to medications that have varied effects on numerous neurologic receptors with the potential for drug interactions that can lead to deleterious effects such as altered mental status, cardiac dysfunction, and seizures. Toxicity in these situations can lead to numerous secondary illnesses, including rhabdomyolysis, pneumonia, and kidney and liver failure. Regardless of the specific drug, neurotransmitter and receptor activity in the central and peripheral nervous systems causes predictable and recognizable patterns of toxicity. Recognition and identification of these patterns, known as toxidromes, are the basis of successful therapy.

Approach for the Poisoned Patient

Treatment of a poisoned patient involves a systematic approach in obtaining a detailed history of exposure and available drugs, and a comprehensive physical examination. Distinct signs and symptoms that are obtained in the assessment can be used to identify the specific toxidrome.

Items to consider in the history include prescription and over-the-counter medications available to the patient and whether the patient has been using any illicit substances. Supplements such as vitamins or dietary substances should be reviewed, as they can also cause drug interactions or toxicity. Finally, it is important to gather information about the scene where the patient was found. What substances were around the patient? In what state was the patient found (e.g., unresponsive, seizing)? What substances were available in the home? As patients are often unable or unwilling to provide accurate information, additional resources, such as pre-hospital providers, family, friends, pharmacy records, and previous medical records, are important resources for identifying potential toxins.

In terms of the physical exam, factors that may guide you to a particular toxidrome include the patient's vital signs, neurological examination, and skin examination. Is the patient tachycardic or bradycardic? Tachypneic or bradypneic? Hyperthermic or hypothermic? Things to note from the neuropsychiatric examination include the patient's level of consciousness, psychomotor agitation or slowing, fluctuating attention and concentration, presence of hallucinations, and altered thought processes. Does the patient have hyperreflexia or clonus? What is the pupil exam: pinpoint or dilated? Finally, in terms of the integumentary exam, does he or she have dry axilla or are they diffusely diaphoretic? Is the patient flushed, pale, or cyanotic? Is his or her capillary refill normal? All of these findings may guide you to a particular toxidrome. At the same time, consideration should be given to non-toxicologic causes of illness.

The differential diagnosis for a patient presenting in such a manner is broad. Things to consider and rule out include the following:

a. Infection (e.g., urinary tract infection, meningitis, sepsis);
b. Neurologic (e.g., seizure and the postictal period, stroke, Pick's disease, spongiform encephalopathy);
c. Toxic/metabolic (e.g., drug overdose, vitamin deficiency, chronic alcohol abuse, liver or kidney failure, hypoxemia, thyrotoxicosis);
d. Cardiac (e.g., myocardial infarction, dysrhythmia);
e. Immunologic/endocrine (e.g., anti–glutamic acid decarboxylase antibody; anti-NDMA antibody, thyrotoxicosis, myxedema);
f. Neoplastic (e.g., malignant myeloma, metastatic lesions to brain);
g. Psychiatric.

Once all of the information has been obtained and the clinical suspicion involves drug ingestion, the findings should be used to identify the presenting toxidrome. Identifying the correct toxidrome is paramount in guiding treatment in the poisoned patient. It is important to stress that toxic physiology is not the same as infectious or septic physiology, and this difference guides the treatments recommended in this chapter.

The major toxidromes that you should be able to identify include the following:
1. Anticholinergic
2. Cholinergic
3. Sympathomimetic
4. Sedative-hypnotic
5. Opioid (see Chapter 16)
6. Withdrawal syndromes (see Chapter 16)
7. Serotonin syndrome (see Chapter 14)
8. Neuroleptic malignant syndrome (see Chapter 14).

Diagnosis of toxicity is primarily clinical. However, diagnostic testing for most toxic patients should include the following:
1. An EKG;
2. Electrolytes, BUN, creatinine;
3. Drug levels; acetaminophen, ethanol, and salicylate levels should be ordered in all intoxicated patients. Additional serum drug levels should be obtained based on drugs available to the patient and clinical presentation. Routine urine testing for drugs of abuse are rarely useful in the identification and treatment of acute toxicity due to the significant false positives and false negatives of the test. Obtaining a comprehensive urine drug screen (which is done via gas chromatography with mass spectroscopy) can confirm most exposures, but the results are rarely available in time to be clinically relevant. However, these tests may be beneficial for subsequent treatment of abuse and dependence.
4. Total creatinine phosphokinase should be considered in patients for whom rhabdomyolysis is a concern.
5. Consider liver function tests and complete blood count depending on the suspected substance exposure.
6. Chest X-ray may be considered for patients in whom clinically significant aspiration is suspected.
7. CT scan of the head may be considered if you are concerned about head Injury.
8. EEGs are generally only useful if you think the patient may have a seizure disorder or may be in status epilepticus, but should not be ordered routinely.

Anticholinergic Syndrome

Clinical Presentation

Physical Exam Findings *"Dry as a bone, Red as a beet, Hot as Hades, Blind as a bat, Mad as a Hatter, Stuffed as a pipe."*

1. Dry mucous membranes and dry axilla
2. Flushing
3. Hyperthermia
4. Blurred vision, mydriasis (late finding up to 24 hours after overdose)
5. Delirium with soft mumbled incoherent speech, unable to complete sentences or attend to a conversation
6. Hallucinations.
7. Urinary retention, absent or hypoactive bowel sounds
8. Agitated or somnolent
9. Hypertension or hypotension may be present
10. Tachycardia
11. Seizure

Mechanism of Action

Antimuscarinic
1. Blocks areas that acetylcholine binds to the muscarinic receptor. While "anticholinergic" is the common nomenclature, antimuscarinic is a more correct characterization of toxicity, as cholinergic nicotinic receptors are unaffected.
2. Includes receptors in the CNS, postganglionic parasympathetic nerve endings, and postganglionic sympathetically innervated sweat glands. Substances and medications which have significant antimuscarinic activity are listed in Table 15.1.

Treatment

1. Good supportive care and prevention of further exposure to antimuscarinic agents (i.e., stop exposure to the offending agent).
2. Avoid physical restraint and opt for chemical treatment of agitation.
   a. Benzodiazepines: Lorazepam 1–2 mg every 20 minutes or Diazepam 5–10 mg every 10 minutes. Aggressively titrate doses with an endpoint of arousable somnolence.
   b. Avoid psychotropic medications, as many have anticholinergic properties and may potentiate toxicity (e.g., olanzapine). *Although psychotropic medications are the mainstay of treatment for undifferentiated agitated delirium, the mechanism for drug-induced delirium is physiologically distinct and should be treated as such.*
3. Treat EKG QRS interval greater than 120 milliseconds due to sodium channel blockade with sodium bicarbonate. Many antimuscarinic agents also have sodium channel blocking properties similar to tricyclic antidepressants (TCAs). Initially treat with 1–3 amps of sodium bicarbonate via bolus. Then infuse 150 MEQ NaHCO3 in 1 liter of D5W with a rate up to twice maintenance to narrow QRS (Sasyniuk & Jhamandas, 1984).

Table 15.1 Antimuscarinic Substances

Class	Common (Based on frequency of reporting on AAPCC database)	Others
Antihistamines	Diphenhydramine Chlorpheniramine Dimenhydrinate	Doxylamine Meclizine Prochlorperazine Promethazine
Muscle relaxants	Cyclobenzaprine Orphenadrine	
Tricyclic antidepressants (TCA)	Amitriptyline Nortriptyline Imipramine	Amoxapine Clomipramine Desipramine Doxepin Trimipramine
Antipsychotics	Olanzapine Quetiapine	Chlorpromazine Clozaril Erphenazine Fluphenazine Loxapine Molindone Perphenazine Thioridazine
Antispasmodics	Dicyclomine	Methantheline bromide
Antiparkinsonian drugs	Benztropine Trihexyphenidyl	Biperiden Procyclidine
Plants	Jimsonweed Deadly nightshade	Angel's trumpet Mandrake Henbane

4. Physostigmine 0.5–2 mg IV push over 5 minutes.
   a. Diagnostic: Acetylcholinesterase inhibitor. Will reverse mental status, but only lasts for about an hour.
   b. Therapeutically, physostigmine may improve severe delirium and agitation management by temporarily improving mental status while allowing time to titrate sedation.

c. Do *NOT* use in patients with known TCA ingestion, seizures, QRS prolongation, or bradycardia. Use has been associated with seizures, bradycardia, and asystole. *If you are uncertain what the patient has ingested, avoid using this drug.*

Special Considerations: Tricyclic Antidepressant Overdoses

The main presentation of tricyclic antidepressant (TCA) overdose is an antimuscarinic syndrome. However, these drugs work on multiple receptors, leading to additional signs and symptoms of toxicity (see Table 15.2).

Table 15.2 Seven Mechanisms of TCA Toxicity

Mechanism	Effect
1 *Antihistaminic*	Sedation
2 *Catecholamine/serotonin reuptake inhibition*	Tachycardia, agitation, hypertension
3 *Antimuscarinic*	Delirium, dry mucous membranes, dry axilla, agitation
4 *Sodium channel blockade*	QRS interval widening
5 *Potassium channel blockade*	QTc interval widening
6 *Alpha receptor blockade*	Hypotension
7 *GABA blockade*	Seizure

Adapted from Mills (2004).

Treatment Considerations

Mortality from TCA overdose is strongly associated with cardiac dysrhythmia due to sodium channel blockade. EKG should be obtained in all patients demonstrating antimuscarinic toxicity.

(Hulten et al., 1992)

If QRS widening does not occur in the first six hours after ingestion, it is unlikely to occur.

(Liebelt et al., 1995)

1. Widened QRS should be treated with sodium bicarbonate (Sasyniuk & Jhamandas, 1984) with the following goals:
   a. QRS < 120 ms
   b. pH 7.5–7.55
   c. Serum sodium to 150–155 mmol
   d. *The patient may require bolus vials of sodium bicarbonate to initially stabilize the patient.*

2. For hypotension, treat with a direct vasopressor such as norepinephrine or epinephrine as dopamine may worsen hypotension (Tran et al., 1997).
3. *Avoid physostigmine in the TCA overdose as it has been associated with bradycardia and asystole* (Pentel & Peterson, 1980).
4. Avoid antipsychotics in particular for this overdose.
   a. Can worsen clinical presentation, as many of the antipsychotic medications have anticholinergic properties (e.g., olanzapine).
   b. Can also contribute to worsening cardiac dysrhythmias, as these medications can have sodium and potassium channel effects.
   c. Potentially may lower the seizure threshold.

Treatment, as with other anticholinergic drugs, consists of supportive care and titrated benzodiazepines for agitation and seizures. Avoid phenytoin for seizure, as it may increase cardiovascular toxicity (Callaham et al., 1988).

Cholinergic Syndrome

Clinical Presentation

Physical Exam Findings: "DUMBBELLS"

1. Diarrhea
2. Urination
3. Miosis/muscle weakness
4. Bronchorrhea/bronchospasm
5. Bradycardia
6. Emesis
7. Lacrimation
8. Lethargy
9. Salivation/sweating/seizure

Mechanism of Action

The mechanism of action is through stimulation of the nicotinic and muscarinic receptors by physiologically increasing acetylcholine available at receptor sites. Symptoms may be purely nicotinic, purely muscarinic, or a combination, depending upon the substance involved (see Table 15.3 for substances with significant cholinergic activity).

Table 15.3 Cholinergic Xenobiotics

Class	Drug
Urinary retention drug	Bethanechol
Acetylcholinesterase inhibitors	Neostigmine Pyridostigmine Physostigmine Rivastigmine
Glaucoma medication	Carbachol Echothiophate Pilocarpine
Alzheimer's disease medications	Donepezil Galantamine Tacrine
Natural substances	Nicotine (*Ingestion*) Clitocybe and Inocybe mushrooms

Note: With the e-cig (vaping) trend, the amount of nicotine ingested and formulation concentration need to be considered. Contact the poison center for specific product information.

Treatment
1. Supportive care and removal of exposure to the offending agent
2. Atropine and/or glycopyrolate for treatment of muscarinic symptoms (Eddleston et al., 2004)
   a. 1 vial = 1 mg boluses as needed
   b. Titrate to treat bradycardia and prevent/reduce diarrhea and bronchial secretions
3. Use benzodiazepines to treat seizures; if refractory, load with phenobarbital (Murphy et al., 1993).

Sympathomimetic Syndrome

Clinical Presentation

Physical Exam Findings: "Fight or Flight"

1. Psychomotor agitation/anxiety/hallucinations/delusions
2. Mydriasis
3. Diaphoresis
4. Tachycardia/hypertension/hyperthermia
5. Seizures
6. Rhabdomyolysis
7. Dysrhythmias.

Mechanism of Action

The mechanism of action stems from increased catecholamine effect at the receptor sites (see Table 15.4). This can occur from the following:

1. Direct agonism of alpha and beta adrenergic receptors (Gold, Geyer, & Koob, 1989);
2. Mixed/indirect action by inducing release of presynaptic norepinephrine;
3. Reuptake inhibition at the synapse, leading to excess stimulation of the adrenergic receptors (Groves et al., 1989);
4. Monoamine oxidase inhibitors (MAOI)/catechol-O-methyl transferase inhibitors (COMTI), which prevent metabolism of catecholamines;
5. Mixed ingestions or single medication overdoses.

Treatment

1. Stop the offending agents;
2. Benzodiazepines for agitation (Derlet et al., 1990);

Table 15.4 Sympathomimetic Xenobiotics

Mechanism of Toxicity	Common	Others
Direct acting	Albuterol Epinephrine	Ergot alkaloids Midodrine Terbutaline
Mixed/indirect acting	Amphetamine "Bath salts" Caffeine Cocaine	Methylphenidate Fenfluramine Dopamine Tyramine
Reuptake inhibitors	Amphetamine Buproprion Tramadol Venlafaxine	Carbamazepine Cyclic antidepressants Duloxetine Trihexyphenidyl

3. Hydration; patients can have high insensible water losses due to psychomotor agitation, diaphoresis, and fever;
4. Active cooling for hyperthermia with ice or cooling blanket; drug-induced hyperthermia is associated with increased morbidity and mortality (Marzuk et al., 1998);
5. Consider a single dose of a typical antipsychotic such as haloperidol (2.5–5 mg) for psychomotor agitation or choreoathetoid movements related to the dopaminergic effects of a stimulant (Espelin & Done, 1968); consider a dose of antipsychotic medication if 10–20 mg equivalents of lorazepam have not controlled the agitation;
6. Treat severe hypertension with phentolamine (2–5 mg IV) (Bieck & Antonin, 1988); *avoid using beta blockers due to a possible unopposed alpha effect.*

Special Consideration: MAOI Overdose

MAOI overdose is relatively uncommon, accounting for 0.22% of all antidepressant overdoses in the 2012 AAPCC database (Mowry et al., 2012).

Mechanism of Toxicity

The mechanism of toxicity is prevention of presynaptic metabolism of monoamine neurotransmitters. See Table 15.5 for a list of substances with MAO inhibition.

Toxicity

Toxicity is frequently biphasic, with the initial presentation of CNS excitation and peripheral sympathetic stimulation followed by coma with cardiovascular collapse. This is thought to be caused by the initial

Table 15.5 MAO Inhibitors

Type	Substances	
1st Generation: Nonselective irreversible inhibition	Phenelzine Isocarboxazid Tranylcypromine	
2nd Generation: Selective and irreversible inhibition	MAO-A Clorgyline	MAO-B Selegiline Rasagiline
3rd Generation: Selective and reversible	Moclobemide Brofaromine Toloxatone	
Other MAOIs	St. John's wort, Linezolid, Ladostigil	

adrenergic crisis, followed by inhibition of norepinephrine release and depletion of catecholamine stores (Gessa, Cuenca, & Costa, 1963).

The patient may be asymptomatic for several hours before showing clinical toxicity. However, toxicity will present within the first 24 hours after the overdose (Linden, Rumack, & Strehlke, 1984).

Treatment

1. Stop the offending agent;
2. Supportive care and fluid resuscitation; treat hyperthermia aggressively with active cooling methods like ice baths or cold water (Marzuk et al., 1998);
3. Avoid use of beta blockers alone due to unopposed alpha effect; phentolamine (2–5 mg IV) or other alpha adrenergic antagonists may be used in the treatment of hypertension (Bieck & Antonin, 1988);
4. For hypotension, aggressively treat with fluid resuscitation and direct acting vasopressors like epinephrine and norepinephrine. Dopamine is contraindicated and can worsen hypotension in these cases (Braverman, McCarthy, & Ivankovich, 1987). Hypotension is thought to occur secondary to catecholamine depletion.
5. Benzodiazepines for muscle rigidity, seizures, and agitation;
6. Life-threatening dysrhythmias require emergent cardioversion, while stable patients with ventricular tachycardia may benefit from antidysrhythmic drugs such as lidocaine.

Special Consideration: Hyperadrenergic Crisis

Monoamine oxidase-A (MAO-A) inhibitors may interact with tyramine-containing foods, resulting in an adrenergic crisis (see Table 15.6). A meal containing 6–8 mg of tyramine can potentially induce this

Table 15.6 Tyramine-Containing Substances

Red Wine

Fava Beans

Smoked, pickled, or aged fish

Sauerkraut

Liver

Figs

Yeast

Avocado/Guacamole

Aged cheeses (cheddar, parmesan, Swiss, blue cheese)

Aged, pickled, and fermented meats (sausages, salami, etc.)

Banana peels or stewed bananas

Distilled alcohol and select beers (tap beers)

Soybean products

Adapted from Walker et al. (1996)

reaction, and a total ingestion of 25–50 mg can produce severe and possibly life-threatening reactions (Walker et al., 1996).

Mechanism of Toxicity

Tyramine is an indirect-acting sympathomimetic with a similar mechanism of action as amphetamine (Youdim & Weinstock, 2004). Normal MAO-A in the intestinal wall and liver prevents dietary amines such as tyramine from entering the circulation. However, with irreversible MAO-A inhibition, the protective mechanism is lost, leading to a massive release of catecholamines and "hyperadrenergic crisis" (Bieck & Antonin, 1988).

Toxicity

The presentation is hallmarked by hypertension, headache, flushing, diaphoresis, mydriasis, neuromuscular excitation, and potential cardiac dysrhythmia. Most patients who follow the dietary restrictions have few side effects, with only up to 10% of patients chronically on MAOIs subjectively reporting reactions (Rabkin et al., 1985).

Treatment

1. Stop the offending agent.
2. Similar to treatment for the sympathomimetic toxidrome and MAOI overdose.
3. Consider using short-acting alpha adrenergic antagonists such as phentolamine (Bieck & Antonin, 1988);
4. Success of blood pressure control has been seen with dihydropyridine calcium channel blockers such as nifedipine and oral alpha adrenergic antagonists such as terazosin (Hesselink, 1991). Caution must be taken to not be overly aggressive in blood pressure reduction, as this may lead to decreased cerebral perfusion.

Patients must wait at least three weeks following discontinuation of their MAOI before it is considered safe to ingest such foods (Thase et al., 1995).

Sedative-Hypnotic Syndrome

Clinical Presentation

Physical Exam Findings: "Sleepy with Normal Vital Signs"
1. Sedated with otherwise benign physical exam;
2. As sedative dose increases, the likelihood of respiratory depression increases.

Mechanism of Action

Presentation can be caused by GABA agonism, N-methyl-D-asparate (NMDA) antagonism, or a combination of both (Criswell et al., 2004), see Table 15.7.

Treatment

1. Supportive care;
2. Intubation for respiratory depression versus antidotal reversal;
3. The antidote for benzodiazepine toxicity is flumazenil. Indicated for respiratory depression, the drug should be used with caution in persons with chronic benzodiazepine use, as it may induce significant withdrawal symptoms including seizures (Spivey et al., 1993).

Table 15.7 Sedative-Hypnotic Substances

Benzodiazepines
Barbiturates
Ethanol
Propofol
Meprobamate/Carisoprodol
Gluththimide
Chloral hydrate
Paraldehyde
Zolpidem

Key Points

1. Obtain a good history and physical examination.
2. Identify the toxidrome.
3. Stop the offending agent(s).
4. Generally, treatment for a poisoned patient is good supportive care.
5. Toxic physiology is not the same as infectious/septic physiology, so don't start any agent that might make the toxidrome worse.
6. Benzodiazepines are generally the safest option for treating agitation in a poisoned patient.
7. If you must start a vasopressor for hypotension, use direct-acting pressors such as epinephrine or norepinephrine.

Disclosures

Dr. Abesamis does not have any conflicts of interest.

Further Reading

Bieck PR, Antonin KH (1988). Oral tyramine pressor test and the safety of monoamine oxidase inhibitor drugs: Comparison of brofaromine and tranylcypromine in healthy subjects. *J Clin Psychopharmacol.*, 8(4), 237–245.

Braverman B, McCarthy RJ, et al. (1987). Vasopressor challenges during chronic MAOI or TCA treatment in anesthetized dogs. *Life Sci.*, 40(26), 2587–2595.

Brent J, Wallace KL, et al. (Eds.) (2005) Critical care toxicology: Diagnosis and management of the critically poisoned patient, Chapters 32, 39, 42, 47, 1st ed. Philadelphia: Elsevier Mosby.

Callaham M, Schumaker H, et al. (1988). Phenytoin prophylaxis of cardiotoxicity in experimental amitriptyline poisoning. *J Pharmacol Exp Ther.*, 245(1), 216–220.

Criswell HE, Ming Z, et al. (2004). Macrokinetic analysis of blockade of NMDA-gated currents by substituted alcohols, alkanes and ethers. *Brain Res.*, 1015(1–2), 107–113.

Derlet RW, Albertson TE, et al. (1990). Antagonism of cocaine, amphetamine and methamphetamine toxicity. *Pharmacol Biochem Behav.*, 36(4), 745–749.

Eddleston M, Buckley NA, et al. (2004). Speed of initial atropinisation in significant organophosphorus pesticide poisoning: A systematic comparison of recommended regimens. *J Toxicol Clin Toxicol.*, 42(6), 865–875.

Espelin DE, Done AK (1968). Amphetamine poisoning: Effectiveness of chlorpromazine. *N Engl J Med.*, 278(25), 1361–1365.

Gessa GL, Cuenca E, et al. (1963). On the mechanism of hypotensive effects of MAO inhibitors. *Ann N Y Acad Sci.*, 107, 935–944.

Gold LH, Geyer MA, et al. (1989). Neurochemical mechanisms involved in behavioral effects of amphetamines and related designer drugs. *NIDA Res Monogr.*, 94, 101–126.

Groves PM, Ryan LJ, et al. (1989). Neuronal actions of amphetamine in the rat brain. *NIDA Res Monogr.*, 94, 127–145.

Hesselink JM (1991). Safer use of MAOIs with nifedipine to counteract potential hypertensive crisis. *Am J Psychiat.*, 148(11), 1616.

Hulten BA, Adams R, et al. (1992). Predicting severity of tricyclic antidepressant overdose. *J Toxicol Clin Toxicol.*, 30(2), 161–170.

Liebelt EL, Francis PD, et al. (1995). ECG lead aVR versus QRS interval in predicting seizures and arrhythmias in acute tricyclic antidepressant toxicity. *Ann Emerg Med.*, 26(2), 195–201.

Linden CH, Rumack BH, et al. (1984). Monoamine oxidase inhibitor overdose. *Ann Emerg Med.*, 13(12), 1137–1144.

Marzuk PM, Tardiff K, Leon AC, Hirsch CS, Portera L, Iqbal MI, et al. (1998). Ambient temperature and mortality from unintentional cocaine overdose. *JAMA*, 279(22), 1795–1800.

Mowry JB, Spyker DA, et al. 2012 Annual Report of the American Association of Poison Control Centers' National Poison Data System (NPDS): 30th Annual Report. *Clin Toxicol (Phila)*, 51(10), 949–1229.

Murphy MR, Blick DW, et al. (1993). Diazepam as a treatment for nerve agent poisoning in primates. *Aviat Space Environ Med.*, 64(2), 110–115.

Nelson L, et al. (Eds.) (2010). *Goldfrank's Toxicologic Emergencies*, Chapters 13, 50, 71, 73 75, 76, 9th ed. New York: McGraw-Hill.

Pentel P, Peterson CD (1980). Asystole complicating physostigmine treatment of tricyclic antidepressant overdose. *Ann Emerg Med.*, 9(11), 588–590.

Rabkin JG, Quitkin FM, et al. (1985). Adverse reactions to monoamine oxidase inhibitors. Part II: Treatment correlates and clinical management. *J Clin Psychopharmacol.*, 5(1), 2–9.

Sasyniuk BI, Jhamandas V (1984). Mechanism of reversal of toxic effects of amitriptyline on cardiac Purkinje fibers by sodium bicarbonate. *J Pharmacol Exp Ther.*, 231(2), 387–394.

Spivey WH, Roberts JR, et al. (1993). A clinical trial of escalating doses of flumazenil for reversal of suspected benzodiazepine overdose in the emergency department. *Ann Emerg Med.*, 22(12), 1813–1821.

Thase ME, Trivedi MH, et al. (1995). MAOIs in the contemporary treatment of depression. *Neuropsychopharmacology*, 12(3), 185–219.

Tran TP, Panacek EA, et al. (1997). Response to dopamine vs norepinephrine in tricyclic antidepressant-induced hypotension. *Acad Emerg Med.*, 4(9), 864–868.

Walker SE, Shulman KI, et al. (1996). Tyramine content of previously restricted foods in monoamine oxidase inhibitor diets. *J Clin Psychopharmacol.*, 16(5), 383–388.

Youdim MB, Weinstock M (2004). Therapeutic applications of selective and non-selective inhibitors of monoamine oxidase A and B that do not cause significant tyramine potentiation. *Neurotoxicology*, 25(1–2), 243–250.

Exercises

1. A 17-year-old male presents with tachycardia, hypertension, dry mouth, dry axilla, and hyperreflexia with a 2–3 beat clonus. He has a medical history of ADHD and on methylphenidate. An empty box of "sleeping pills" was found next to him. He has no other injuries. Vital signs are only remarkable for the tachycardia of 130 bpm and a fever of 38.9C. Laboratory studies show a mild metabolic acidosis and the EKG shows sinus tachycardia with a QRS of 102 ms. Which toxidrome best matches this presentation?
   a. Sympathomimetic
   b. Hyperadrenergic crisis
   c. Cholinergic
   d. Anticholinergic

2. This same patient was treated with 3 mg of lorazepam over the next 6 hours in the ICU. He is still agitated and pulling on his soft restraints. They request additional treatment for his agitated delirium. Which is the most appropriate drug for treatment?
   a. Carbamazepine
   b. Additional lorazepam
   c. Olanzapine
   d. Quetiapine

3. A 24-year-old former IV heroin abuser presents hypertensive, tachycardic, and diaphoretic. She has been under treatment for infective endocarditis and on Linezolid due to medication allergies. She was out drinking wine with her friends when her symptoms suddenly started. She denies any chest pain or shortness of breath. She is currently taking clonazepam, birth control pills, baclofen, and linezolid. What is the most likely cause of her presentation?
   a. She is having a hypertensive crisis.
   b. She is experiencing withdrawal.
   c. She has a blood clot.
   d. She has gone back to abusing drugs.

4. A 4-year-old child gets into his grandparent's pill box. He presents bradycardic with vomiting, profuse salivation, and diarrhea. The grandparent is currently on quetiapine, donezepil, buproprion, aspirin, and carisoprodol. Which of these drugs is likely causing this presentation?
   a. Aspirin
   b. Buproprion
   c. Quetiapine
   d. Carisoprodol
   e. Donezepil

Answers: (1) d (2) b (3) a (4) e

Substance Intoxication and Withdrawal States in the General Medical Setting

Jody Glance, Priya Gopalan, and Kurt D. Ackerman

Substance Use Disorders in the General Medical Setting

Substance use disorders (SUDs) are a frequent reason for psychiatric consultation in the medical setting. Because addiction is a chronic, relapsing, and remitting disease, patients with SUDs often struggle with repeated hospital admissions for intoxication and withdrawal, as well as for medical conditions related to substance use such as liver disease, cardiac abnormalities, and pancreatitis. Additionally, withdrawal symptoms may arise unexpectedly in patients without a known SUD who are admitted for other medical problems. Early warning signs may be missed if the medical team does not anticipate their occurrence.

Comorbid behavior patterns frequently seen in patients with SUDs may result in hospital staff having difficulty approaching patients with objectivity. Valid pain complaints may be dismissed as drug-seeking behaviors, leading to further stigmatization, poor medical care, and potential misdiagnosis of injuries or illness. Further, frustration toward patients who are perceived to have caused their illnesses (e.g., cirrhosis, HIV, hepatitis C) may lead to inadequate history-taking and missed diagnoses of SUDs, which could in turn delay diagnosis and treatment.

Additionally, patients with SUDs may have psychiatric disorders that must be managed appropriately. Psychiatric illness increases the risk for SUDs, with highest rates seen in patients with bipolar disorder, followed by schizophrenia, anxiety disorders, and major depression. While consultation may be requested for managing intoxication or withdrawal, a comprehensive approach is required in order to identify treatment needs and motivate patients to pursue further treatment.

Screening and Assessment

Screening for substance use in the medical setting is an important first step in identifying SUDs. There are several validated screening tools for detecting alcohol use disorders (AUDs), with many taking ≤ 10 minutes to complete. The best-known and most widely used are the CAGE questionnaire (Ewing, 1984) and the Alcohol Use Disorders Identification Test (AUDIT; Babor et al., 2001).

CAGE is an acronym for asking about (1) feeling a need to Cut down on drinking; (2) feeling Annoyed when others comment on use; (3) feeling Guilty about use; and (4) requiring an Eye-opener (i.e., drinking alcohol in the morning to avoid withdrawal symptoms). A score of ≥ 2 suggests excessive drinking, warranting further evaluation (Dhalla & Kopec, 2007).

The AUDIT is a 10-question screen scored 0–40, with scores of ≥ 8 for men (7 for women) suggesting a high likelihood of hazardous drinking behaviors (e.g., binge drinking), and scores of ≥ 15 (13 for women) indicating a severe AUD. Some clinicians may find the AUDIT too lengthy and prefer the AUDIT-C (Bradley et al., 2007), a three-item validated screening test using questions from the AUDIT, which has been found to have similar sensitivity and specificity. The AUDIT-C, scored 0–12, inquires how often the person has an alcoholic beverage, how many drinks they have on a typical drinking day, and how often they have ≥ 6 drinks on one occasion. Scores of ≥ 4 (3 for women) are suggestive of problem drinking.

Perhaps lesser known are screening instruments for determining other SUDs. The simple question, "How many times in the past year have you used an illegal drug or used a prescription medication for non-medical reasons?" detects SUDs in primary care settings with 100% sensitivity and 73.5% specificity (Smith, 2010). A corresponding version of the AUDIT has also been developed. The Drug Use Disorders Identification Test consists of 11 self-administered items measured from 0 to 44 (Berman et al., 2005) and takes ~10 minutes to complete. The National Institute on Drug Abuse (NIDA) has developed a modified screening tool for identifying substance use in medical settings, the Alcohol, Smoking, and Substance Involvement Screening Test (NM-ASSIST), and may be administered by a clinician on a paper form (http://www.drugabuse.gov/sites/default/files/files/QuickScreen_Updated_2013%281%29.pdf) or online (http://www.drugabuse.gov/nmassist/), which can be integrated into the electronic medical record.

A positive screen detects the possibility that an SUD exists and indicates the need for more comprehensive evaluation. *DSM-5* has combined the criteria for previous diagnoses of "Substance Abuse" and "Substance Dependence" into one category termed "Substance Use Disorders," whereby meeting even one of the 11 criteria results in a diagnosis of SUD. This approach focuses on severity and how use negatively affects patients' lives. Brief interventions aimed at educating patients about the potential dangers of substance use, suggesting ways to reduce use, and providing information on social norms and what is considered "safe" use (e.g., one drink/day for women and two drinks/day for men) may help patients develop an internal discrepancy about use and consider decreasing or ceasing use.

Primary medical teams, social workers, and nursing staff may utilize screening tools to identify patients in need of withdrawal monitoring and management, to refer for further evaluation and treatment of SUDs, and to identify and guide management of patients at high risk for withdrawal. For delirious patients with unclear etiology, a simple screen may help to differentiate the etiology. Risk factors for developing complicated withdrawal include: BAL > 100 mg/dL on admission, history of withdrawal seizures or delirium tremens (DTs), autonomic hyperactivity, and concomitant use of benzodiazepines or barbiturates. While most institutions have withdrawal screening tools in place, few have been validated for use in medically ill populations. The Prediction of Alcohol Withdrawal Severity Scale (PAWSS) has been developed to help identify patients at risk of developing complicated alcohol withdrawal, with pilot data demonstrating 100% sensitivity, specificity, and positive and negative predictive values (Maldonado et al., 2014).

Urine Drug Screens

Urine drug screening (UDS) is a useful tool in the clinical setting. Urine samples are easily collected and can provide rapid results in emergent situations. UDS involves immunoassays that use antibodies to detect drugs or their metabolites. Results are always presumptive and must be interpreted in the context of the patient's medical and substance use histories, and recent use of other medications, vitamins, and supplements. Many substances cross-react with immunoassays, leading to false positive results (see Table 16.1). Conversely, laboratory cutoff values may be too high to detect lower concentrations, leading to false negatives. Sensitivity of drug selection also varies (e.g., an assay may detect alprazolam but not clonazepam at the same amount of use). Thus, a clinician may wish to confirm immunoassay results using gas or liquid chromatography/mass spectrometry, especially in situations where presenting symptoms do not concur with patient history or initial UDS results.

Table 16.1 Urine Drug Screen Detection Times and Potential False Positives

Substance Tested	Length of Detection Time in Urine	Agents Potentially Contributing to False Positives
Amphetamine/ Methamphetamine	48 hours	Antihistamines, decongestants, bupropion, trazodone, chlorpromazine, ranitidine
Benzodiazepines	3–30 days, depending on half-life	Sertraline
Cocaine	2–4 days (metabolites)	None likely
Cannabis	Single use: 3 days Moderate use (4x/wk): 5–7 days Daily use: 10–15 days Chronic use: > 30 days	Ibuprofen, naproxen
Opioids	Heroin, codeine, morphine: 48 hours Hydromorphone, oxycodone, methadone: 2–4 days	Quinolone antibiotics Methadone only: Diphenhydramine, doxylamine, clomipramine, chlorpromazine, quetiapine, thioridazine, verapamil
Phencyclidine (PCP)	8 days	Dextromethorphan, ibuprofen, venlafaxine

Alcohol and Other GABA-agonists

Intoxication and withdrawal states for alcohol, benzodiazepine, and other GABA-agonists have characteristic signs and symptoms that may overlap with those of other medical disorders. A typical presentation of acute intoxication may include slurred speech, reddened conjunctivae, dilated and sluggishly reactive pupils, loss of motor coordination, and ataxia. Behavioral manifestations include decreased attention span, mood changes, disinhibition, and poor judgment (see Table 16.2).

Between 25% and 50% of dependent drinkers will experience withdrawal upon alcohol cessation. Of these, 20%–25% experience moderate-severe symptoms requiring close monitoring, suggesting a 5%–12% risk of significant withdrawal in patients with alcohol dependence, with approximately 5% progressing to DTs and 3% developing seizures. In patients with high tolerance, withdrawal symptoms may appear before the blood alcohol level approaches zero. Conversely, symptoms may not emerge for several days due to variability in individual pharmacokinetics and any concurrent administration of GABA-agonists. For example, some patients experience withdrawal following cessation of prolonged intubation with propofol, as it exhibits similar receptor effects to recreational alcohol.

Withdrawal from alcohol and other GABA-agonists may be conceptualized as a series of high-risk periods, with alcohol withdrawal having a more predictable time course than other GABA-agonists. Within the first 24 hours of cessation or significant reduction of use, the patient may develop flushing and tremors. Hallucinations (visual or tactile) may develop in 24–48 hours. The primary treatment is benzodiazepines, *not* antipsychotics, as these hallucinations are due to GABAergic withdrawal

Table 16.2 Clinical Manifestations at Increasing Breath Alcohol Concentration Levels

Breath Alcohol Concentration	Clinical Manifestations*
0.01–0.1	Disinhibition, euphoria, mild deficits in attention and coordination, increased reaction time
0.1–0.2	Increasing deficits in attention, coordination and reaction time, mood lability, impaired judgment, dysarthric speech, ataxic gait
0.2–0.3	Confusion, incoherent thoughts, severely impaired coordination, nausea/vomiting
0.3–0.4	Stupor, loss of consciousness, possible death
> 0.55	Death likely

* Effects may vary based on level of tolerance

(and antipsychotics can lower seizure threshold). Alcohol withdrawal seizures are generally tonic-clonic, with the highest risk period occurring ~48 hours after the last drink.

DTs may develop within the first five days of cessation. DTs are seen in ~5% of patients undergoing withdrawal and are identified by delirium and autonomic instability (i.e., unpredictable vital signs). Mortality rates can be as high as 40%, but with intensive medical treatment rates are reduced to 5%–15%, with death occurring due to aspiration pneumonia or cardiac arrhythmias. High-level monitoring is critical in patients who develop early signs of DTs. Other GABA-agonists (e.g., benzodiazepines) can produce similar withdrawal syndromes, with more severe withdrawal observed in patients using drugs with shorter half-lives (see Table 16.3 for relative half-lives and dose equivalency).

Table 16.3 Pharmacology and Dose Equivalency of Common Benzodiazepines

Medication (Trade Name)	Dose Equivalent	Time to Peak (hours)	Elimination Half-Life (hours)	Active Hepatic Metabolites
Alprazolam (*Xanax*)	0.5 mg	1–2	6–18	+
Chlordiazepoxide (*Librium*)	25 mg	1–4	5–30 (parent) 28–200 (metabolites)	+
Clonazepam (*Klonopin*)	0.25–0.5 mg	1–4	18–60	–
Diazepam (*Valium*)	5–10 mg	PO: 1–2 IM: 1 IV: 6–10 min	14–100 (parent) 30–200 (metabolites)	+
Lorazepam (*Ativan*)*	1 mg	PO: 1–4 IM: 1 IV: 5–10 min	8–24	–
Oxazepam (*Serax*)*	15 mg	1–4	3–20	–
Temazepam (*Restoril*)*	10 mg	2–3	8–22	–

Psychosomatic Medicine Pocket Cards, ©2014, University of Pittsburgh and UPMC. Reprinted and used with permission; all rights reserved.

Options for Managing GABA Withdrawal

Medical facilities differ in admission standards, use of withdrawal protocols, and access to treatment following stabilization. However, benzodiazepines are generally considered first-line agents for treating and preventing withdrawal. Choice of agent varies, depending on the patient's history and medical condition. Lorazepam is often preferred due to the availability of IV administration and the ability to prescribe to patients with hepatic insufficiency. Longer-acting agents may be preferable if the patient will continue with outpatient detoxification. For example, the patient may be given a loading dose of diazepam, with fast absorption and a long half-life that will gradually self-taper.

Potential non-benzodiazepine treatments for GABA withdrawal are being studied, including valproic acid, baclofen, gabapentin, and alpha-2 agonists such as clonidine. These agents focus on correcting the relative imbalance of GABA versus glutamate/N-methyl-D-aspartate (NMDA) systems during withdrawal and limiting the autonomic instability that leads to adverse outcomes during DTs. Because these agents have not been thoroughly studied for use in withdrawal, we do not yet recommend their use as first-line treatment. Similarly, ethanol should not be used to manage withdrawal due to a lack of evidence supporting its use, difficulty in monitoring and titration, significant risk of continued damage to end organs, and an unspoken message to the patient that the SUD does not merit appropriate treatment.

Benzodiazepines may be used in a number of ways for managing withdrawal. In order of increasing acuity, these include the following:

- Symptom-triggered administration based on a withdrawal assessment scale
- Gradual taper over a three- to five-day period
- Taper combined with symptom-triggered management
- Front-loaded administration of long-acting benzodiazepines with subsequent monitoring
- Continuous IV infusion (reserved for severe cases).

Table 16.4 describes characteristics of each approach and optimal use. Factors influencing protocol choice include symptom severity, history of seizures or DTs, patient's ability to communicate effectively, and likelihood that concurrent psychiatric illness or medical delirium will create false positives on withdrawal assessment.

Monitoring vital signs and sedation, along with assessment using a standardized scale, such as the Clinical Institute Withdrawal Assessment of Alcohol Scale, Revised (CIWA-Ar; Sullivan et al., 1989), is critical to determine whether the patient is receiving effective treatment. Most withdrawal instruments assess subjective symptoms such as agitation and anxiety, in addition to objective findings such as tremors, flushing, and autonomic signs. The CIWA-Ar is well validated, and the most commonly used instrument; however, the lack of vital sign monitoring may decrease its sensitivity for complicated withdrawal.

Table 16.4 Standardized Approach to Management of GABA-Agonist Withdrawal Using Benzodiazepines

Protocol	Description	Optimal Uses
Symptom-triggered administration	A standardized assessment scale (e.g., CIWA-Ar) is administered approximately q4h Benzodiazepines are administered if score exceeds threshold	• Surveillance and initial treatment of patients at risk for withdrawal • Treatment of mild to moderate withdrawal in patients with relatively intact cognition (if non-withdrawal delirium will not create false positives)
Benzodiazepine taper	Administer a standing dose of BZD and decrease by approximately 20%–25% per day • e.g., Day 1: chlordiazepoxide 50 mg every 6 hours • Day 2: 50 mg every 8 hours • Day 3: 50 mg every 12 hours • Day 4: 50 mg at bedtime only then d/c *Withdrawal symptoms may arise as taper decreases; assessments should be done routinely along with taper to monitor effectiveness *May need slower taper for benzodiazepine withdrawal than alcohol withdrawal	• Management of benzodiazepine withdrawal • Management of alcohol withdrawal in patients who have altered mental status unrelated to alcohol (e.g. psychosis), or cannot effectively communicate

Benzodiazepine taper with symptom-triggered breakthrough administration	Benzodiazepine taper as above along with additional PRN benzodiazepines if patient scores above threshold on assessment scale during withdrawal monitoring *May be optimal treatment for a Behavioral Health/Inpatient Detox setting where risk of false positive is low	• Initial treatment for patients with history of complicated withdrawal • Management of moderate-severe withdrawal • Management of withdrawal that gradually worsens despite initial treatment
Loading dose (aka "front-loading")	A long-acting benzodiazepine with rapid onset (e.g., diazepam) is administered in frequent, small boluses until the patient is sleepy but arousable • e.g., diazepam 10 mg IV every 10 minutes until mildly sedated May use oral or IV medication; risk of over-sedation is higher with oral administration due to delayed absorption Requires continuous pulse-oximetry and high-level monitoring during administration Withdrawal should be closely monitored for at least 48h after treatment	• Patients presenting with significant withdrawal symptoms and/or at high risk for complicated withdrawal • Patients not responding to other treatment (including those showing signs of impending DTs)
Continuous IV infusion	Reserved for the most severe cases (typically DTs) Lorazepam is commonly used Patient should be under constant monitoring in intensive care unit Risk of propylene glycol toxicity with prolonged use	• Patients in active DTs

Other Treatment Considerations

Wernicke's Encephalopathy/Korsakoff Syndrome

Wernicke's encephalopathy is a potential consequence of long-term alcohol use, and can be at least partially reversed by administering thiamine (vitamin B_1). IV or IM administration is preferred, as oral absorption may be decreased in long-term alcohol users. With few known side effects, it is advisable to give high doses (e.g., 500 mg IV tid) to any patient with known AUD and cognitive impairment until withdrawal and cognition have stabilized.

Wernicke's encephalopathy is characterized by sudden onset of the classic triad of ataxia, ocular signs (e.g., ophthalmoplegia or nystagmus), and altered mental status. However, only 15% of patients present with all three symptoms, requiring empiric treatment of the syndrome in high-risk patients without full criteria. Conventional teaching asserts that if not reversed with thiamine, Wernicke's encephalopathy will lead to Korsakoff syndrome with permanent memory loss (anterograde and retrograde). In reality, memory deficits often persist even with repletion of thiamine, as alcohol has selective adverse effects on mammillary bodies and the hippocampus.

Table 16.5 Medical Complications of Chronic Alcohol Use

Organ System	Complication of Chronic Use
Gastrointestinal	Variceal bleeding
	Hepatitis/cirrhosis of the liver
	Gastroesophageal reflux disease
	Peptic ulcer disease
	Acute/chronic pancreatitis
Cardiac	Hypertension
	Coronary artery disease
	Cardiomyopathy
	Peripheral artery disease/claudication
Central nervous system	Wernicke's encephalopathy/Korsakoff syndrome
	Alcohol-induced cognitive impairment
Peripheral nervous system	Peripheral neuropathy
Endocrine	Hyponatremia
	Hypoglycemia
	Diabetes mellitus
Hematologic	Macrocytic anemia

Medical Complications of Alcohol Use

Chronic alcohol users are at high risk of many other medical complications (see Table 16.5). A careful substance use history should be obtained in patients presenting with these symptoms.

Psychosocial Interventions

While managing acute substance withdrawal is essential, it is usually insufficient for assuring positive long-term health outcomes. Providers must also facilitate further SUD treatment, including residential programs, outpatient programs, and self-help groups (e.g., Alcoholics Anonymous). Addressing mood, anxiety, or other psychiatric disorders is critical. CBT can be adapted to treat SUDs as well by its incorporating elements of brief motivational interviewing (see Chapter 7).

Opioids

Acute symptoms of opioid overdose are typically managed by non-psychiatric providers. However, a solid understanding of opioid intoxication and withdrawal helps with toxidrome recognition and management. This represents a frequent psychosomatic consult for patients, including those with suicide attempts that are associated with opiate use, or who experience opiate withdrawal during other medical treatment. Withdrawal can be safely managed in inpatient or outpatient settings.

Opioid intoxication is characterized by initial euphoria, impaired judgment, and psychomotor changes. Physical signs and symptoms include pupillary constriction, drowsiness, slurred speech, and impairment in attention and/or memory.

The classic triad of opioid overdose includes **pinpoint pupils, respiratory depression**, and **coma**. For patients who are found to be unresponsive, respiratory depression (e.g., rate < 12) is the most sensitive indicator for overdose, especially with other stigmata of abuse such as fresh track marks. Treatment includes initial stabilization of the airway, breathing, and circulation with concomitant administration of naloxone (Narcan) 0.4–2 mg every 2–3 minutes until the respiratory depression is reversed.

A characteristic syndrome helps in differentiating opioid withdrawal from that of other substances the patient might also be abusing. **Opioid withdrawal** symptoms include rhinorrhea, lacrimation, piloerection, yawning, diaphoresis, heat/cold intolerance, myalgias, nausea/vomiting, abdominal cramping, diarrhea, and autonomic hyperactivity. Patients also frequently complain of insomnia, anxiety, and dysphoria.

Opioid withdrawal is generally not associated with increased risk of mortality; thus, symptomatic management is common. Clonidine, an alpha-2 adrenergic agonist, dampens norepinephrine outflow, reducing symptoms of withdrawal, including rhinorrhea, agitation, and anxiety. Hydroxyzine may be used for anxiety at doses of 25–50 mg every 4–6 hours. Trazodone 50–100 mg may be used for insomnia. Diarrhea may be treated with loperamide or diphenoxylate. Some centers use a buprenorphine taper for a more comfortable withdrawal. However, this may precipitate more severe withdrawal in patients who have very recently used opioids; thus, the patient should exhibit visible signs of withdrawal (as outlined above) prior to taper initiation.

Following detoxification, some patients may do well with **long-term opioid maintenance therapy (MT)** with methadone or buprenorphine. Substitution of long-acting opioid receptor agonists or partial agonists blocks the high from heroin and other shorter-acting agents and helps deter illicit drug use by preventing withdrawal and cravings. MT has been shown to reduce HIV and hepatitis co-infection, improve overall health outcomes, increase employment rates, and decrease crime rates. While methadone is a full opioid agonist, buprenorphine is a partial agonist at the μ opioid receptor, giving it a better safety profile, with little chance of fatal overdose when taken alone. Though there is less abuse potential than other opiates, there is nonetheless the potential for misuse, abuse, and diversion.

For patients on MT admitted to the hospital, the dose MUST be confirmed with the outpatient provider prior to ordering the medication, as mistakenly dosing a patient can result in over-sedation or respiratory compromise. Additionally, methadone may prolong the QTc interval and lead to risk of arrhythmia, especially if given in the context of an electrolyte imbalance or along with other medications that may cause QTc prolongation. Patients on MT admitted for injuries or surgeries should be provided with additional medications for pain relief. Management with MT alone is NOT sufficient for analgesic control.

Methadone treatment is the gold standard for pregnant patients with opiate addiction (see Chapter 17). Buprenorphine is increasingly being used as an alternative to methadone, with possible improvement in birth outcomes (Jones, 2010).

Mixed Withdrawal States

Psychiatric consultants may be challenged by managing withdrawal from multiple substances. When a patient undergoes simultaneous withdrawal from opioids and GABA agonists, management is guided by both subjective complaints and objective data (see Table 16.6). Similarly, patients with comorbid medical illness such as an active infection may present with symptoms such as agitation and a clouded sensorium, which can confuse the evaluation and result in falsely elevated scores on withdrawal assessment tools. Primary teams and nursing staff should be educated regarding proper use of benzodiazepines for clear indicators of GABAergic withdrawal. While first-line treatment, benzodiazepines should be administered with caution in medically high-risk patients (e.g., respiratory illness or concurrently taking prescribed opioids), particularly when given in IV form. **Antipsychotics should be avoided for treating agitation in an acute intoxication or withdrawal state due to their tendency to lower seizure threshold** (though they may be considered for extreme agitation not responding to benzodiazepines).

Table 16.6 Identification of Mixed Withdrawal States

Signs and Symptoms	Alcohol/Benzodiazepine Withdrawal	Opioid Withdrawal
Vital Signs	Autonomic instability (tachycardia, hypertension)	Mild vital sign changes
Pupils	Mild mydriasis	Marked pupillary dilation
Skin	Flushing, paroxysmal sweats	Piloerection, hot/cold flashes
GI	Gastritis, nausea/vomiting	Abdominal cramping, diarrhea, nausea/vomiting
Neuro	Tremors, seizures, headache, photophobia, phonophobia, disorientation, visual/tactile hallucinations	Tremors
Other	Restlessness/anxiety	Restlessness/anxiety, myalgias/joint pain, lacrimation, rhinorrhea, yawning

Other Drugs of Abuse

Cocaine and Other Stimulants

Cocaine, amphetamines, and other stimulants present similarly during intoxication and withdrawal, and are thus discussed as a group. Stimulants are sympathomimetic drugs that act via reuptake inhibition of serotonin, norepinephrine, and dopamine, with some also contributing to presynaptic dopamine release. Signs of stimulant intoxication include pupillary dilation, psychomotor agitation or retardation, diaphoresis, chills, nausea/vomiting, muscle weakness, chest pain. Patients are often admitted to the medical hospital after a stimulant overdose because of dangerous medical complications, including autonomic instability, respiratory depression, cardiac arrhythmias, seizures, delirium, and coma. Cardiac monitoring is essential in patients with autonomic or cardiac symptoms to prevent death from myocardial infarction or arrhythmias (such as ventricular fibrillation). Stroke may also occur.

Management of stimulant intoxication is frequently non-pharmacologic. It is often sufficient to observe patients in a quiet environment and to provide reassurance that distressing symptoms are a direct result of drug use and will soon subside. Benzodiazepines (e.g., lorazepam, diazepam) may be used for acute agitation, which will also help decrease blood pressure. If an antihypertensive agent is required, phentolamine is recommended. Dexmedetomidine (Precedex), a central alpha-2 agonist, may treat agitation from amphetamine overdose (Spiller et al., 2013), and may also treat comorbid autonomic symptoms. Adrenergic-blocking medications such as propranolol should not be used, as they may exacerbate stimulant-induced vasoconstriction. Antipsychotics should be used with caution, as they can lower seizure threshold and increase autonomic instability. If antipsychotics are required, haloperidol or risperidone are good choices, as they have minimal anticholinergic activity and thus contribute less to delirium and hyperthermia. Supportive care with cardiac monitoring and fluid support may be necessary.

Psychoactive effects of cocaine and stimulants include euphoria, anxiety, insomnia, hyperactivity, paranoid ideation, hypervigilance, and hallucinations (auditory, visual, and tactile) that may lead to dramatic behavior changes, including violent or aggressive behaviors. Stimulant-induced psychotic disorders are difficult to distinguish from primary psychotic disorders such as schizophrenia without history, collateral information, or lab work. Cocaine-induced psychosis is usually shorter in duration than that of other stimulants. Any psychosis lasting more than a few weeks after cessation of use suggests an underlying etiology other than substance use (e.g., an "unmasking" of a primary psychotic disorder in a vulnerable individual). Unfortunately, clinical guidelines are lacking regarding when to initiate treatment with antipsychotic medications and duration of treatment in patients with suspected substance-induced psychosis. One approach is to start medications if the psychotic symptoms are causing significant impairment, continue treatment for at least one month (assuming the patient has stabilized and is no longer using the stimulant), then taper and discontinue the antipsychotic with close monitoring for return of symptoms.

Treatment of withdrawal is symptomatic. There is no need to taper stimulants. Stimulant withdrawal is often associated with a "crash," characterized by lethargy, dysphoria, and at times, suicidal ideation. Thus, patients who are withdrawing from these substances may require psychiatric hospitalization until their mood has stabilized. Hypersomnia and increased appetite are also common following cessation of chronic cocaine use. Because stimulants suppress REM sleep, patients may notice vivid dreams due to REM rebound.

Currently there are no clearly effective pharmacologic treatments for stimulant use disorders, though many are being studied. As with any SUD, patients with stimulant use disorders should be referred to substance abuse treatment with concurrent psychiatric treatment if needed. Mutual self-help programs (e.g., 12-step groups) should also be encouraged.

Hallucinogens

Hallucinogens (e.g., LSD, psilocybin mushrooms) are drugs that cause alterations in perception, thought, and mood. As they do not typically lead to outcomes requiring hospitalization, psychiatrists are rarely consulted for hallucinogen-related problems. However, primary teams might request assistance with situations that indirectly involve these substances (e.g., a young patient presenting with agitation and psychosis of unknown etiology).

Intoxication states for hallucinogens include an array of symptoms, including autonomic hyperactivity, ataxic gait, hyperreflexia, nystagmus, bruxism, trismus, dry mouth, nausea/vomiting, mood lability, paranoia, and hallucinations.

Acute medical complications may occur, including liver damage, rhabdomyolysis, and acute renal failure. Generally speaking, hallucinogens are not believed to cause cravings or addiction, and there is no clear withdrawal syndrome.

Designer Drugs

Consults for use of designer drugs are increasing, with variability across regions. It is important to possess a basic understanding of these substances because of increasing prevalence, especially among young adults. Designer drugs are a heterogeneous class of synthetic substances that have been developed specifically for their psychoactive effects. While there are hundreds of different compounds that fit this definition, three commonly encountered designer drugs are synthetic cannabinoids (e.g., "Spice"), synthetic cathinones (e.g., "bath salts") and 3,4-methylenedioxymethamphetamine (MDMA, aka "Ecstasy" or, in its purer form, "Molly").

Synthetic cannabinoids do not contain cannabis, but act on the same brain receptors and cause similar effects. Because of higher potency, they may cause psychoactive effects at lower doses. **Synthetic cathinones** are stimulants that enhance the activity of dopamine, norepinephrine, and serotonin and produce effects similar to cocaine or amphetamines. **MDMA** is a stimulant with weak hallucinogenic properties. It is similar in structure to the synthetic cathinones but has more serotonergic activity, and thus may lead to psychotic symptoms more readily than other stimulants. At lower doses MDMA is considered to be "entactogenic" in that it promotes empathy, increases self-confidence, and creates a sense of well-being and connectedness to others. However, at high doses it may cause severe anxiety and paranoid ideation. It is also neurotoxic to serotonergic neurons, which can lead to persistent mood disturbances and cognitive impairment. Concurrent use of MDMA with antidepressants may cause serotonin syndrome.

Treatment of intoxication and withdrawal for designer drugs is symptomatic, as described above for stimulant intoxication and withdrawal. At this time, most clinical laboratories do not routinely test for synthetic cannabinoids and cathinones. Thus, detection is frequently via clinical history. If a patient with negative toxicology testing presents with unexplained psychiatric and neurological symptoms, such as new onset of psychotic symptoms, severe irritability, agitation, aggression, sedation, or confusion, then use of these drugs should be considered (especially when there is a known history of substance use or the patient is required to undergo frequent drug testing for work purposes, legal situations, methadone clinics, etc.).

Key Points

- SUDs are common, with high rates of psychiatric and physical comorbidity.
- SUDs are critical to identify because of the need to address use and withdrawal management, and can be quickly and easily identified using screening tools.
- Withdrawal management varies by substance: benzodiazepines for GABA agonists, buprenorphine-naloxone taper or symptomatic management for opioids, supportive management for stimulant and designer drugs, and so on.
- Urine drug screening is a useful clinical tool that must be interpreted in the clinical context, with unexpected positive results requiring further investigation.
- The psychiatric consultant has an obligation to refer patients with SUDs for specialized treatment, preferably to a treatment program that utilizes a multidisciplinary approach, including group and individual therapy, family involvement, treatment of co-occurring psychiatric disorders, medications, and 12-step or other mutual self-help groups.

Disclosures

Dr. Glance has no conflicts of interest to disclose.

Dr. Gopalan has no conflicts of interest to disclose.

Dr. Ackerman has no conflicts of interest to disclose.

Further Reading

Babor TF, Higgins-Biddle JC, et al (2001). AUDIT: The Alcohol Use Disorders Identification Test: Guidelines for use in primary care, second edition. Retrieved from http://whqlibdoc. who.int/hq/2001/WHO_MSD_MSB_01.6a.pdf.

Berman AH, Bergman H, et al. (2005). Evaluation of the Drug Use Disorder Identification Test (DUDIT) in criminal justice and detoxification settings in a Swedish population sample. *Eur Addict Res.*, *11*, 22–31.

Bradley KA, DeBenedetti AF, et al. (2007). AUDIT-C as a brief screen for alcohol misuse in primary care. *Alcohol Clin Exp Res.*, *31*(7), 1–10.

Dhalla S, Kopec J. (2007). The CAGE questionnaire for alcohol misuse: A review of reliability and validity studies. *Clin Invest Med N Am.*, *30*(1), 33–41.

Ewing JA (1984). Detecting alcoholism: The CAGE questionnaire. *JAMA*, *252*(14), 1905–1907.

Jones HE, Kaltenbach K, et al (2010). Neonatal abstinence syndrome after methadone or buprenorphine exposure. *New Engl J Med.*, *363*(24), 2320–2331.

Maldonado JR, Sher Y, et al. (2014). The "Prediction of Alcohol Withdrawal Severity Scale" (PAWSS): Systematic literature review and pilot study of a new scale for the prediction of complicated alcohol withdrawal syndrome. *Alcohol*, *48*(4), 375–390.

Moeller KE, Lee KC, et al. (2008). Urine drug screening: Practical guide for clinicians. *Mayo Clin Proc.* *83*(1), 66–76.

National Institute on Drug Abuse. (2009). NIDA-Modified Alcohol, Smoking and Substance Involvement Screening Test (NM-ASSIST). "NIDA-Modified ASSIST V2.0." Website accessed May 24, 2014.

Smith PC, Schmidt SM, et al. (2010). A single-question screening test for drug use in primary care. *Arch Intern Med.*, *170*(13), 1155–1160.

Spiller HA, Hays HL, et al. (2013). Overdose of drugs for attention-deficit hyperactivity disorder: Clinical presentation, mechanisms of toxicity, and management. *CNS Drugs*, *27*(7):531–543.

Sullivan JJ, Sykora K, et al (1989). Assessment of alcohol withdrawal: The revised clinical institute withdrawal assessment for alcohol scale (CIWA-Ar). *Br J Addict.*, *84*, 1353–1357.

Exercises

1. Which of the following scales can be used to screen for alcohol use disorders?
   a. CAGE questionnaire
   b. AUDIT questionnaire
   c. PHQ-2
   d. a and b
   e. None of the above

2. Alcohol and benzodiazepine withdrawal may be managed using which of the following approaches?
   a. Symptom-triggered
   b. Benzodiazepine taper
   c. Front-loading
   d. Continuous IV infusion
   e. All of the above

3. The classic triad of opioid overdose includes:
   a. pinpoint pupils, respiratory depression, coma
   b. respiratory depression, pupillary dilation, tachycardia
   c. disinhibition, slurred speech, gait ataxia
   d. gait ataxia, confusion, nystagmus
   e. gait apraxia, urinary incontinence, confusion

4. Variceal bleeding, cardiomyopathy, cognitive impairment, and pancreatitis are all complications of long-term use of:
   a. Opioids
   b. Inhalants
   c. Alcohol
   d. Cocaine
   e. None of the above

5. Chronic use of cannabis results in urine drug screens that remain positive for:
   a. 24 hours
   b. 3 days
   c. 1 week
   d. 10 days
   e. > 30 days

Answers: (1) d (2) e (3) a (4) c (5) e

Part V

Special Topics in Psychosomatic Medicine

Chapter 17

Perinatal Psychiatry

Priya Gopalan and Jody Glance

Introduction and Approach to Perinatal Psychiatry

Perinatal psychiatry focuses on treatment of psychiatric conditions in women of childbearing age during the preconception, antepartum, and postpartum periods. Few national guidelines exist in this area, with reports issued on the management of depression in pregnancy by the American Psychiatric Association and the American College of Obstetricians and Gynecologists (Yonkers et al., 2009) and on bipolar management in pregnancy (Yonkers et al., 2004). In this chapter, we will outline the general approach to managing psychiatric illness in pregnancy and postpartum periods, followed by the specifics of treating mood, anxiety, and psychotic disorders, substance use disorders, hyperemesis gravidarum, perinatal loss, and decision-making capacity.

The Perinatal Consult

As half of all pregnancies are unplanned, the ideal time to discuss with patients the effects of psychiatric medications in pregnancy is at medication initiation prior to conception. Thorough sexual and medical histories of women of childbearing age should be obtained as part of routine medical care, including use of contraceptives and psychotropic medications. Pharmacological studies pertaining to perinatal psychiatry are difficult to interpret, as the "gold standard" study in research—the double-blinded placebo-controlled trial—is unavailable in pregnancy. Clinical management of pregnant patients is largely guided by retrospective and prospective case-control studies, registry data, and expert consensus, thus making generalizations difficult.

The perinatal psychiatric evaluation includes all of the standard components of a psychiatric evaluation (reviewed in Chapter 2) with a few additional considerations:

- Previous pregnancies and the courses of psychiatric illness and treatment response
- Previous postpartum periods with any concurrent psychiatric symptoms
- Previous lethality, specifically thoughts to harm self or baby in the antepartum or postpartum periods
- Past medication trials
- Current symptoms
- Plans for breastfeeding
- Anticipated psychosocial supports in the postpartum period, including the baby's father.

Reproductive toxicity is grouped into various domains, all of which should be taken into account in the treatment of perinatal psychiatric conditions.

Risks to the pregnancy include the following:
- Miscarriage/spontaneous abortion
- Preterm delivery
- Preeclampsia, hypertension

Risks to the baby include the following:
- Fetal malformations
- Effects on birth weight
- Neonatal withdrawal
- Developmental effects

When considering treatment of perinatal mood, anxiety, and psychotic disorders, it is imperative to discuss each of the relevant domains against the 1%–3% baseline population risk of birth defects. In addition, risks of exposure are contingent on trimester and stage of fetal development. For example, since organogenesis occurs in the first trimester, often the time period for most physical malformations has passed by the time a patient is seen in consultation:

- Neural tube development occurs within the first two weeks of pregnancy.
- Heart, lip/palate, other organs form within the first 10–11 weeks.

- Lung development occurs at the end of the third trimester.
- CNS development continues throughout pregnancy (and beyond).

Risk-Benefit Discussions in Pregnancy

US Food and Drug Administration (FDA) pregnancy drug classes (A–X) are of limited utility for clinical discussions in pregnancy, and have been removed from the FDA's Pregancy and Lactation Labeling Rule. Instead, a thorough risk-benefit discussion with pregnant patients is of the utmost importance. Thoughts, concerns, and values regarding pharmacologic treatments during pregnancy vary greatly between individuals. When discussing treatment options with the patient, many factors must be considered, including risks of treatment with psychotropic medications to fetus and mother, potential benefits of pharmacotherapy, risks to fetus and mother of leaving the psychiatric illness untreated, and available alternative treatment modalities. Literature-based risk discussions should be adjusted according to each individual's history and response to treatment. Risks of specific abnormalities should be stated explicitly when known, but should be discussed in understandable terms and framed against the general population risk and the risk of non-treatment (Wisner et al., 2000).

Physiologic changes associated with pregnancy present challenges for the prescribing physician:

- Increased fluid volumes combined with increased rates of hepatic metabolism (particularly the cytochrome P450 system) result in decreased blood levels of most psychotropic medications, especially in the second and third trimester. These effects reverse during the postpartum period, requiring close attention.
- The placenta, which allows free passage of most psychiatric medications (except antipsychotics), is fully developed around 18–20 weeks of pregnancy.
- Fluid shifts during pregnancy require close monitoring of renally excreted medications such as lithium.
- Release of estrogen and relaxin during pregnancy results in loosening of ligaments, which could lead to increased risk of falls if combined with psychiatric medications associated with sedation and orthostatic hypotension.

Practical Considerations

A few practical guidelines are helpful in treating psychiatric disorders in pregnant women. Consider non-pharmacological alternatives first. Psychotherapy is an established method of treatment for mild to moderate depression and anxiety, and randomized placebo-controlled trials are available in antepartum and postpartum women. Of these treatments, interpersonal therapy has the largest evidence base, though randomized studies have also found cognitive behavioral therapy (CBT) to be effective. Light therapy, fish oil supplements, exercise, yoga, and acupuncture may also be beneficial for mood regulation, though varying levels of evidence exist for their use in pregnancy. Electroconvulsive therapy is a viable option with minimal risk for women with moderate to severe illness for whom medications have not been effective, or who opt for this modality to avoid fetal exposure to multiple medication trials.

If opting for treatment with psychotropic medications, the following general guidelines can help to minimize risk to both mother and baby:

- Choose a medicine that has been effective in the past.
- Use the lowest effective dose for treatment.
- Avoid poly-pharmacy whenever possible.
- Do not prescribe known teratogens.

Psychiatric Disorders in Pregnancy: Approach and Management

Perinatal Depression

While pregnancy was historically thought to be protective for the development of mood disorders, the perinatal period is high risk for the development and exacerbation of depression and mania. Depression affects up to 15% of women during the pregnancy and postpartum period. Conflicting study results make interpretations of data difficult; thus, practitioners in psychosomatic medicine and women's mental health need to critically synthesize the literature and communicate clearly with patients.

Untreated depression has been implicated in conditions such as preeclampsia, maternal obesity, fetal cardiac defects, fetal growth restriction, low-birth-weight infants, and preterm birth (Yonkers et al., 2009). Meta-analyses identify late preterm delivery, growth restriction, and low birth weight as the primary consequences of depression in pregnancy (Grote et al., 2010). Poorly treated depression is associated with poor prenatal care, poor nutritional status, and an increased risk of alcohol and other substance use (including cigarettes). An increased risk of attempted or completed suicide associated with untreated depression can also have dire results for both mother and baby.

Antidepressant medications have been studied extensively in pregnancy, and data suggest that women who discontinue their antidepressants during pregnancy are at higher risk of relapse. Up to 68% experience a recurrence of major depressive disorder (MDD), and of those women, 90% relapse by the end of the second trimester (Cohen et al., 2006). Many women struggle with weighing the risks and benefits of treatment, and psychiatrists struggle with interpreting studies in an area that is rapidly changing and difficult to synthesize.

Perinatal psychiatrists generally view antidepressant use as conveying minimal risk to the fetus. However, clinical decision-making must be made on a case-by-case basis. While SSRIs and TCAs have been thoroughly studied, many questions remain unanswered. SSRIs were once thought to be associated with cardiac defects and persistent pulmonary hypertension of the newborn, but inconsistent results across studies and large prospective studies no longer support this notion. In studies finding an association, the absolute risk of these disorders remains low (e.g., 6/1,000 for persistent pulmonary hypertension compared to a 1/1,000 general population risk); confounds included maternal obesity, mode of delivery, and symptom burden of depression (Occhigrosso et al., 2012). While third trimester discontinuation was once considered a strategy to mitigate the risk of pulmonary hypertension, this is no longer recommended, as mothers are then without treatment during the vulnerable postpartum period. Associations have not been found between SSRIs and miscarriages or congenital abnormalities such as oral clefts and neural tube defects. While some studies have found associations between antidepressants and preterm delivery and low birth weight, these findings have not been consistent across trials, and untreated depression is also associated with these conditions, making it even more difficult to establish causality.

Developmental effects of antidepressants are unclear. While antidepressants have been reported to result in a post-delivery neonatal withdrawal syndrome, characterized by mild irritability, jittery behaviors, and possible increased difficulty with feeding, this syndrome is usually transient, seemingly without long-term risks to the newborn (Chambers et al., 1996). To our knowledge, deaths associated with this syndrome have not been reported. Studies of motor and behavioral developmental effects have largely shown that children born to mothers who used SSRIs during their pregnancy develop normally, show low-normal motor and behavioral development, or have slower motor development that catches up with no long-term delays (Nulman et al., 2012). These studies are limited by difficulties in controlling for effects of underlying maternal mood dysregulation. Studies controlling for underlying depression found no significant differences in development between SSRI-treated depressed mothers and those with untreated depression. Thus, long-term effects of SSRIs are not thought to be of clinical concern, though this area is still being closely studied. See Table 17.1 for a summary of risks.

Venlafaxine and bupropion use during pregnancy appear to have effects consistent with those of SSRIs and TCAs. Studies involving duloxetine,

Table 17.1 Risks of Untreated Depression Compared to Risks of SSRI Use in Pregnancy

Fetal Toxicity Domain	Untreated Depression	SSRIs
Miscarriage/ Spontaneous abortion	Case reports of associations	Unlikely to be associated
Preterm delivery	Likely	Likely
Fetal malformations	Case reports of associations	Unlikely (some studies report higher rates of cardiac defects and persistent pulmonary hypertension of the newborn)
Effects on birth weight	Likely low birth weight	Likely low birth weight
Neonatal withdrawal	N/A	Likely but transient
Developmental effects	Unknown	Unknown but unlikely (studies show catch-up with initial delays)

mirtazapine, and desvenlafaxine are limited; potential outcomes can only be inferred based on what is known about other antidepressants. Continuing one of these agents may be preferred if it is particularly effective for that patient.

The evaluation and treatment of perinatal depression include the following:

- Thorough history-taking, examination, and appropriate formulation/ diagnosis to determine appropriate treatment course;
- Discussion of known risks of antidepressant medications with the mother;
- Discussion of known risks of untreated depression during pregnancy;
- Discussion of alternate treatment options (e.g., psychotherapy as sole treatment);
- Discussion of alternate treatment strategies (e.g., delay of medication use until the postpartum period), along with discussion of benefits (decreased exposure) and risks (delay in treatment effect).

Perinatal Bipolar Disorder

Bipolar disorder is heavily influenced by hormonal factors and requires close monitoring during the perinatal period. Discontinuing mood-stabilizing medications results in a twofold increased risk of recurrence. Further, women with bipolar disorder have a 23-fold increased risk of psychiatric admission in the postpartum period. Limited data suggest that patients may not return to their previous baselines when mood-stabilizing medications are re-initiated.

The choice to use a mood stabilizer during pregnancy should be made with careful consideration of risks of untreated illness versus risks of medication use, as well as risks and benefits of alternative, non-pharmacologic options that may be safer but less effective. Lithium use has long been considered an effective treatment option for bipolar disorder in pregnancy (Llewellyn et al., 1998). While lithium is associated with an increased risk of cardiac defects (specifically a 1/1,000 or lower risk of Ebstein's anomaly compared to a general population risk of 1/10,000–20,000), the absolute risk of these malformations remains low. Babies born to mothers on lithium are at increased risk of preterm delivery, increased birth weight, neonatal hypotonicity, and cyanosis. Neonatal Apgar scores may be affected by lithium dose, with lower scores for higher doses (Newport et al., 2005). See Table 17.2 for a summary of risks.

Management of lithium includes the following:

- Titration of lithium is similar in pregnant and non-pregnant patients (starting dose of 300 milligrams per day with upward titration as tolerated and to treatment effect).
- Careful education on the effects of fluid shifts on lithium levels is important, especially with patient's vomiting.
- Increased renal clearance of medications may require dose increases of lithium throughout the course of the pregnancy.
- Divided dosing (2–3 times per day) may be required if the patient is unable to tolerate the gastrointestinal side effects.

Table 17.2 Reproductive Toxicity Risks with Lithium

Fetal Toxicity Domain	Lithium
Miscarriage/Spontaneous abortion	Unlikely to be associated
Preterm delivery	Likely
Fetal malformations	Higher relative risk of Ebstein's anomaly with first trimester exposure
Effects on birth weight	Large for gestational age
Neonatal withdrawal	Decreased APGARs, neonatal hypotonicity
Developmental effects	Unlikely

- Expert consensus recommends suspension of lithium either at onset of labor or, if possible, 24–48 hours prior, to counter rapid fluid contraction that occurs post-delivery.
- Careful dose reduction in the two weeks prior to delivery is recommended, though guidelines do not exist.
- Similarly, re-initiation at half of the third trimester dose will potentially prevent toxicity with postnatal fluid contraction, though the amount of reduction should be tailored to the patient.

Of the anticonvulsants, valproate and carbamazepine are considered known human teratogens with increased risk of neural tube defects. Additionally, both agents are associated with potential cognitive and developmental deficits in the neonate and should be avoided as first-line agents. Valproate, in particular, has been linked to increased risk of autism and lower IQ scores compared to controls. Known teratogenic agents should be avoided in women of childbearing age when possible, unless reliable birth control methods are available.

Lamotrigine and gabapentin have fewer studies investigating their effects during pregnancy. Limited data suggest an association of lamotrigine with oral clefts, though this is likely confounded by use of multiple anticonvulsants. Data on both of these agents are limited to self-reported registries.

Perinatal Psychotic Disorders

Historically, women with schizophrenia and especially those on first-generation antipsychotics were found to have decreased fertility. With the advent of second-generation antipsychotics, with less prominent effects on prolactin and other reproductive hormones, rates of pregnancy have increased to numbers consistent with the general population, and it is thought that 50%–60% of women with schizophrenia will become pregnant.

The management of pregnant patients can be especially challenging, depending on the severity of the schizophrenia. The risk-benefit conversation regarding treatment during pregnancy depends on the patient's ability to provide adequate informed consent. Discontinuation of medications among non-pregnant patients leads to high rates of relapse, with up to 50% relapsing within a year and 90% in two years. Schizophrenia may be associated with obstetrical risks such as placental abruption, preterm delivery, low birth weight, stillbirth, and neonatal death (Vigod et al., 2014), either due to the illness itself or poor prenatal care related to illness severity.

Antipsychotic medication management during pregnancy is challenging due to limited data on perinatal effects of second-generation agents. First-generation phenothiazine antipsychotics may convey an increased risk of teratogenicity, though the malformation rate of 2.4% is only marginally higher than the general population risk of about 2%. Based on limited data, no consistent malformations have been noted for second-generation agents, unique among antipsychotics in their variability in placental transfer due to protein-binding effects. Quetiapine has the least amount of placental transfer (23%), while olanzapine likely has the most (75%), with risperidone (42%) and haloperidol (60%) showing intermediate placental crossing (Newport et al., 2007). Data implicate these medications in the higher likelihood of preeclampsia, gestational diabetes, and large-for-gestational-age babies. The FDA has issued a warning for all antipsychotics that may cause withdrawal dyskinesias for neonates after delivery. See Table 17.3 for a summary of risks.

Guidelines for antipsychotic use in pregnancy include the following:

- Determine the most effective antipsychotic medication; use this as first line.
- If the patient is already on an antipsychotic and has good symptom control, do not change the agent.
- If starting a new agent, discuss the known risks of first-generation versus second-generation antipsychotics, including perinatal risks and maternal risks of movement disorders and metabolic side effects.
- Consider antipsychotics with decreased placental transfer if possible.
- Avoid the newest antipsychotics (e.g., asenapine, iloperidone), as safety data are limited.

Perinatal Anxiety Disorders

Anxiety disorders, trauma, and stress-related disorders are understudied areas in perinatal psychiatry. In animal models, stress and anxiety have been associated with variable outcomes, including impaired cognitive development attributed to *in utero* cortisol levels, and subsequent impairment in the quality of the mother-infant relationship (Glover et al., 2010). Chronic stress during the perinatal period has potential adverse effects on the development of the fetus; human studies have implicated untreated anxiety in preterm delivery and low birth weight (Dunkel Schetter & Tanner, 2012). Evidence suggests that anxiety during pregnancy may interfere with development of the hypothalamic-pituitary-adrenal axis. Specific vulnerability periods for stress and anxiety during pregnancy have not been established.

Table 17.3 Risks of Untreated Psychosis Compared to Risks of Antipsychotics Use in Pregnancy

Fetal Toxicity Domain	Untreated Schizophrenia	Antipsychotics
Miscarriage/ Spontaneous abortion	Possible association with placental abruption, stillbirth, neonatal death	Unlikely to be associated
Preterm delivery	Likely	Likely
Fetal malformations	Unlikely	1st generation: Unlikely 2nd generation: No consistent malformations reported
Effects on birth weight	Likely low birth weight	Unclear: Studies with low and high birth weight for 2nd generation
Neonatal withdrawal	N/A	FDA warning for withdrawal dyskinesias
Developmental effects	Unknown	Unknown

As pregnancy is a time of elevated risk of interpersonal violence toward women, worsened by comorbid substance use, a careful screen for trauma is necessary. PTSD is associated with complications such as preterm delivery and low birth weight. Providers should be aware that a delivery may be experienced as traumatic due to loss of control and overt physical injury. PTSD has arisen from traumatic deliveries, C-sections, and preeclampsia, with symptoms such as difficulty interacting with the newborn due to avoidance of reminders of the delivery.

Perinatal Addiction

Fetal Effects of Substances of Abuse

Perinatal addiction has an estimated prevalence of 5.5%, independent of age, race, and socioeconomic class. However, women of lower socioeconomic classes and African-American women are more prone to illicit substance use (especially cocaine), while Caucasian women, women of higher socioeconomic classes, and women of higher education levels have higher rates of alcohol use.

Pregnancy provides a unique window of opportunity to promote behavioral change. Pregnant women often feel a new sense of responsibility associated with raising a child, combined with a sense of self-worth and feelings of hope and connectedness with the future. Conversely, failure to achieve abstinence during pregnancy can lead to guilt and a sense of failure, and can have social and/or legal consequences. Women report many barriers to care, including a sense of stigma from family members, social networks, medical professionals, and society at large; transportation; or financial limitations. Finally, pregnant addicts may avoid the healthcare system, fearing legal ramifications or being reported to child protective agencies.

Each substance of abuse has a unique profile and varying levels of teratogenic effects:

- The impact of **alcohol use** during pregnancy is often debated, and the periods of vulnerability and quantity of alcohol required for adverse effects to the baby are not well established. Fetal alcohol syndrome is well described with the following neonatal features: facial abnormalities (smooth philtrum, thin vermillion, and small palpebral fissures), growth retardation (height, weight, and microcephaly), and central nervous system impairment (cognition, attention, behavior, motor skills, and other effects). Fetal alcohol syndrome develops in about 0.5 to 2 per 1,000 live births. Neonatal withdrawal symptoms from alcohol include tremors, seizures, inconsolable crying, abnormal reflexes, and hypertonia, with management aimed at symptom management and assisting neonates with proper sleeping and feeding. Treatment of the mother's withdrawal during pregnancy usually requires inpatient medical admission.

- **Cigarette smoking** increases risk of miscarriage, intrauterine fetal demise, preterm birth, and intrauterine growth retardation. Infants born to mothers who are smokers have more than a threefold risk of dying from sudden infant death syndrome. Long-term effects are also being studied, and the Maternal Lifestyles Study (Bauer et al., 2005) found an association with smoking and childhood sleep problems that lasted through age 12. Women are more likely to stop smoking during pregnancy, providing a window of opportunity for intervention, although only a third successfully quit long-term.

- **Cannabis use** has not been associated with major birth defects, miscarriage, or stillbirth. Infants may show increased tremulousness, hyper-startle response, high-pitched cries, and altered response to visual stimuli (perhaps suggesting neurological impairment). There may also be long-term neurological effects of prenatal cannabis use, with exposed school-aged children found to have impaired memory, attention, problem-solving, and learning.

- **Cocaine use** carries an increased risk of miscarriage, premature rupture of membranes, meconium-stained amniotic fluid, and especially placental abruption. The developmental effects are not clearly established. As there are no effective medications for treatment of cocaine use, close psychosocial management and treatment of co-occurring conditions are vital.
- There are limited data on the effects of the use of **methamphetamine** and **other stimulants** during pregnancy.
- **Opioid dependence** poses a different set of problems. Withdrawal from opioids during pregnancy is potentially fatal to the fetus, resulting in such complications as miscarriage and premature labor. While opioids have no known teratogenic effects, relapse rates for opioid dependence seem particularly high during pregnancy, leading to a dangerous cycle of use and withdrawal. Methadone maintenance treatment remains the gold standard for opioid replacement therapy in pregnancy, helping patients maintain abstinence from illicit substances throughout pregnancy, reducing withdrawal symptoms, reducing risk of relapse, and preventing extreme withdrawal symptoms.
- **Sedative-hypnotics, hallucinogens**, and **dissociative medications** have limited data regarding their effects in pregnancy.

Management of Substance Withdrawal

Withdrawal management of all substances requires careful monitoring of both mother and fetus. There are no established guidelines for management of alcohol and benzodiazepine withdrawal during pregnancy. As benzodiazepines are the mainstay of treatment for **GABAergic withdrawal**, these are preferred in managing alcohol and benzodiazepine withdrawal in pregnancy. The clinician must balance the need for minimizing pharmacologic exposure to the neonate with ensuring a smooth detoxification process. Studies looking at non-pregnant patients suggest that symptom-triggered protocols reduce total benzodiazepine dosing in withdrawal states, so this may be attempted with close monitoring of maternal vital signs and fetal heart tones.

Opioid maintenance treatments are considered the safest option for mother and baby during pregnancy due to the unstable nature of the cycle of intoxication and withdrawal; therefore, conversion to methadone is standard clinical practice for the management of opioid withdrawal states. Methadone maintenance results in fewer premature births, less intrauterine growth retardation, fewer low birth weight babies, decreased maternal use of opiates and other drugs of abuse, fewer co-occurring infections such as HIV and hepatitis, decreased overdose fatalities, decreased criminal activity, and improved prenatal care. Methadone induction can be done in any trimester, but is generally done inpatient to allow for close monitoring of mother and fetus during titration. As the pregnancy progresses, higher methadone doses are often required due to physiologic changes such as increased blood volume, changes in liver metabolism of the drug, and variations in how the placenta metabolizes methadone during the course of pregnancy and between individuals. These changes reverse after delivery.

Methadone is not considered dangerous to the fetus, with only mild slowing of fetal heart rate and less fetal movement in the hours after dosing; after delivery, however, neonates require observation in the ICU for withdrawal symptoms known as the neonatal abstinence syndrome (NAS). Some clinical centers have used conversion to buprenorphine as an alternate management strategy. In the MOTHER study, buprenorphine was found to have similar beneficial effects to the mother but with potentially shorter lengths of ICU stays for infants; however, this is confounded by higher dropout rates for the buprenorphine-maintained mothers (Jones et al., 2010).

Lactation

Most psychiatric medications are generally considered safe for use during lactation. If mothers have been on medications throughout their pregnancy, the quantity of medication conferred to babies through breast milk is significantly lower than in utero exposure. Certain medications such as lithium, benzodiazepines, and methadone require close monitoring of the newborn by a pediatrician; adequate coordination of care is vital. Aripiprazole has been linked to decreased milk production and should be avoided if the mother plans to nurse. Otherwise, no medications are absolutely contraindicated for breastfeeding. Lactmed (www. toxnet.lactmed.com) and the website of the American Association of Pediatrics can serve as guides for prescription and as the basis for risk-benefit discussions.

Postpartum Syndromes

Postpartum depression affects 10%–15% of women after delivery and is associated with low mood, anhedonia, hopelessness, and neurovegetative symptoms. Diagnostically, symptoms must begin within four weeks of delivery, though onset may be peripartum. Women remain at increased risk of depressive illness for up to two years postpartum, so careful screening and follow-up are required. Postpartum depression must be distinguished from the syndrome of "maternity blues," which affects up to 80% of women after delivery. Symptoms of maternity blues include mood swings and tearfulness, generally without anhedonia and hopelessness, and are time-limited to the first one to two weeks post-delivery. If symptoms continue beyond this time or worsen, additional evaluation and treatment may be indicated.

Untreated postpartum depression has implications for maternal-infant bonding and the development of secure attachment, and could thereby convey a higher risk of developing mood disorders in the child. Screening for postpartum depression is imperative, and the Edinburgh Postnatal Depression Screen (Cox et al., 2014) is a validated screening tool that is self-administered. Many studies have investigated treatment options for postpartum depression, including pharmacotherapy and psychotherapy. Prophylactic treatments of postpartum depression using SSRIs, nortriptyline, and various hormonal treatments have been investigated and are reasonable options for high-risk patients.

Management of postpartum depression includes the following:

- Screen for postpartum depression within one month of delivery.
- Consider evidence-based psychotherapy options for mild-to-moderate depression, including interpersonal therapy and CBT.
- Moderate-to-severe depression should be managed with pharmacologic treatments including SSRIs and TCAs.
- For patients with a history of recurrent depression or past episodes of postpartum depression, consider prophylaxis of postpartum depression with initiation of SSRIs or TCAs immediately after delivery.

Postpartum psychosis occurs in approximately 1/1,000 live births, requiring the psychiatrist to screen and counsel carefully. Considered a psychiatric emergency, postpartum psychosis can be rapid in onset and often involves quick deterioration from prior functioning. The syndrome is heterogeneous, with clinical features including delusions (paranoid, grandiose, or bizarre), mood lability, confusion, and disorganized behavior. Infanticide rates in the United States are low, but about a quarter are associated with psychosis. In postpartum psychosis, approximately 4% of mothers will engage in infanticide, emphasizing the importance of screening and intervention. Most cases of infanticide, however, are *not* due to mental illness but other psychosocial factors. Postpartum delirium (with potential etiologies including but not limited to postpartum thyroiditis or seizures) must be ruled out, as it can present similarly, but with fluctuating arousal and inattention. Postpartum psychosis is strongly associated with bipolar disorder (approximately 75% of cases).

Management of postpartum psychosis includes the following:
- Screen patients carefully for personal and family history of postpartum psychosis (risk factors).
- Counsel all patients regarding the presentation of postpartum psychosis.
- Consider prophylaxis in high-risk patients with lithium or an antiepileptic agent.
- For symptomatic patients, begin pharmacologic management with lithium, antiepileptics, or antipsychotics.
- Consider hospitalization for severe symptoms such as disorganized thought processes, poor self-care, paranoid ideation toward the infant, and infanticidal thoughts.

Obsessions and compulsions (especially checking) are common in the postpartum period; harming obsessions may be more common than in non-postpartum OCD. Women with postpartum depression are at especially high risk for this syndrome, and in one study, 87% of postpartum women presenting to a mental health clinic presented with intrusive thoughts. Postpartum obsessions need to be differentiated from postpartum psychosis, as women with harming obsessions are not more prone to infanticide (Abramowitz et al., 2003).

While SSRI treatment and CBT (specifically, exposure-response prevention [ERP]) are the standards of care in the treatment of OCD, pregnancy data are limited. Despite the scarcity of studies, postpartum OCD should be managed similarly to OCD in non-pregnant patients, and the combination of ERP and SSRIs is recommended.

Special Topics

Hyperemesis Gravidarum

Hyperemesis Gravidarum (HG) is a syndrome of persistent nausea and vomiting throughout pregnancy. While depressive disorders commonly develop in women with HG, several studies indicate that anxiety disorders are even more prevalent, with a rate of up to 35%. Conversely, depression and anxiety may be risk factors for developing HG. Adequate symptom control of hyperemesis may also help to alleviate comorbid psychiatric symptoms.

Capacity in Pregnancy

Assessments of decision-making capacity in pregnancy must also consider the rights and medical well-being of the fetus. Evaluations often involve determining the patient's ability to consent to or refuse C-sections. Models outlining maternal versus fetal rights may guide the healthcare provider, and state-specific legislation must be considered, though there is no universal consensus on how much weight should be given to maternal rights versus fetal rights in these evaluations.

Perinatal Loss

Perinatal loss is typically a devastating event for both parents, yet few studies guide psychiatric consultants on how to approach these encounters. Patients should be approached with empathy, and staff should be advised of the heterogeneous responses to loss and grief. Patients should be referred to support groups in the immediate period following the loss, and for psychiatric follow-up if depressive symptoms or signs of complicated grief emerge.

Conclusion

The perinatal period is a time of vulnerability for women with psychiatric conditions. Treatment of mental illness during this time requires the provider to be thoughtful and measured, assisting the mother in weighing numerous factors, including maternal and neonatal risks of medications and untreated psychiatric illness, in order to make informed decisions regarding her mental health. Appropriate and thorough discussions of risks and benefits of all treatment options during pregnancy versus risks of untreated behavioral and substance use disorders are imperative. Pharmacotherapy, as well as psychotherapy, should be discussed with confidence and without bias in order to provide the pregnant patient with the best available information to make a well-informed decision regarding her own health, as well as that of her baby.

Key Points

- Psychiatric disorders in the perinatal period are associated with numerous adverse outcomes for both mother and baby.
- Treatment of psychiatric disorders in pregnancy should always be based on an analysis of the risks of untreated illness versus the potential risks of medications, with consideration of the likely benefits of treatment. The difference in perinatal psychiatry is helping the mother to understand and weigh the risks to both herself and the fetus.
- FDA categories (A, B, C, D, X) are of minimal utility in choosing pharmacologic agents for management of perinatal psychiatric conditions and have been removed from the FDA's Pregnancy and Lactation Labeling Rule.
- Fetal domains of toxicity include miscarriage/spontaneous abortion, preterm delivery, fetal malformations, effects on birth weight, neonatal withdrawal, and developmental effects.
- Psychiatric consultants may encounter other concerns related to perinatal illness such as HG, capacity in pregnancy, lactation, and perinatal loss.

Disclosures

Dr. Priya Gopalan has no conflicts to disclose.

Dr. Jody Glance has no conflicts to disclose.

Further Reading

Abramowitz JS, Scwhatrz SA, et al. (2003). Obsessive-compulsive symptom in pregnancy and the puerperiu: A review of the literature. *J Anxiety Disord.*, 17, 461–478.

Bauer CR, Langer JC, et al. (2005). Acute neonatal effects of cocaine exposure during pregnancy. *Arch Pediatr Adolesc Med.*, 159(9), 824–834.

Chambers CD, Johnson KA, et al. (1996). Birth outcomes in pregnant women taking fluoxetine. *New Engl J Med.*, 335, 1010–1015.

Cohen LS, Altshuler LL, et al. (2006). Relapse of major depression during pregnancy in women who maintain or discontinue antidepressant treatment. *JAMA*, 295(5), 499–507.

Cox J, Holden J, Henshaw C (2014). *Perinatal Mental Health: The Edinburgh Postnatal Depression Scale Handbook*, 2nd ed. London: RCPsych Publications.

Dunkel Schetter C, Tanner L. (2012). Anxiety, depression and stress in pregnancy: Implications for mothers, children, research and practice. *Curr Opin Psychiatr.*, 25, 141–148.

Glover V, O'Connor TG, et al. (2010). Prenatal stress and programming of the HPA axis. *Neurosci Biobehav Rev.*, 35, 17–22.

Grote NK, Bridge JA, et al (2010). A meta-analysis of depression during pregnancy and the risk of preterm birth, low birth weight, and intrauterine growth restriction. *Arch Gen Psyhicat.*, 67(10), 1012–1024.

Jones HE, Kaltenback K, et al. (2010). Neonatal abstinence syndrome after methadone or buprenorphine exposure. *New Engl J Med.*, 364(24), 2320–2331.

Llewellyn A, Stowe ZN et al. (1998). The use of lithium and management of women with bipolar disorder during pregnancy and lactation. *J Clin Psych.*, 59, s57–64.

Newport DJ, Calamaras MR, et al. (2007). Atypical antipsychotic administration during late pregnancy: Placental passage and obstetrical outcomes. *Am J Psychiat.*, 164, 1214–1220.

Newport DJ, Viguera AC, et al. (2005). Lithium placental passage and obstetrical outcome: implications for clinical management during late pregnancy. *Am J Psychiat.*, 162(11), 2162–2170.

Nulman I, Koren G, et al. (2012). Neurodevelopment of children following prenatal exposure to venlafaxine, selective serotonin reuptake inhibitors, or untreated maternal depression. *Am J Psychiat.*, 169, 1165–1174.

Occhigrosso M, Omran SS, et al. (2012). Persistent pumonary hypertension of the newborn and selective serotonin reuptake inhibitors: Lessons from clinical and translational studies. *Am J Psychiat.*, 169, 134–140.

Robinson GE. (2012). Psychopharmacology in pregnancy and postpartum. *Focus*, X(1), 3–14.

Vigod SN, Kurdyak PA, et al. (2014). Maternal and newborn outcomes among women with schizophrenia: A restrospective population-based cohort study. *BJOG*, 12(5), 566–574.

Wisner KL, Zarin DA, et al. (2000). Risk-benefit decision making for treatment of depression during pregnancy. *Am J Psychiat.*, 157, 1933–1940.

Yonkers KA, Wisner KL, et al. (2009). The management of depression during pregnancy: A report from the American Psychiatric Association and the American College of Obstetricians and Gynecologists. *Obstet Gynecol.*, 114(3), 703–713.

Yonkers KA, Wisner KL, Stowe Z, et al. (2004). Management of bipolar disorder during pregnancy and the postpartum period. *Am J Psychiat.*, 161, 608–620.

Exercises

1. Domains of fetal toxicity to consider in the management of perinatal psychiatric disorders include:
   a. Preterm delivery
   b. Fetal malformations
   c. Neonatal withdrawal
   d. Developmental effects
   e. All of the above

2. SSRIs are contraindicated in pregnancy and should be avoided at all cost.
   a. True
   b. False

3. A discussion of treatment of perinatal psychiatric disorders should include:
   a. Thorough history-taking, examination, and appropriate formulation/diagnosis to determine appropriate treatment course
   b. Discussion of known risks of antidepressant medications with mother
   c. Discussion of known risks of untreated depression during pregnancy
   d. Discussion of alternate treatment options (e.g., psychotherapy as sole treatment)
   e. All of the above

4. Which of the following statements is correct?
   a. Perinatal addiction has an estimated prevalence of substance use disorders in pregnancy of 25%.
   b. Postpartum depression affects 1% of women after delivery and is associated with low mood, anhedonia, hopelessness, and neurovegetative symptoms.
   c. Discontinuation of medications in schizophrenia in the general population leads to high rates of relapse in illness, with up to 90% relapsing within a year.
   d. There is a 1%–3% baseline population risk of birth defects.

5. Which of the following second-generation antipsychotics crosses the placenta the least?
   a. Quetiepine
   b. Risperidone
   c. Haloperidol
   d. Olanzapine

Answers: (1) e (2) b (3) e (4) d (5) a

Psycho-Oncology

Kevin R. Patterson

Introduction

Acknowledging and addressing psychiatric symptoms in cancer patients is a relatively recent (1970s) development. Improvements in cancer care have made cancer not only an acute and terminal condition but also a chronic condition, leading to an increasing focus of patients, family members, and practitioners on quality of life.

Psychiatric symptomatology occurs at many points along the time course of cancer diagnosis and treatment. Psychiatric symptoms may pre-exist the cancer diagnosis, and cancer and cancer care complicate the management of these premorbid conditions. For other patients, psychiatric symptoms may emerge at the time of diagnosis and initial treatment for cancer, while still others may experience symptoms following recovery or during remission. Recurrence, expansion of metastatic disease, and when treatment is no longer available or advisable are often times of great distress when psychiatric symptoms may emerge.

Treatment of pre-existing psychiatric conditions needs to be maintained, and often symptoms need to be treated more aggressively, during the course and after cancer treatment and care. The prevalence of schizophrenia, bipolar disorder, and substance abuse can be the same in cancer patients as in the general population, and their management can significantly impact the course of cancer care and adherence to treatment plans.

It is important to note that traditional diagnostic labels may be less useful at this time than careful attunement to patient symptoms. Areas of overlap between psychiatric symptomatology and symptoms emerging more directly from the medical illness (of cancer) include fatigue, sleep disturbance, pain, neuropathy, nausea, anorexia, cognitive changes, and hot flashes. Under these circumstances it can be difficult to determine a specific psychiatric diagnosis, but that should not inhibit providers' intervention for symptom improvement.

Medical oncologists and psychiatric care providers can improve patient quality of life by examining and understanding comorbidity, organic considerations, and the psycho-social impacts of cancer. Symptoms resulting from oncologic treatment should be addressed, independent of whether they meet criteria for traditional psychiatric diagnoses. For example, a physician might treat fatigue and amotivation rather than diagnosing the patient newly with depression.

Epidemiology

In meta-analysis, Miovic and Block demonstrated that comorbidity of cancer and psychiatric symptomatology is considerable. Fifty percent of patients in advanced stages of cancer have met or do meet criteria for *DMS-IV-TR* diagnosis, and many patients have multiple psychiatric presentations during the course of their care (see Table 18.1).

Accurate measurement of the epidemiology of psychiatric symptomatology during cancer care may be undermined by the important distinction between strict diagnostic criteria and observed symptom set. Diagnosis of previously undiagnosed or non-emergent psychiatric illness, or determination of the extent of psychiatric symptomatology, can be biased in two directions. Patients struggle to determine for themselves what constitutes a "normal" reaction to cancer diagnosis and treatment, and this is complicated by familial and social pressures toward the "power of positive thinking" and the notion that grief and trauma responses are automatically pathological. The patient may struggle to sort out what is "normal" and/or to tolerate symptoms for which relief is available for fear of the stigma that still attends psychiatric illness and symptomatology, and the medical oncologist and oncology team may share this reluctance. Alternatively, providers who are using strict criteria can overdiagnose as a result of overlapping vegetative symptoms. Thus, others—*including providers*—may under-recognize treatable symptoms *or* overpathologize them.

Table 18.1 Prevalence of Psychiatric Comorbidity with Advanced Cancer

DSM-IV-TR Diagnosis	Prevalence in Advanced Cancer Patients
Adjustment Disorder	14%–37.5%
Major Depression	5%–26%
Generalized Anxiety	3.2%–5.3%
Panic Disorder	4.2%
Post-Traumatic Stress Disorder	2.4%
Delirium	≥ 15%–30%

Adapted from Miovic & Block (2007).

Presentation

Depression

Depression is *more* likely in certain cancers, including breast cancer, pancreatic cancer, oropharyngeal cancer, CNS tumors, and neuroendocrine tumors (see Table 18.2). Neurovegetative symptoms are prominent, and cancer patients frequently demonstrate low energy, low motivation, and anhedonia. Depression is also a side effect of common cancer treatments, including corticosteroids, interferon, Tamoxifen, anti-androgens, and chemotherapies (including vincristine, vinblastine, and procarbazine) due to direct stimulation of neurotransmitter receptors or via their effect on the endocrine system (see Table 18.3). The importance of an early discussion about these possible responses to treatment cannot be overestimated.

Data from a large national survey showed a 0.314% suicide rate among cancer patients, twice the risk of the general population's rate of 0.167% (167 deaths/100,000 people per year). Suicides are more common in the first five years after diagnosis, and rates are higher for white, unmarried men (as in the general population), and are elevated for men diagnosed at a later stage of the disease. Cancers of the lung, stomach, and head and neck also carry greater risk (Misono et al., 2008). This is consistent with the increased prevalence of depression with these cancers, and increases in *suicidal ideation* seem to be further correlated with anxiety and post-traumatic stress disorder (PTSD; Spencer et al., 2012).

Determining and responding to suicidality is complicated in the course of a life-threatening illness. What might otherwise be considered a passive death wish could be a "normal" expression of a shifting understanding of mortality and/or the time course of the illness, while what might otherwise be perceived as suicidal ideation can be an expression of a need for control. The expression itself can provide a sense of relief over

Table 18.2 Prevalence of Depression with Cancer Subtypes

Cancer Subtype	Prevalence
Oropharyngeal	22%–57%
Pancreatic	33%–50%
Breast	1.5%–46%
Lung	11%–44%
Colon	13%–25%
Gynecological	12%–23%
Prostate	14%–18.5%
Lymphoma	8%–19%

Adapted from Masie (2004).

Table 18.3 Prevalence of Depression as Side Effect of Common Cancer Treatments

Agent	Effect	Prevalence	Treatment
Interferon	MDD, mood lability, anxiety, suicidal ideation	Up to 70%	SSRI or SNRI
Tamoxifen	MDD, anxiety	15%	Venlafaxine (other SSRI/SNRI may effect Tamoxifen efficacy, as below)
Androgen deprivation therapy	MDD	12%	Buproprion (given lower risk sexual side effects than SSRI/SNRI) or venlafaxine (if hot flashes are present)

Heinze et al. (2010); Massie (2004); Grossmann et al. (2011).

the unknown (the future), including pain and loss of function. So while we normally distinguish between passive death wish and suicidal ideation, it is also possible to observe a third form of expression in advanced cancer patients: a patient wishing to postulate a future point where irreversible decline would mark the end of his desire to live. Thus, when a late stage cancer patient states, "I feel better knowing I can kill myself when the pain becomes unbearable" or "before I am no longer myself" (both patient-defined parameters), a psycho-oncologist can perceive a greater need for palliation, and an opportunity for discussion of end-of-life planning rather than imminent suicidal risk. Here, time is the key. Given the elevated suicide risk, a sensitive, thoughtful, and attentive provider must parse out such statements and respond proactively rather than reactively.

In patients with a history of depression preceding the cancer diagnosis, or in patients experiencing moderate to high levels of symptoms, antidepressants have been found to be efficacious. Psychopharmacological intervention can improve both non-iatrogenic and iatrogenic psychiatric symptoms, enabling the patient to continue the course of treatment recommended by the oncologist and to increase adherence. Thus, for patients with a prior history of mood disorder, a provider can have a lower threshold for initiating antidepressant therapies. Psychostimulants can be added when energy, motivation, or cognitive function are felt to be particularly problematic (see further discussion in Cognitive Change and Special Considerations sections). In addition, it is reasonable to recommend some form of modified exercise to all patients, even quite ill patients, for its antidepressant and anxiolytic effects (Herring et al., 2012).

Anxiety

Anxiety during cancer care may be triggered by the diagnosis itself or the medical symptoms that led to diagnosis. Symptoms associated with anxiety include pain, shortness of breath, diarrhea, and unanticipated physical symptoms, with the highest correlation (unsurprisingly) to pain. This anxiety frequently responds well to education and access to providers for normalization and reassurance. However, responses to unpredictable but recurring physical symptoms may require additional treatment with anxiolytics.

Persistent low-level anxiety and moderate to high levels of anxiety are more common in patients with a history of anxiety disorders or PTSD. If a patient has a premorbid anxiety disorder of any type, the patient is predisposed to developing worsened anxiety in response to the new stressors. In a patient with a premorbid history of anxiety, anxiety during cancer care is likely to take an intensified form of the prior expression of anxiety. Thus, a patient with generalized anxiety may experience "familiar" but worsened symptoms. While low-level anxiety and adjustment disorder respond well to CBT, moderate to high anxiety or more persistent anxiety symptoms may require SSRIs or SNRIs.

Although most features of anxiety are similar in patients with cancer and the general population, patients may have increased somatic symptoms, including nausea, pain, and neurological complaints such as headache and dizziness. These can be difficult to tease apart from organic pain, and nausea and neurological concerns arising from cancer and cancer treatment. Frequently pain and nausea symptoms go hand in hand with anxiety, and both show improvement with the down-regulation provided by benzodiazepines. In particular, chronic management that includes the long-acting clonazepam can reduce symptoms and decrease opiate dosing.

Patients experiencing specific phobias and panic responses to cancer care–related stimuli, including needles, recurrent scans, and even approach to the clinic or hospital itself, can also benefit from pre-medication with short-acting benzodiazepines. For example, a patient who feels panic and nausea prior to chemotherapy can be pre-medicated with lorazepam for symptom relief and re-establishment of a sense of control. This enables her to comply with her chemotherapeutic regimen until such time that behavioral strategies can be implemented.

Post-Traumatic Stress Disorder

A patient with a prior history of PTSD may be "triggered" by the proximal awareness of his or her mortality that a cancer diagnosis or major medical episode brings. Indeed, as we are coming to understand, a patient with no history of PTSD may report the full set of symptoms associated with that disorder as a result of the acuteness of thoughts about death and the disruptive experience of treatment, diagnosis, or an intense episode of medical illness and hospitalization, remembered delirium episodes, and surgical procedures.

PTSD (both initial experience and recurrence) is responsive to education, supportive therapy, and psychopharmacological interventions.

Therapy should focus on appreciating the life-changing quality of diagnosis and treatment and integrating the experience and information into the patient's life.

One difference between PTSD in the cancer setting and PTSD resulting from other causes is the chronic rather than acute nature of the stressor. Another is the future—rather than past—orientation of intrusive thoughts. Thus, while a veteran with PTSD may experience the intrusive thought of a moment of heightened risk of death, a cancer patient's intrusive thoughts may be characterized more by thoughts of future suffering or death. Continuing with this example, a veteran with a history of PTSD and subsequent threat to life via cancer may experience powerful symptoms of PTSD, including intrusive thoughts of the past and future. (This circumstance is not uncommon in practice and will be expected to be observed more as the veteran population ages and as veterans of recent wars present for cancer care.) The same could be said for patients with other prior causes of PTSD. They may need more aggressive management, and antidepressants and/or benzodiazepines should be considered. Antipsychotics would only be appropriate if psychotic symptoms are present or if dual-purpose prescribing is warranted, as described later in this chapter.

Cognitive Changes

Cognitive changes primarily exhibit as changes in levels of attention and concentration, as well as short-term memory dysfunction. This is patient-reported as well as measurable by neuro-psychological testing (Ahles et al., 2012). Unfortunately, the degree of loss is frequently subtle, and may not be observable by bedside neuropsychological testing, instead requiring the use of long-form instruments. These changes are commonly and casually described by patients using terms such as "chemo-brain," and while there is some evidence that a subset of patients who have been treated with chemotherapy are vulnerable to cognitive effects that persist after treatment concludes, it is less clear how and under what circumstances chemotherapeutic agents cause cognitive changes. The most convincing studies have shown both anatomic and physiologic changes to the brain after exposure to chemotherapy (McDonald & Conroy, 2010; Deprez et al., 2012). For patients experiencing this cognitive dysfunction, function can be improved by psycho-stimulants (typically starting with methylphenidate 5 mg at morning and midday) and cognitive exercise (multilevel puzzles such as sudoku or crosswords, as well as more structured brain-training programs).

Specific cognitive changes can be anticipated with the direct effect of both primary and secondary brain tumors, and intervention (surgical and radiological) for brain tumors. These tumors can also lead to personality change and increased impulsivity, both of which may respond to antipsychotics. These symptoms are particularly prominent when damage is in the frontal lobe or the parieto-frontal region. In addition, neuro-endocrine tumors can effect personality changes and cognitive changes.

Delirium

Delirium, elucidated in Chapter 10, is very common among hospitalized advanced cancer patients (15%–30%), terminal cancer patients (40%–85%), and patients undergoing chemotherapy. Hypoactive, hyperactive, and mixed forms are observed. Hypoactive delirium may be more common, but hyperactive delirium is more likely to be observed and treated (Bush & Bruera, 2009). As indicated in Chapter 10, a first episode of delirium is predictive of subsequent episodes when a patient experiences subsequent delirium triggers, including anticholinergic medications, electrolyte imbalance, infections, and anemia. Advanced cancer patients have a high likelihood of experiencing ongoing or multiple episodes of medical illness and/or provoking chemotherapeutic treatments. Thus, for patients who have experienced an episode of delirium, there may be some benefit to preventative treatment with a low-dose antipsychotic. The data for prescribing delirium prevention presurgically is increasingly convincing; however, in the special condition of advanced cancer, more chronic prophylaxis may be warranted. Given that overlap exists between medications used as antipsychotics and medications used for nausea, the choice to treat patients experiencing nausea and at risk for delirium with a medication such as haloperidol or olanzepine is well considered and may offer some delirium prevention as well. In practice, it is reasonable to use 5 mg olanzapine at night or 0.5–1 mg of risperidone twice daily, principally based on the patient's risk of recurrent delirium.

Special Concerns for Pharmacologic Intervention

In the setting of cancer care, physicians can often make excellent use of secondary characteristics or side effects of a pharmacologic agent to maximize outcomes and minimize medications (see Table 18.4).

Cancer care necessitates special consideration of pharmacologic interventions:

- SSRIs and SNRIs increase bleeding time, and while this is rarely a consideration in the general population, it can be of significant concern for cancer patients, who may also be on other agents that affect bleeding time.

Table 18.4 Making the Most of the Psychopharmacologic Agent

Psychiatric Symptomatology	Alongside	Favors Use of
Anxiety	Insomnia	Clonazepam
Anxiety	Nausea	Benzodiazepine
Depression or anxiety	Pain	SNRI (venlafaxine, duloxetine), tricyclic antidepressants
Depression or anxiety	Neuropathy	SNRI, tricyclic antidepressants
Depression or anxiety	Tamoxifen	Venlafaxine (see special concerns below)
Depression or anxiety	Hotflashes	Venlafaxine
Depression or anxiety	Fatigue	Augment with psycho-stimulant
Depression	Insomnia	Mirtazapine
Depression	Anorexia, weight loss, cachexia	Mirtazapine
Delirium	Nausea	Antipsychotics (haloperidol, olanzepine)
Cognitive change	No delirium	Psycho-stimulant
Personality change/ Increased impulsivity	Brain Tumor	Atypical antipsychotics

- Rare reports of bone marrow suppression with mirtazapine (0.1%–1%) indicate a need for monitoring for this complication in immunocompromised patients.
- As with other conditions that increase seizure risk, bupropion should be avoided for patients with primary and secondary brain tumors.
- Some antidepressants, including paroxetine and fluoxetine, have been shown to decrease the efficacy of Tamoxifen, which is used to decrease the recurrence of breast cancer after active treatment (Sideras et al., 2011). Others are assumed to have similar effects in relation to their 2D6 binding properties. Venlafaxine, a non-2D6 metabolizer, has been shown to have no effect on Tamoxifen efficacy.
- Psycho-stimulant use in the setting of advanced cancer is not well studied. Most of the research on psycho-stimulant use for cognitive change in this context derives from research on the use of these agents in post-traumatic brain injury, where they have been shown to improve acute function and hasten recovery. Studies show long-standing psycho-stimulants only negatively impact the most severe arrythmia patients, and that most cardiac patients will tolerate them well. As a considered alternative, most recent studies show that modafinil is no better than placebo for cancer fatigue (Spathis et al., 2014).
- Pre-existing substance abuse may impact prescription decision-making, but treatment decisions should also be reflective of the setting. The goal for substance abuse treatment during cancer should be a decrease in negative impact and an increase of functionality as opposed to total sobriety. For example, a patient with a remote history of opioid dependence may require higher doses of pain medication to achieve relief, but should be monitored closely for use-as-prescribed. A patient with a recent history or active use may still require opiate pain management, but will fare better in the structured context of methadone maintenance.

Key Points

- Psychiatric symptoms occur at many points along the timeline of cancer diagnosis, treatment, and post-treatment care. Recognizing and treating these symptoms is essential for quality-of-life care.
- Many symptoms that are associated with depression and anxiety are also symptoms of cancer and side effects of cancer treatment. These include anergia/fatigue, insomnia, anorexia, and amotivation.
- Treatment decision-making should include a consideration of secondary effects of medications, problematic interactions, and rapidity of action.
- Direct effects of cancer on brain function can be observed in cancer patients in relationship to primary and metastatic brain tumors, neuroendocrine tumors, radiation, and chemotherapy. These effects can last well past the point of active cancer.

Disclosures

Dr. Patterson has no conflicts of interest.

Further Reading

Ahles T, Root J, et al. (2012). Cancer and cancer treatment–associated cognitive change: An update on the state of the science. *J Clin Oncol.*, *30*(30), 3675–3686.

Bush S, Bruera E (2009). The assessment and management of delirium in cancer patients. *Oncologist*, *14*(10), 1039–1049.

Deprez S, Amant F, et al. (2012). Longitudinal assessment of chemotherapy-induced structural changes in cerebral white matter and its correlation with impaired cognitive functioning. *J Clin Oncol.*, *30*(3), 274–281.

Grossmann M, Zajac J. (2011). Management of side effects of androgen deprivation therapy. *Endocrin Metab Clin N Am.*, *40*(3), 655–671.

Heinze S, Egberts F, et al. (2010). Depressive mood changes and psychiatric symptoms during 12-month low-dose interferon-alpha treatment in patients with malignant melanoma: Results from the multicenter DeCOG Trial. *J Immunother.*, *33*(1), 106–114.

Herring MP, Puetz T, et al. (2012). Effect of exercise training on depressive symptoms among patients with a chronic illness: A systematic review and meta-analysis of randomized controlled trials. *Arch Intern Med.*, *172*(2), 101–111.

Massie MJ. (2004). Prevalence of depression in patients with cancer. *J Natl Cancer I Monog.*, *2004*(32), 57–71.

McDonald B, Conroy S (2010). Gray matter reduction associated with systemic chemotherapy for breast cancer: A prospective MRI study. *Breast Cancer Res Tr.*, *123*, 819–828.

Miovic M, Block S (2007). Psychiatric disorders in advanced cancer. *Cancer*, *110*(8), 1665–1676.

Misono S, Weiss N, et al. (2008). Incidence of suicide in persons with cancer. *J Clin Oncol.*, *26*(29), 4631–4638.

Sideras K, Ingle J, et al. (2011). Coprescription of tamoxifen and medications that inhibit CYP2D6. *J Clin Oncol.*, *28*(16), 2768–2776.

Spathis A, Dhillan R, et al. (2014). Modafinil for the treatment of fatigue in lung cancer: A pilot study. *Palliative Med.*, *23*(4), 325–331.

Spencer RJ, Ray A, Pirl WF, Prigerson HG (2012) Clinical correlates of suicidal thoughts in patients with advanced cancer. *Am J Geriat Psychiat.*, *20*(4), 327–336.

Exercises

1. Which of the following cancer subtypes is among those that carry the highest risk of depression according to current research?
   a. Colon cancer
   b. Prostate cancer
   c. Pancreatic cancer
   d. Lymphoma
   e. Uterine cancer

2. In a patient with a history of delirium while hospitalized, and chronic nausea associated with chemotherapy, which of the following would be the best choice for nausea management?
   a. Lorazepam 0.5 mg prn nausea
   b. Ondansetron 4 mg tid
   c. Ziprasidone 20 mg bid
   d. Haloperidol 0.5 mg bid
   e. Metoclopramide 5 mg bid

3. Which of the following medications is the best choice for treating depression in a patient with neurovegetative symptoms and neuropathy who is taking Tamoxifen for breast cancer relapse prevention?
   a. Fluoxetine
   b. Venlafaxine
   c. Paroxetine
   d. Bupropion
   e. Mirtazapine

4. Which of the following is least likely to cause cognitive change in a cancer patient?
   a. Primary brain tumor
   b. Focal radiation for vertebral metastases
   c. Lung cancer with brain metastases
   d. Systemic chemotherapy for breast cancer
   e. Carcinoid tumor (neuroendocrine tumor in the gut)

Answers: (1) c (2) d (3) b (4) b

Organ Transplantation Psychiatry

Andrea F. DiMartini, Donna M. Posluszny, Traci D'Almeida, and Mary Amanda Dew

Introduction

The Role of Psychosomatic Medicine Specialists

With over 250 organ transplant programs in the United States, psychosomatic medicine (PM) specialists typically play an important role in the evaluation of patients under consideration for transplant. Additionally, PM psychiatrists are consulted to address psychiatric and behavioral issues as they arise pre- and post-transplant. In this chapter we cover PM issues relevant to solid organ transplantation for adults.

Transplant Epidemiology

Organ transplantation is the accepted treatment for many chronic or acute organ diseases and certain types of cancer. Unfortunately, although the transplant wait list continues to lengthen, the number of transplants is static (~ 28,000 recipients/year) and over 130,000 candidates (about 80% kidney candidates) currently are on the US transplant wait list (2014). Most transplant candidates wait a year or more for an organ, while many kidney candidates wait three to five years; 10%–18% of all candidates will not survive to transplant. Transplant recipients face long-term complications, including recurrent organ disease, graft dysfunction/rejection, and the development of immunosuppressive medication complications (e.g. diabetes, renal failure, cancer), making adherence to treatment and surveillance directives imperative to successful long-term outcomes.

Phases of Transplantation

The transplantation process is a continuum demarcated by transitions into specific phases, from evaluation, to waiting on the national list, to early recovery and long-term adaptation to life as an organ recipient. Each phase is associated with different stressors requiring differing skills and resources from patients, their caregivers, and their behavioral health clinicians (Figure 19.1). It is helpful to consider the patient in the context of this continuum, recognizing that while the development of advanced organ disease heralds the beginning of the transplant process, many patients have dealt with chronic illness for years.

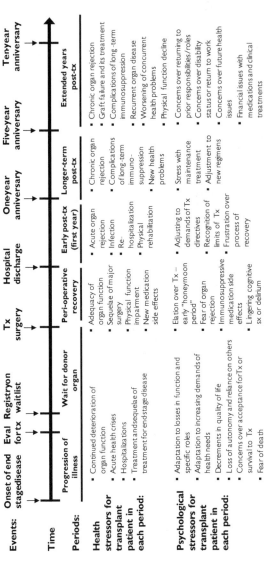

Events: Time	Onset of end stage disease	Eval for tx	Registry on wait list	Wait for donor organ	Tx surgery	Peri-operative recovery	Hospital discharge	Early post-tx (first year)	One year anniversary	Longer-term post-tx	Five-year anniversary	Extended years post-tx	Ten year anniversary
Periods:	Progression of illness					Peri-operative recovery		Early post-tx (first year)		Longer-term post-tx		Extended years post-tx	
Health stressors for transplant patient in each period:	• Continued deterioration of organ function • Acute health crises • Hospitalizations • Treatment and sequelae of treatment for end-stage disease					• Adequacy of organ function • Sequelae of major surgery • Physical function impairment • New medication side effects		• Acute organ rejection • Infection • Re-hospitalization • Physical rehabilitation		• Chronic organ rejection • Complications of long-term immuno-suppression • New health problems		• Chronic organ rejection • Graft failure and its treatment • Complications of long-term immunosuppression • Recurrent organ disease • Worsening of concurrent health problems • Physical function decline	
Psychological stressors for transplant patient in each period:	• Adaptation to losses in function and specific roles • Adaptation to increasing demands of health needs • Decrements in quality of life • Loss of autonomy and reliance on others • Concerns over acceptance for Tx or survival to Tx • Fear of death					• Elation over Tx – early "honeymoon period" • Fear of organ rejection • Immunosuppressive medication side effects • Lingering cognitive sx or delirium		• Adjusting to demands of Tx directives • Recognition of limits of Tx • Frustration over process of recovery		• Stress with maintenance treatment • Adjustment to new regimens		• Concerns over returning to prior responsibilities/roles • Concerns over disability status or return to work • Concerns over future health issues • Financial issues with medications and clinical treatments	

Figure 19:1 Organ Transplant Timeline: Critical Events and Time Periods for Transplant Patients.

Abbreviations: tx = transplantation; eval = evaluation.

Source: Adapted from Dew et al. (2007) and reprinted with permission from Elsevier.

Pre-Transplant Phase

Psychosocial Evaluation: Approach and Purpose

PM specialists are frequently requested to assist in the evaluation of prospective transplant candidates. Limited organ availability and the extensive healthcare resources and degree of personal responsibility required of recipients and caregivers for successful outcomes necessitate careful candidate assessment. The primary goal of a pre-transplant psychosocial evaluation is to determine whether patients have cognitive, behavioral, psychological, or social issues that may negatively affect post-transplant outcomes such as the ability to adjust to transplantation or to adhere to medical directives. It is noteworthy that even complicated patients (e.g., those with severe and persistent mental illness or intellectual disabilities) can have successful post-transplant outcomes if they have good social supports, expert psychiatric management, and a collaborative relationship with the transplant team. While most transplant evaluations occur in the outpatient setting, inpatient evaluations are often urgent, and time to address psychosocial issues may be limited.

Although there are published guidelines on the basic components for the psychosocial evaluation (see Box 19.1 for evaluation goals), there are no national psychosocial criteria for candidate listing in the United States. Additionally, there are considerable differences between programs regarding the purpose and details of the psychosocial evaluation, who performs it (clinical social workers versus behavioral health clinicians), and how such information will be used in candidacy determinations. There is no consensus on psychosocial characteristics that make patients unsuitable for listing or lead to poorer post-transplant outcomes; evidence to support the use of specific criteria is either lacking or equivocal. Due to these complexities, the consultant must be knowledgeable of his or her team's approach to psychosocial issues so that the needs of the transplant team and patient, as well as mandatory requirements for transplant listing, are met. In many programs the sheer volume of patients precludes a comprehensive psychiatric evaluation for all candidates, and other health professionals often screen patients, with referrals to PM consultants if specific behavioral health issues are identified. Therefore, it is prudent to determine if there is a specific issue that prompted the evaluation request.

The potential dual roles of the PM consultant can be challenging in addressing the needs of the transplant team while assisting patients to prepare for transplant (if issues are identified). In addition, PM consultants may need to advocate, if appropriate, on a patient's behalf because transplant teams may not be knowledgeable about the availability of effective treatments for many behavioral health disorders and may underestimate the patient's prognosis post-transplant. Patients also generally recognize the importance of the PM evaluation, although some fear that it may lead to their disqualification and may withhold pertinent mental health information. Often it is possible to allay fears by explaining that the purpose of the evaluation is to identify potential mental health issues and to assist patients before transplant in order to foster

Box 19.1 Goals of the Pre-transplant Psychosocial Evaluation

1. Develop individualized treatment plans for patients, including requirements for transplant listing.
2. Establish working relationships with patients and family/caregivers and assess their ability to collaborate with the transplant team.
3. Assess patients' coping strengths and weaknesses/vulnerabilities.
4. Diagnose and provide options for treatment of active psychiatric disorders and maintenance plans for chronic or remitted behavioral health disorders.
5. Assess substance use/abuse history, treatment, and recovery, and ability to maintain lifelong abstinence.
6. Assess adherence and identify factors (including lifestyle characteristics, e.g., poor diet, lack of exercise, lack of structured schedule) that may interfere with adherence.
7. Establish baseline mental status and cognitive functioning.
8. Evaluate availability and stability of social support systems.
9. Facilitate the informed consent process for patients.
10. Educate patients on transplant-specific expectations and prepare them for transplantation.
11. Provide input to transplant team regarding potential obstacles for candidacy and recommended treatment plan for addressing difficulties.

Adapted from Levenson & Olbrisch (2000) and used with the permission of Cambridge University Press. Reprinted with the permission of Cambridge University Press.

optimal post-transplant outcomes. Developing a working alliance with the patient allows the PM consultant to both explain and address transplant expectations with the patient and communicate a mental health management plan to the transplant team.

Typically, the PM consultant works with the patient to minimize behavioral health symptoms and to prepare the patient for transplant, rather than recommending outright denial of candidacy. The PM consultant may make recommendations (e.g., addiction counseling, psychiatric treatment, behavioral changes, establishing an adequate support system), which the transplant team may adopt as requirements for listing. However, listing decisions are always team decisions in formal candidacy meetings, and the surgeons typically have the final determination. Nevertheless, information obtained from the PM evaluation may be used to uphold or deny listing, and caution must be taken regarding comments on a patient's lack of suitability for transplant. Fortunately, many programs do not decline candidates outright for psychosocial issues, but allow a period for these issues to be addressed or resolved, followed by candidacy reassessment. In rare circumstances a PM consultant may suggest additional consultations with medical ethics teams, risk management, or the hospital's legal department (e.g., when a candidate/family is challenging candidacy requirements or the team decision). Thorough documentation is essential to delineate the issues involved, the rationale for specific recommendations, and efforts to work with the patient/family.

Psychosocial Evaluation: Specific Areas of Transplant Assessment

Pre-transplant psychosocial evaluations also focus on transplant-specific areas. A PM consultant may employ rigorous scrutiny of data to uncover pertinent information for the evaluation (e.g., examining medical records to look for inconsistencies in history and treatment engagement, reviewing toxicology screening and pharmacy records, and discussing adherence to treatment directives with other treatment providers).

Informed Consent

The PM consultant can assess how well the patient understands his or her illness, prognosis, treatment options, and the need for transplant, as well as the post-transplant requirements for lifelong adherence to treatment directives and follow-up with the transplant team. Patients should be aware of the risks of transplant surgery and both early and long-term complications. However, it can be challenging to assess a patient's understanding of these issues in the face of life-threatening illness where transplant is the only option for extension of life or when other treatment options become intolerable (e.g., dialysis) or are a bridge to transplant (e.g., ventricular assist devices). Patients may perceive the situation as desperate and may view transplant as a procedure that will rescue them. Given the enormous stresses in considering a life-preserving therapy, patients may not fully appreciate or comprehend the requirements for transplantation or the significant alterations that transplantation would necessitate in their lives. Interactive decision aids based on personal values have been created for scenarios in which the benefits of transplant may be less certain (e.g., patients with cystic fibrosis considering lung transplantation).

Substance Use

Substance use is an area of special concern for transplant teams, especially when the substance has contributed to organ disease and the need for transplantation (e.g., smoking for lung/heart transplant or alcohol in liver transplant). The PM consultant will likely be the clinician relied upon to most thoroughly review the addiction history and make treatment recommendations. Tobacco use (smoked/chewed) has long been a prohibition for cardiothoracic transplant, and abdominal transplant programs are increasingly requiring tobacco cessation pre-transplant due to evidence of poorer outcomes for recipients who use tobacco (e.g., higher rates of oropharyngeal cancers and lung infections). Currently, there is no consensus among transplant teams regarding the recreational use of marijuana. PM consultants should evaluate the use of marijuana, providing their best clinical advice on the need for abstinence and/or rehabilitation, while recognizing that their team may not require a "casual" marijuana user to be abstinent. Patients stable on opioid agonist therapy should not be required to stop these therapies as a condition for transplant eligibility because it may increase relapse risk, especially during the stressful pre-transplant period.

Transplant programs aim to select patients with low risk for substance use relapse. Many programs require a period of abstinence before evaluation referral or transplant listing (6 months at many centers). No single risk factor except short length of abstinence strongly predicts future use, although poor social support, family history of addiction, polysubstance use, and failed rehabilitation have been associated with increased risk. While risk for relapse increases in the presence of multiple risk factors, it is important to note that no risk factor indicates inevitable relapse, and many patients even with multiple risk factors do not relapse post-transplant. Relapse prevention is best achieved by providing the patient with the necessary skills to stay sober. Many patients have some period of abstinence but no addiction rehabilitation, and often do not perceive a need for addiction treatment. Many have not incorporated the skills or strategies to stay sober and may be abstinent at the time of evaluation, primarily due to being ill. Many require basic recovery education and maintenance treatment to prepare for continued abstinence post-transplant. Motivational interviewing is a key tool for assisting those reluctant to engage in treatment. In some cases, outright mandating of treatment as a requirement for transplant listing is needed. Traditional addiction rehabilitation may be complicated by (a) the severity of the patient's medical illness and possible encephalopathy, (b) limited insurance coverage and availability of local rehabilitation resources, and (c) medical deterioration, which might result in death or ineligibility for listing if too much time is taken. If full completion of goals is not possible due to medical deterioration, patients should be scheduled to return and demonstrate that rehabilitation objectives have been at least initiated.

Social Support

Social workers focus on social/caregiver supports, but the PM consultant can also evaluate the adequacy of support. Especially during pre-transplant and in the early recovery period, patients may be too physically or cognitively impaired to care for themselves and often require assistance with medications, clinic attendance, activities of daily living, transportation, and specialized treatments (e.g., dressing changes, IV medications). Caregivers should demonstrate both the willingness to take on the responsibilities and the ability (physically and cognitively) to manage complex transplant tasks (e.g., managing multiple medication schedules and dose/timing, adjustments, possibly dressing changes, being able to monitor and report symptoms to the team, etc.).

Adaptation to and Stresses of the Evaluation and Wait Period

A patient's adaptation to the diagnosis of terminal, advanced organ disease and the need for transplantation may depend on the chronicity of the disease and the patient's expectations about transplantation. Patients with chronic disease may have psychologically accommodated to gradual decrements in functioning and may view transplant as an opportunity for improved quality of life. With an acute illness (e.g., acute MI, hepatocellular carcinoma), a patient may be in disbelief, denial, or shock about the recent diagnosis of terminal disease and possible transplant. These patients often feel a heightened sense of unexpected vulnerability. They may not have been ill or required much healthcare prior to their diagnosis, and they often view transplant with apprehension as an unwelcomed event. They may hope that the transplant team will deem surgery unnecessary and may be devastated to be recommended for transplantation. In either case, patients must adjust to decrements in physical health with attendant losses in physical, mental, and social functioning and roles, losses of independence with increasing reliance on caregivers, and possible financial hardships. While patients may experience the news that they are on the transplant list with elation and relief, they still face the uncertain waiting list duration, continued declines in functioning, and the uncertainty of surviving to receive a transplant. The inherent stresses in waiting for transplantation challenge the adaptive skills, character style, coping behaviors, and social supports of all patients and their caregivers. Additionally, wait list candidates may develop contraindications to transplant (e.g., stroke, excessive medical decline, addiction relapse) and may be removed from the wait list. Psychological counseling can be useful in aiding patients to successfully adapt to these challenges, deal with grief and losses, maintain hope or, if needed, prepare for death.

Early Post-Transplant Phase and Adjustment to Recovery Process

Following transplantation, patients may have a sense of elation at surviving. This optimism can be heightened by the typically short postoperative hospital stays and transition to home. Some patients may require more extensive physical rehabilitation, and others with long-standing encephalopathy may experience cognitive impairment that persists through the early recovery period. Those with mental disorders who were stable on psychotropic medications before transplant may be destabilized by the transplant process and medication changes that occur perioperatively. Psychological issues can emerge with some patients who experience difficulties incorporating the organ and who may experience guilt over the loss of life that saved their own. Psychological rejection of the organ may lead to poorer survival, and interventions should focus on acceptance and incorporation of the transplanted organ. While information about the deceased donor is not revealed to the recipient, the patient may write anonymously to the donor's family through official channels, which can provide a measure of peace and closure. Some patients develop acute stress disorder and PTSD due to the wait-list process, transplant surgery, intensive care unit, or other experiences, and will require treatment to prevent the development of avoidance behaviors that can interfere with transplant care or clinic attendance.

Patients often believe that following transplant their health will be quickly restored; they may be discouraged to discover that they will need to rebuild the health and vitality that was lost, sometimes over a period of years. High-dose corticosteroids sometimes used for adjunctive immunosuppression in the early postoperative period may be tapered off, so any steroid-induced energy and feelings of well-being may be lost, adding to patients' sense of slowed recovery. Patients and caregivers are educated by treatment teams on an extensive range of transplant-related directives, including taking medications regularly, obtaining bloodwork, monitoring vital signs and measures of organ function (e.g., spirometry for lung transplant), diet and exercise recommendations, attendance at clinic, and other tests and procedures as indicated. Reliance on caregivers is essential at this time, and caregivers may feel anxious or overwhelmed by their responsibilities in dispensing medications and monitoring the recipient for any health concerns. Recipients must adjust to immunosuppressive medications which can have unpleasant side effects (see discussion later in this chapter); these symptoms may further impede a sense of recovery and return to normalcy. Common complications during the early recovery period, including acute organ rejection episodes and infections, can further add to patients' concern over losing their transplanted organs and a diminished sense of well-being.

The likelihood of developing mood or anxiety disorders, as well as relapsing to substance use, is highest in the first year following transplantation and decreases over time. PM consultants may be called on to manage these problems. Periodic monitoring to identify prodromal symptoms during routine transplant clinic follow-up may be the best strategy to avoid development of disabling symptoms. Recurrent substance use has been linked to poorer transplant outcomes (e.g., graft failure and death). Mood disorders have also been increasingly linked to poorer post-transplant outcomes (e.g., graft loss, decreased survival); whether treatment to improve psychiatric outcomes will improve transplant outcomes is likely, but not yet established.

Long-Term Post-Transplant Phase

Beyond the early recovery, patients must work to reintegrate back into as normal a lifestyle as possible. Although the post-transplant phase provides improvements in health and quality of life compared to the pre-transplant phase, transplant recipients usually do not rate their health on par with normal healthy individuals. For patients who have been ill for years before transplant, what constitutes a normal lifestyle may no longer be familiar. Some may become psychologically stuck, functioning in a sick role even though physically capable of achieving more. For some, recovery may mean attempting to return to work or school. Others who are unable to perform these roles may worry about maintaining their disability status. Health insurance and financial issues can also become problematic.

Special Issues

Emergency Evaluation

In acute organ failure (e.g., fulminant liver failure or acute cardiomyopathy), patients may participate minimally in their evaluation due to coma/stupor or mechanical ventilation. Patients and families will likely be overwhelmed with the seriousness of the situation, and the need to learn and decide about transplantation. The urgent situation demands quick assessment, often with limited time to address mental health issues if present, thus making an adequate psychosocial evaluation challenging. For those with identified mental health issues, understanding prior psychiatric treatment course, adherence, and stability, based on input from current/prior psychiatric care providers, may be critical to estimating the prognosis and making treatment recommendations. Families already distraught over the situation may be the only source of information if time does not allow identification of and access to psychiatric care providers. Existence of a stable support system is essential. With acetaminophen or other toxic ingestion/overdoses, it is important to determine if it was accidental or intentional and, if intentional, to obtain information such as whether it was impulsive or planned, prior history of suicide attempts or other self-destructive behaviors, substance abuse, active psychiatric disorders, presence of character pathology, current stressors, and additional risk factors and protective factors for future suicide attempts. In addition to assessing current prognosis and future risk, PM consultants, along with the transplant team and caregivers, can develop individualized post-transplant psychiatric care plans focused on relief of patient distress, modifying factors for future suicide attempts, and development of a safety plan.

Adherence

The post-transplant regimen is complex and multifaceted, with patients required to take multiple medications on a daily basis, self-monitor for a variety of symptoms, attend clinic appointments, undergo diagnostic tests, and adhere to substance use restrictions. The rates of non-adherence are discouraging; nearly 30% of transplant recipients are non-adherent to immunosuppressants, contributing up to 50% of late acute rejection, graft dysfunction, and loss. Even a few missed doses can result in organ damage. Many factors contribute to non-adherence, including medication side effects, behavioral factors (e.g., poor planning, poor health responsibility), and social issues (e.g., insurance coverage, copayments, transportation). Patients often do not experience any immediate effects of non-adherence and thus do not perceive the danger. Re-education about the treatment regimen and its rationale can be helpful. Identification and treatment of depression and/or substance use may improve adherence. PM consultants may additionally recommend problem-solving, CBT, or other behavioral therapies. Patients traumatized by the transplant experience may require psychotherapy.

Medications

Immunosuppressants

Calcineurin inhibitors (e.g., tacrolimus and cyclosporine), the main-stays of transplant immunosuppression, have similar neuropsychiatric side effects, with 40%–60% of patients experiencing mild symptoms (tremors, insomnia, vivid dreams/nightmares, headache, restlessness, hyperesthesia/dysesthesias, agitation, and anxiety). These effects are most pronounced in the early post-transplant period, when drug levels are typically higher, and they may spontaneously resolve over time with dose reduction and often require minimal or temporary psychotropic management. Moderate-severe neuropsychiatric side effects (e.g., delirium, seizures, coma, focal neurologic deficits, dysarthria, corti-cal blindness, and cognitive impairments) are experienced by up to 20%–30% of patients. Posterior reversible encephalopathy syndrome is a rare (1%–2%) but serious syndrome characterized by headache, altered sensorium, seizures, and visual disturbances, or other neuro-logical symptoms, depending on the location of the lesion. Diagnosis is made by identification of characteristic cortical/subcortical white matter changes, typically in parietal or occipital lobes on radiographic imaging with MRI, with diffusion weighted imaging (DWI) being supe-rior to CT. Moderate to severe side effects may require switching to a different immunosuppressive agent. Immunosuppressants have signifi-cant metabolic side effects (e.g., weight gain, hyperlipidemia, glucose intolerance), which must be considered in choosing which psychotro-pics to prescribe.

Psychotropics

Although no psychotropic medication is absolutely contraindicated, cau-tion is recommended, with lower doses and closer monitoring for side effects in the pre-transplant and perioperative periods. Some drugs are not ideal for use in transplant populations (e.g., lithium due to its nar-row therapeutic window and fluid shifts associated with organ disease and surgery) or may be relatively contraindicated due to potential organ toxicity (see Chapter 6 for details of pharmacologic management in the setting of organ dysfunction).

Following transplant, physiologic function is restored for most patients, and normal therapeutic drug dosing can be used, assuming recovery from immediate postoperative complications (e.g., sedation, delirium, ileus, ability to take oral medications). However, delayed graft functioning or episodes of acute rejection are common and affect pharmacokinetics, and thus should be considered. Psychotropic medi-cations prescribed at lower dosages pre-transplant may need to be increased. Drug-drug interactions should be carefully considered, as patients often take a wide variety of medications in addition to immu-nosuppressants. Psychotropics that can significantly inhibit or induce cytochrome P450 3A4 (e.g., inhibitors: nefazodone, fluvoxamine, and to some degree fluoxetine; inducers: St. John's wort, carbamazepine/oxcarbazepine, phenytoin, armodafinil, and modafinil) may have clinically meaningful interactions with many immunosuppressant medications (e.g., calcineurin inhibitors, mycophenolate, sirolimus/everolimus, and glucocorticoids/corticosteroids) that are metabolized by CYP3A4. Calcineurin inhibitors also inhibit CYP3A4, and tacrolimus can prolong Qt intervals.

Conclusions

Transplantation is a challenging process for patients, caregivers, and medical professionals alike. Identification and amelioration of potential psychosocial risk factors for poor outcomes are a major focus of the PM consultant's role in evaluating patients for candidacy. Appreciation of acute and chronic pathophysiologic changes and concomitant psychological stress and lifestyle adjustments associated with each phase of transplantation is critical.

Key Points

- There are no national psychosocial criteria for transplant listing; each program makes individual decisions.
- Behavioral health issues can often be addressed to better prepare a patient for transplant listing.
- Patients with complex or serious behavioral health disorders can often be successfully transplanted with appropriate psychiatric and psychosocial management.
- No psychotropic medications are absolutely contraindicated, but PM consultants should carefully consider each case based on the type of organ disease, drug, dosage, and potential for side effects and drug-drug interactions.

Disclosures

Dr. DiMartini receives funding from the National Institutes of Health for research related to living liver donor transplantation.

Dr. Posluszny receives funding from the National Institutes of Health for research related to hematopoietic cell transplantation.

Dr. Dew receives funding from the National Institutes of Health for research related to living liver and kidney transplantation, palliative care, and late life mood disorders.

Further Reading

Dew MA et al. (2007). Stress of organ transplantation. In Fink G (Ed.), *Encyclopedia of Stress*, 2nd ed., vol 3, pp. 35–44. Oxford: Academic Press (Elsevier).

DiMartini A, Dew MA, Crone C. Organ transplantation. (2009). In Kaplan, Saddock (Eds.), *The Comprehensive Textbook of Psychiatry*, 9th ed., vol. II, pp. 2441–2456. Philadelphia: Lippincott Williams & Wilkins.

DiMartini A, Sotelo J, Dew MA (2011). Organ transplantation. In Levenson J (Ed.), *The American Psychiatric Press Textbook of Psychosomatic Medicine: Psychiatric Care of the Medically Ill*, 2nd ed, pp. 725–758. Washington, DC: American Psychiatric Publishing.

DiMartini A, Crone C, Fireman M. (2010). Psychopharmacology in organ transplantation. In Ferrando, Levenson, Owen (Eds). *Psychopharmacology of the Medically Ill*, pp. 469–500. Washington, DC: American Psychiatric Publishing.

Levenson J, Olbrisch ME. (2000). Psychosocial screening and selection of candidates for organ transplantation. In Trzepacz PT, DiMartini AF (Eds.), *The Transplant Patient* (p. 23, pp. 21–41). Cambridge: Cambridge University Press.

Exercises

1. Which of the following is true?
   a. Patients with complex psychiatric disorders cannot be successfully transplanted.
   b. Any alcohol or substance use is an absolute contraindication to transplant listing.
   c. A patient turned down at one center for psychosocial issues may be considered at another transplant program.
   d. Transplant teams rely on national criteria for transplant listing.

2. Which of the following IS an important goal of the psychosocial screening of potential transplant candidates?
   a. Establish the occupational history to determine the candidate's social worth.
   b. Evaluate coping skills and psychosocial strengths and weaknesses.
   c. Determine if the candidate is well liked by the transplant team.
   d. Confirm that the candidate does not have a prison record.
   e. Confirm that the candidate plays an essential role in his or her family or community.

3. Risk for psychiatric disorders post-transplant include:
   a. Appears to be greatest in the first year post-transplant.
   b. Increases with each year post-transplant.
   c. Is equal across all years post-transplant.
   d. Is low unless the recipient faces graft loss.

Answers: (1) c (2) b (3) a

Psychiatric Evaluation and Management of Pain

Ronald M. Glick and Pierre N. Azzam

Introduction

Pain is the most common symptom described by patients who present for medical hospitalization. Often, as in the case of cardiac pain, treatment of the underlying condition results in the resolution of pain. However, many individuals experience severe pain that does not respond to acute therapies, necessitating alternative measures. Psychiatric comorbidities may complicate pain and increase disability. Targeting these conditions provides a unique opportunity for mental health clinicians to ameliorate pain-associated distress. As with other conditions in psychiatry, self-report establishes severity and quality of pain. A nonjudgmental stance allows clinicians to connect with ailing patients. Pain has a bidirectional relationship with psychiatric symptoms, each amplifying the other. With appropriate knowledge and sensitivity, the psychiatry consultation service is in a unique position to help mitigate distress and suffering.

Knowledge of four concepts related to pain physiology may strengthen the consultation psychiatrist's capacity to facilitate the holistic management of pain:

- Gate-control theory
- Endogenous opioid pathways
- Serotonergic and noradrenergic pain pathways
- Pain windup.

Gate control theory provides a schema to integrate pain modulation from afferent stimulation and descending pathways. Much like a pain thermostat, efferent pathways from the midbrain and medulla directly modulate pain regulation at a spinal cord level. Consequently, neural signaling in times of emotional distress can amplify pain at its source. Mind-body approaches that mitigate affective distress can diminish pain perception.

Endogenous opioid pathways provide another approach to active pain relief via physical activity (e.g., "runner's high"). Moderate aerobic activity can have a substantial impact on the psychological and physical distress associated with depression, anxiety, and pain.

The analgesic effect of tricyclic antidepressants (TCAs) alerted neuroscientists to the pain-mediating effects of monamines. Independent of **serotonergic and noradrenergic** effects on anxiety and depression, these pathways are key in descending inhibition of pain. The nucleus raphe magnus is a hub of serotonergic activity, and the locus coeruleus is a major noradrenergic center. Both are tied in with descending inhibition, overlapping with endogenous opioid pain-modulating pathways.

Pain windup describes the amplification of pain via repetitive nociceptive stimulation. This can progress to extreme and enduring pain in the absence of painful stimulation, such as in post-herpetic neuralgia. NMDA and glutamate mediate what can become lasting changes in neuronal membranes and firing, "winding-up" pain. Perhaps it is possible to "wind down" these neurons. Anticonvulsants, TCAs, and SNRIs can have substantial impact on pain control via these mechanisms.

Maintaining an appreciation for the neural underpinnings of pain permits the clinician to synthesize subjective findings with physiologic and neuropsychiatric factors to offer practical approaches to analgesic care.

Assessment of Pain

As pain is a subjective experience, assessment relies primarily on self-report. For infants, nonverbal, or cognitively impaired patients, assessment is based on observation and physiologic signs, such as grimacing and tachycardia. Most patients, including children and those with communication or cognitive problems, can provide a reliable gauge using one of the standard faces scales such as the Wong-Baker FACES® Pain Rating Scale (Figure 20.1).

For a verbal patient, pain severity is commonly assessed with a verbal rating scale. The patient is asked to rate pain on a scale of 0–10, with 0 being no pain and 10 being the most severe pain possible. It may help to ask about current pain, as well as the best and worst pain on an average day. While this assesses severity, it is equally important to determine the level of functional impairment related to pain. Scales such as the Brief Pain Inventory can assess impairment, or one can ask the patient qualitatively to what extent pain interferes with daily life.

One common issue is the occasional disparity between the patient's self-report and visible signs of comfort or distress. Pain behavior can be a *no-win scenario*, as a patient writhing in pain may be seen as overly dramatic, whereas someone conversing calmly may be seen as exaggerating the pain rating. Even if pain is not the primary reason for consultation, it may be helpful to introduce the topic of pain and discomfort early in the interview. Another pragmatic guide is to err on the side of assuming that the patient's experiences are real and not embellished, at least at the outset. This enhances rapport and may facilitate future attempts to steer the patient toward behavioral change.

Wong-Baker FACES® Pain Rating Scale

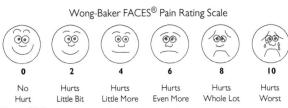

0	2	4	6	8	10
No Hurt	Hurts Little Bit	Hurts Little More	Hurts Even More	Hurts Whole Lot	Hurts Worst

Figure 20.1 Wong-Baker FACES Pain Rating Scale.
©1983 Wong-Baker FACES® Foundation. Reprinted with permission.

Acute versus Chronic Pain

We are wired to perceive pain for protection from injury. In the case of a Charcot joint, an individual lacking protective sensation may walk on an injured ankle, resulting in further damage. Between three to six months following the onset, pain is considered chronic. With chronicity, duration of pain symptoms exceeds the expected time of tissue healing following an acute event or injury. Individuals with chronic pain conditions have a much greater likelihood of developing a host of psychosocial difficulties. Concerns may include loss of employment or decreased work productivity, family stressors, financial difficulties, development of anxiety or depression, sleep problems, and propensity for alcohol or other substance abuse.

Regardless of the etiology, the approach to acute versus chronic pain is different. For acute pain, one is generally liberal with analgesics. Commonly, clinicians advise rest, lest the individual compound the injury. The medical or surgical focus is on treating the underlying condition. In chronic pain, clinicians advise patients that they are not harming themselves by progressing activity. Rather, this return to activity helps a person increase quality of life and daily functioning. In a hospital setting, pain may be primarily acute, chronic, or a combination.

Psychiatric and Behavioral Comorbidities

Psychiatric conditions that accompany and/or complicate pain commonly fall into four categories:

• Mood and anxiety disorders
• Personality disorders
• Substance use disorders
• Behavioral styles or reactions.

Mood and Anxiety Disorders

Individuals with chronic pain are more likely than the general population to experience distressing or impairing dysphoria, particularly when pain halts an otherwise active lifestyle. An epidemiological study in Canada found a sevenfold greater risk factor for suicide in older adults with severe chronic pain (Juurlink et al., 2004). Anxiety disorders are slightly more prevalent than depression among individuals with chronic pain. Both anxiety and depression tend to reverberate with pain.

Personality Disorders

Personality disorders are over-represented among individuals with chronic pain, raising the question of whether character pathology reflects cause or effect of pain. Additionally, when psychiatrists are called for consultation, cluster B traits may contribute to challenging interactions between patients and their primary medical team.

Substance Use Disorders

Moving away from the distinction between substance abuse and dependence, *DSM-5* recognizes that tolerance and withdrawal are not, in themselves, pathologic. For instance, patients who are prescribed narcotics for chronic cancer-related pain may experience physiologic opioid tolerance, and withdrawal upon discontinuation. Patients with chronic pain are at risk for developing addictive behaviors and aberrant use patterns with prescribed medications. They are also more likely to overuse alcohol, marijuana, non-prescribed opioids or sedatives, and other substances. As with personality disorders, individuals with substance issues may try the patience of the primary service. Substance use disorders are further discussed in Chapter 16.

Behavioral Styles or Reactions

Patients with chronic pain often experience a loss of sense of control; in behavioral medicine terms, this experience is associated with an **external locus of control** and **limited self-efficacy**. The pattern of **fear-avoidance** experienced by many patients with chronic pain can also precipitate more generalized anxiety symptoms and limit activities. A tendency toward **pain-catastrophizing** is a common reaction, noted in the literature and seen every day in the care of these patients. Rather than suggesting a specific psychiatric diagnosis, these constructs can be helpful in understanding a patient and in developing a cognitive-behavioral approach. The goals center around engaging the patient to improve functioning, decrease affective distress, and improve behavioral self-management strategies.

Approach to the Patient with Pain

As in psychosomatic medicine consults more generally, the first task is to clarify the question, issue, or problem. When it is not reflected fully in the consult order, the primary concern of the referring team typically becomes clear in talking to physicians or nursing staff.

Common psychiatric questions or concerns include assessment and management around the following:

- Comorbid psychiatric conditions
- A "psychogenic" component to the patient's pain
- Opioid tolerance and drug-seeking behavior
- Challenging patient-team interactions.

Managing Comorbid Conditions

Common psychiatric comorbidities to pain include depression, anxiety, insomnia, fatigue, and irritability. We commonly recommend psychotherapy, utilizing CBT with an integrative mind-body orientation provided by a clinician who is knowledgeable about chronic health conditions and pain. As part of the cognitive approach, one helps the patient to identify behavioral patterns that may perpetuate distress, mood disturbance, sleep difficulties, and interpersonal conflicts. Additionally, it is helpful to draw attention to factors that increase pain perception and limit functioning, such as all-or-nothing thinking and fear avoidance. Instruction on relaxation techniques can be a vehicle to connect with a patient and impact pain and distress.

Regarding pharmacologic management, we commonly consider antidepressant agents (Dharmshaktu et al., 2012). TCAs and SNRIs have greater analgesic efficacy than SSRIs.

TCAs have been studied most extensively for neuropathic pain, migraines, and fibromyalgia with consistent efficacy demonstrated. In addition to mild analgesia, TCAs may confer benefits for sleep, mood, and anxiety. As compared to SSRIs, TCAs have a worse side-effect profile, more potential for drug interactions, and greater risk for lethal overdose. Analgesia typically occurs at low to moderate antidepressant doses (e.g., 100–150 mg/day for amitriptyline and 30–75 mg/day for nortriptyline. In a medical setting, one would typically start at one-third to one-quarter of the anticipated low therapeutic dose and titrate to effect every three to four days. Common adverse effects include orthostasis, anticholinergic symptoms, and blurred vision. Patients on antihypertensives may experience greater dizziness. Patients with urinary difficulties, such as benign prostatic hyperplasia, may see worsening of symptoms. TCAs are worse offenders than SSRIs in terms of appetite stimulation and weight gain. Cardiac conduction disturbance, particularly atrioventricular (AV) block, is seen with higher doses and may be a concern for patients with heart disease and in pediatrics. Serum levels have been used to titrate the antidepressant effect, but less is known about their value in analgesia.

Of the **SNRIs**, duloxetine and venlafaxine have had the greatest research basis and clinical usage in the setting of depression comorbid with pain. Duloxetine is approved for dosing up to 120 mg/day, but 60 mg/day is used more typically and titration typically begins at lower doses. For fibromyalgia, greater analgesic efficacy may occur with the full 120 mg dosage, whereas for neuropathic pain, the effect appears to max out at 60 mg/day. Venlafaxine combines reasonable analgesic efficacy with energizing properties. As the analgesic effect of venlafaxine is partially mediated by its noradrenergic activity, titration to doses of 150 mg/day or greater is recommended. The side-effect profile of this family is similar to that of the SSRIs, with the most common concern being nausea on initial titration. Venlafaxine at higher doses may raise blood pressure. Newer agents include milnacipran (approved for treating fibromyalgia) and levomilnacipran (approved for treatment of depression).

Although our preference in treating patients with comorbid depression and pain is to utilize agents with combined psychotropic and analgesic effect, the clinical situation may guide us differently. For example, an individual with heart disease, diabetic neuropathy, and insomnia may not be a candidate for an analgesic dosage of a tricyclic. For this patient, venlafaxine may be used for depressive symptoms along with trazodone for insomnia. It is important to remember that some analgesic agents, such as meperidine and tramadol, have serotonergic effects as well. The combination of two or more serotonergic agents should be minimized to prevent the development of serotonin syndrome (see Chapter 14).

Assessment for Psychogenic Component to Pain

Modern medical training has veered away from a Cartesian model for pain. When asked if pain is in the mind or the body, the short answer is "yes." The absence of "hard findings" on MRI or EMG does not preclude a physical condition that may be generating pain. Conversely, for patients with chronic and potentially terminal diseases such as cancer or unstable angina, psychological or family and social factors may impact the experience of pain and the ability to cope. In this setting, the consultation psychiatrist can help the patient, family, and treatment providers refocus energy on alleviating suffering on all fronts, rather than exclusively concentrating on justifying the patient's reported magnitude of pain.

The C-L psychiatrist is frequently asked to evaluate patients who experience physical symptoms that do not fall into a typical physiologic pattern, commonly involving pain, as well as neurologic symptoms such as numbness, weakness, or abnormal movements. Often, the request from primary providers is to determine if these symptoms are "psychogenic." From the standpoint of the patient, the symptoms are real, and labeling them otherwise can create an adversarial clinician-provider relationship. The term **"medically unexplained symptoms"** does not exist within *DSM-5*, but this concept can be helpful pragmatically in discussing management with the patient. Somatoform disorders are discussed further in Chapter 5.

The consultation psychiatrist's objective is to help engage the patient in a productive way to manage symptoms. The first step is to convey an understanding that will help to build a therapeutic alliance. Non-judgmental evaluation of the patient elicits information about psychosocial factors and stressors, permitting treatment providers to formulate a plan and provide holistic care. In discussion with the patient, the consulting psychiatrist may note that the medical workup has found no physical source of the problem; that this is fortunate, as all parties can be confident that no serious medical condition requires further treatment; and that stress is often a component in such cases, citing patient-specific circumstances. Finally, the psychiatric consultant can direct the patient to an appropriate level of physical and psychiatric care.

Management of the Opioid-Tolerant Patient

Opioid tolerance is seen in three scenarios: chronic opioids prescribed for pain management, illicit drug use, and opioid replacement therapy. From a physiologic standpoint, the issues are similar. First, one needs to ensure that the patient's baseline opioid requirement is accounted for. Opioid requirement to treat acute medical or surgical pain is likely to be greater than for the opioid-naïve patients. Collaboration with a hospital's pain service is very helpful in such cases.

A common scenario is the care of a postoperative patient on a chronic opioid regimen receiving morphine via patient-controlled analgesia (PCA). In this case it is preferable to add a continuous infusion, at a dose-equivalent level to make up for the home usage, with additional bolus dosing of intravenous morphine for breakthrough pain. Similarly, for an individual receiving oral medication for acute pain, a provider may opt to utilize a sustained-release oral agent to cover the baseline use, supplemented by as-needed (prn) dosing of a short-acting agent such as oxycodone.

Psychiatric consultants are often drawn into contentious situations that center on the administration of opioid medications. Longitudinal opioid use, whether prescribed or illicit, may lead to a higher tolerance to this family of medications. As such, patients who use opioids chronically may demonstrate altered psychological responses to pain, cross-tolerance to other opioid agents, and physiologic hyperalgesia. They may require higher than average doses of analgesic medications to alleviate pain, and reports of persistent pain despite opioid therapies should not be interpreted reflexively as drug-seeking behavior.

For patients receiving methadone maintenance therapy for opioid dependence, once-daily dosing may curb opioid cravings but may not confer sustained analgesic control. Consequently, the consulting psychiatrist may recommend splitting an established daily methadone regimen into three times daily (tid) administration, and either augmenting with a short-acting agent or adjusting the methadone dose to compensate for acute pain. It is important to keep in mind that at the time of discharge, responsibility for management will fall back on the methadone program, in all likelihood with return to the prior dosage.

Individuals receiving buprenorphine as replacement therapy also require special consideration. In the setting of acute pain requiring significant opioids, buprenorphine should be discontinued, as its mixed agonist/antagonist effect may diminish the analgesic effects of other opioid agents. This is particularly important if the patient is receiving *Suboxone*, which includes naloxone in addition to buprenorphine. Extended release naltrexone is available in a monthly injectable form, *Vivitrol*, for management of opioid addiction-related cravings. As with buprenorphine, this can interfere with acute pain control via opioid receptor blockade.

Patients who experience pain while treated with intramuscular naltrexone require behavioral and non-opioid analgesics until opioid antagonistic effects from naltrexone have subsided. In the surgical setting, alternate efforts to manage pain, such as regional nerve blockade, may be necessary.

Assessment and Management of Challenging Patient Interactions

The most challenging encounters include dealing with patients with acute pain conditions in the setting of chemical dependence, mood or anxiety disorders, and character pathology. With these patients, the role of the consulting psychiatrist shifts to providing support for the patient and treatment team, working the primary team (e.g., nursing staff and physicians) to set consistent limits with the patient, and rebuilding a non-confrontational framework. Care of these patients may cut across inpatient and outpatient settings when there are repeated admissions for pain control. In complex cases, it may help to have a meeting to discuss care; when possible, this should involve the inpatient medical and nursing services as well as outpatient medical, mental health, and pain service teams.

Basic principles of managing challenging pain-related patient interactions include the following:

- Maximizing the patient's understanding of pain-associated medical conditions, indications for specific analgesic regimens, and limitations associated with opioid use for chronic pain;
- Ensuring that treatment providers maintain focus on standard pain management principles, avoid excessive or unnecessary use of opioids for individuals with a tendency for habit-formation, and, at the same time, avoid hindering care due to addiction-related stigma;
- Collaborating with various members of the treatment team, patient, and family (as appropriate) to prevent miscommunication and to ensure a unified patient-centered approach to optimizing pain control while minimizing the risk for habit-formation and medication misuse.

Discussion of Specific Pain Conditions

Table 20.1 lists brief guides to pharmacologic treatment for specific pain syndromes.

Fibromyalgia

Although fibromyalgia does not typically precipitate hospitalization, given its prevalence and comorbidity with mood and anxiety disorders, the condition afflicts many patients seen in psychiatric consultation. Sleep disturbance is a frequent part of the condition, and a TCA such as nortriptyline is a reasonable first choice, titrating by 10 mg every three to four days. Although greater efficacy might be seen with full antidepressant dosing, given the side-effect profile, a target range of 30–50 mg/day is reasonable for the initial titration. If fatigue is more of a problem, the more energizing SNRIs, such as venlafaxine or milnacipran, may be preferable. Duloxetine appears to be intermediate in its energizing versus sedating effects.

Migraines

Patients admitted for management of migraines often experience progression from episodic headaches to a chronic daily pattern. In the inpatient setting, primary analgesics and other abortive agents may be used to "break" acute headache pain. Ongoing use of these agents should be limited to avoid rebound phenomena. This leaves two primary approaches to the management of migraines: prophylactic medications and mind-body therapies. Prophylactic agents include antidepressants, anticonvulsants (e.g., valproate and topiramate), and antihypertensives (e.g., propranolol and verapamil). While TCAs and SNRIs appear most

Table 20.1 Treatment Options for Specific Pain Conditions

Fibromyalgia	TCAs: may help for sleep and pain
	SNRIs: duloxetine (at 60–120 mg/day), Milnacipran
Migraines	Antidepressants: TCAs, SNRIs, SSRIs
	Anticonvulsants: valproate, topiramate
	Antihypertensives: propranolol, verapamil
	Biofeedback
Neuropathic Pain States	Antidepressants: TCAs,
	SNRIs: duloxetine (up to 60 mg/day);
	Anticonvulsants: gabapentin, pregabalin

efficacious, SSRIs also show benefit for migraine prophylaxis. Choice of agent typically falls to the medicine or neurology services. Although C-L psychiatrists are not typically the prescribers, our familiarity with these agents may be helpful in addressing side effects, particularly when polypharmacy is involved. Of the non-pharmacologic approaches, biofeedback has the greatest research support, and constitutes a reasonable referral for outpatient care. Limitations include the scarcity of biofeedback practitioners in many communities and limited insurance coverage. Referral to psychotherapists versed in combined CBT/stress-management approaches may offer some benefit.

Visceral Pain Conditions

Pain constitutes a core component of many chronic health conditions. With time, patients may experience an uncoupling between disease progression and severity of pain or other discomfort. For example, a patient who has chronic pancreatitis or Crohn's disease may experience severe gnawing pain and other GI symptoms in the absence of physiologic signs of disease activity. Many such patients cycle through the emergency room and inpatient service. Ensuring consistent pain management requires collaboration between the hospital's pain service and the inpatient and outpatient physicians.

Neuropathic Pain States

The two most common neuropathic pain conditions, diabetic neuropathy and post-herpetic neuralgia, are more prevalent in older populations and are frequently associated with depressive and anxiety symptoms. Treatment relies principally on pharmacologic therapies, including anticonvulsant and antidepressant medications (Attal, 2012). Physicians often prescribe low doses of gabapentin, TCAs, or SNRIs; when pain persists, physicians must gain comfort with titrating these medications to full clinical effect. Gabapentin dosing up to 3,600 mg/day may be required to demonstrate a full effect. In the same way, pregabalin, commonly used in doses of 25–50 mg PO three times a day, shows its greatest effectiveness at 600 mg/day. Studies of TCAs also found that moderate antidepressant doses, for example amitriptyline 150 mg daily, are optimal for neuropathic pain states.

Musculoskeletal Pain

Admission for musculoskeletal pain is often precipitated by acute exacerbation of an otherwise chronic condition. In such circumstances, surgical intervention is reserved for rare cases such as cauda equina syndrome. More commonly, the onus is on the medical team to provide acute relief of pain, allowing the patient to return home and continue rehabilitation in the ambulatory setting.

Low back pain is the most common musculoskeletal condition to require inpatient admission for analgesia. The involvement of psychiatry becomes especially valuable when other factors coexist, including negative imaging studies, prominent affective distress, and strong requests for medication. Given the prevalence of positive radiologic findings in asymptomatic individuals, the presence of mild disc disease does not imply a specific pathophysiology for the back pain. Patients with prior back surgeries can present a challenge, given presumed epidural scarring and mixed mechanical and radicular pain. As with other forms of non-cancer pain, psychiatry and other members of the medical team can provide reassurance that the condition does not present a danger or warrant surgical intervention. The goal is to transition to outpatient physical rehabilitation and mental health services if needed.

Cancer Pain

In the setting of cancer, pain can be either disease-related or treatment-related.

Disease-related pain may present in the form of one or a combination of the following types of pain:

- Somatic-nocioceptive—as in the case of sarcomas or bony involvement from metastatic disease;
- Visceral—as in the case of local invasiveness of ovarian carcinoma;
- Nerve-related or neuropathic—as with a spinal tumor resulting in nerve root impingement.

Treatment-related pain also falls into several categories:

- Somatic-nocioceptive—for example, from surgery;
- Mucositis—from either chemotherapy or radiation therapy;
- Neuropathic—from radiation, surgery, or chemotherapeutic agents, such as cisplatin or taxanes.

Consultation psychiatrists can optimize their support to the patient and treatment providers by addressing pain alongside affective, behavioral, and cognitive syndromes. Typically, there are not the same concerns for limiting opioid medication as with other health conditions. From a pharmacologic standpoint, we can help with the management of depression, anxiety, insomnia, and somnolence. For those with advanced disease, our efforts tie in closely with the palliative care service and resources for hospice care (see Chapters 18 and 21 for details of psychiatric treatment in oncology and palliative care).

Multiple Sclerosis and Spasticity-Related Pain

For individuals with multiple sclerosis, or those who have experienced stroke, traumatic brain injury, or spinal cord injury, pain may be related to CNS-induced spasticity. The primary treatment is anti-spasticity agents, including baclofen, tizanidine, or long-acting benzodiazepines, such as diazepam. Interventional procedures such as neurolytic blocks, botulinum toxin injections, and intrathecal pumps may be used when pain and spasticity are severe and disabling. Typically, the primary approach is directed to the spasticity, rather than pain per se.

Relaxation 101

Among the wide array of behavioral relaxation options, simple breathing techniques are the easiest to undertake and teach. From a physiologic standpoint, slowed regular breathing augments respiratory sinus arrhythmia, providing a shift from sympathetic to parasympathetic predominance. A young healthy patient may be instructed to breathe in for five seconds and then out for five seconds, repeating the cycle as needed to mitigate discomfort. Someone who has never taken a yoga class or engaged in paced breathing may tend to hyperventilate, so instruction should encourage slow sustained breathing, while breathing alongside the patient. Older and medically ill patients will require a shorter duration of inspiration and expiration, and patients with respiratory problems may fare better with a prolonged expiration (e.g., three seconds in and five seconds out). When altering breathing patterns is not clinically feasible (e.g., in patients with severe COPD), patients can be instructed to attend mindfully to normal breathing, or can be instructed in progressive muscle relaxation.

Before engaging in a mindfulness or relaxation exercise, patients should be asked to rate their pain severity, as well as their level of distress. The same measures may be repeated after two to three minutes of practice. Any response is a useful one. If pain decreases, the clinician can remark, "With just three minutes of breathing, you brought your pain level down by two points out of ten." If distress eases, but pain does not, the clinician may explain that there are different components, and that even though the pain level is unchanged, the patient has the capacity to mitigate suffering. If the patient seems calm and relaxed, but pain scores do not change, the clinician may comment that, even though the pain level has not yet changed, the patient appears more relaxed and comfortable. Finally, if pain severity worsens, the clinician may indicate with confidence that, paradoxically, if the patient can increase pain by breathing, with practice he or she will be able to decrease it as well.

Conclusions

Pain represents an area of significant overlap between physical and psychological distress, and its evaluation and management epitomize the holistic nature of psychosomatic medicine. Armed with knowledge of physiologic pain mechanisms, pharmacologic treatments, and behavioral approaches, the consultation psychiatrist is uniquely positioned to mitigate patient suffering, to maximize clinical support for fellow physicians and nursing staff, and to solidify therapeutic relationships between patients and their providers.

Key Points

- Pain is a common condition seen in medical and surgical inpatients, often comorbid with psychiatric and chemical dependency issues.
- These comorbidities can adversely affect the care of these patients.
- Understanding issues common to patients with acute and chronic pain is essential to C-L psychiatry.
- The C-L psychiatrist is in a unique position to offer assistance and recommendations to enhance the care of patients with pain and to assist in the primary service's medical management.
- TCAs and SNRIs may be especially helpful, given their benefits for pain, mood, and anxiety.

Disclosures

Dr. Glick has no conflicts of interest to disclose.

Dr. Azzam has no conflicts of interest to disclose.

Further Reading

American Society of Anesthesiologists Task Force on Chronic Pain Management & American Society of Regional Anesthesia and Pain Medicine (2010). Practice guidelines for chronic pain management: An updated report by the American Society of Anesthesiologists Task Force on Chronic Pain Management and the American Society of Regional Anesthesia and Pain Medicine. *Anesthesiology, 112*(4), 810–833.

Attal N (2012). Neuropathic pain: Mechanisms, therapeutic approach, and interpretation of clinical trials. *Continuum, 18*(1), 161–175.

Dharmshaktu P, Tayal V, et al. (2012). Efficacy of antidepressants as analgesics: A review. *J Clin Pharmacol., 52*(1), 6–17.

Eccleston C, Morley SJ, et al. (2013). Psychological approaches to chronic pain management: Evidence and challenges. *Br J Anaesth., 111*(1), 59–63.

Fornasari D (2012). Pain mechanisms in patients with chronic pain. *Clin Drug Investigat., 32*(Suppl 1), 45–52.

Juurlink DN, Herrmann N, et al. (2004). Medical illness and the risk of suicide in the elderly. *Arch Intern Med., 164*(11), 1179–1184.

Srinath AI, Walter C, et al. (2012). Pain management in patients with inflammatory bowel disease: Insights for the clinician. *Therap Adv Gastroenterol., 5*(5), 339–357.

Exercises

1. Increased perception of pain following a stressful experience is an example of:
   a. Malingering
   b. Gate control theory
   c. Pain catastrophizing
   d. Need for a tricyclic antidepressant

2. A patient on 60 mg/day of methadone is hospitalized for acute pancreatitis. Which of the following is **not** an appropriate intervention:
   a. Split the methadone dosage into tid.
   b. Advise the patient that he should have sufficient analgesia with his current methadone and that any additional medication would likely become addictive.
   c. Provide additional prn opioid medication at a higher than normal dosage.
   d. If he is NPO, provide IV opioids.

3. A patient with a diagnosis of irritable bowel syndrome requests a third endoscopy in three months due to his certainty that the doctor missed something. In addition to this distress, he is experiencing hot flashes, palpitations, and dizziness. Which diagnosis is most appropriate?
   a. Somatic symptom disorder
   b. Pain disorder associated with psychological factors
   c. Conversion disorder
   d. Factitious disorder

4. Under-medicating is common in the treatment of neuropathic pain states. Which of the following is an example of medication used below a typical effective level for neuropathic pain?
   a. Pregabalin 200 mg tid
   b. Gabapentin 1,200 mg po tid
   c. Duloxetine 60 mg po q day
   d. Amitriptyline 25 mg po q HS

5. Which of the following agents would be expected to offer the greatest benefit for a patient with multiple sclerosis and lower extremity pain associated with hyper-reflexia?
   a. Extended-release oxycodone
   b. Sertraline
   c. Baclofen
   d. Venlafaxine

Answers: (1) b (2) b (3) a (4) d (5) c

Chapter 21

Psychiatry in Palliative Care

Kevin R. Patterson

Introduction

Palliative care is the field that specializes in preventing and relieving suffering in the context of major medical illness. It is frequently confused with *hospice*, which is defined in the United States as care in the anticipated last six months of life (a Medicare requirement), but palliative care is far broader in its aims and can be applied during any major medical illness. Hospital-based palliative care teams can include members from a variety of disciplines with the shared aim of managing troubling symptoms. The Center for the Advancement of Palliative Care cites a perceived need for emotional support for patients and families as one of the principal reasons that palliative care teams are consulted, making collaboration with psychiatry a natural fit. In hospitals or outpatient settings where no formal palliative care service exists, psychosomatic medicine specialists can play a large part in recognizing and directing treatment for quality of life–based care. Palliative care is also a natural field for exploring integrated care models where mental health professionals work as part of multidisciplinary care teams.

Recent position papers from palliative care teams and institutions have indicated several scenarios in which psychiatrists' participation would be especially beneficial for patient care. Among these are distinguishing delirium from depression, anxiety, psychosis, and dementia, differentiating normal grief from syndromal depression, aiding in complicated capacity assessments, advising on patient care in the context of substance abuse, and enhancing communication with difficult patients and families.

Nevertheless, significant barriers exist to the effective integration of psychiatry and palliative care, including finances and provider availability. Other barriers are related to physician perception of differing goals of care and modes of interacting with patients between disciplines (Patterson et al., 2014). One area of agreement across disciplines, however, is the focus on rapid and effective treatments and the concern that some psychopharmacological interventions require a relatively long time course before symptom remission. We should reflect to the palliative care team our understanding of the need for rapid response and improvement of acute symptoms experienced by palliative care patients, and note that this urgency provides opportunity for successful intervention as well. We should also consider that, in places where a formal palliative care team does not exist, the psychosomatic specialist can work to hasten symptom relief in the severely medically ill, and furthermore, potentially can apply this approach to care across a broader range of patients.

This chapter begins with a discussion of special considerations for assessing and stabilizing mood and anxiety in palliative care patients, noting both the similarities and the differences between palliative care and other clinical settings. It then considers delirium progression and management in the palliative setting. Next, we discuss palliative and internal medicine physicians' expectations for the consulting psychiatrist in evaluating a patient's capacity to elect—and to refuse—medical treatment. Finally, we discuss various therapeutic modalities that can help patients in traversing grief and loss.

Psychiatric Symptomatology in the Palliative Care Setting

Psychiatric symptoms are commonly experienced by palliative care patients. A recent study of patients in Japan found that 70% of patients referred for palliative care met criteria for psychiatric diagnoses (Ogawa et al., 2010), while a study by Delgado-Guay et al. (2009) found that 81% of palliative care patients met criteria for delirium and 65% for anxiety.

As palliative care needs cut across all demographics, and psychiatric illness increases the likelihood of hospital admission, it is reasonable to expect similar premorbid incidence of psychiatric diagnoses as in the general population. Thus, palliative care patients include a substantial number of individuals who may need ongoing or revised psychiatric care in concert with broader symptom management. The exacerbation of anxiety and depression in the palliative care setting should not be dismissed—particularly for patients with a history of anxiety, major depression, adjustment disorder, or post-traumatic stress disorder (PTSD). There can be a tendency among medical and surgical providers to normalize a patient's experience of depression or anxiety given their medical circumstances, but this sentiment can serve to minimize troubling and treatable symptoms in the best cases, and can lead to the development or worsening of major psychiatric disorders in the worst cases.

Palliative care patients also include many who experience psychiatric symptoms for the first time as a result of their medical illness, associated treatment, and the stresses and trauma related to illness and hospitalization. Psychiatric symptomatology brought about by underlying medical illness is discussed throughout this text, though especially useful information about intervention in the palliative care setting is discussed later in this chapter. Palliative care physicians have expressed comfort in treating palliative care patients experiencing psychiatric symptoms for the first time (Patterson et al., 2014), although frequently they seek assistance to distinguish delirium from depression, anxiety, schizophrenia, or dementia. These scenarios provide a natural opportunity for consulting psychiatrists to integrate into the palliative care landscape.

Special Considerations for Mood-Related Symptoms in the Palliative Setting

Depression

In the past, the difficulty of distinguishing between normal grief and major depressive disorder (MDD), compounded by not wanting to further complicate the medical situation, has resulted in antidepressants being under-prescribed in the palliative care setting (Rhondali et al., 2012). Indeed, in the *DSM-IV*, bereavement of two months or less operated as an exclusionary criterion for MDD. However, the *DSM-5* recognizes multiple possible relationships between MDD and bereavement. For palliative purposes, the most salient approach is this: some symptoms associated with bereavement, including insomnia, anorexia, and rumination, respond to the same interventions as MDD, and treating such symptoms can stave off a major depressive episode in patients with a history of mood disorders or other significant risk factors. While recent studies have established the efficacy of a variety of SSRIs and SNRIs for treating depression and anxiety in relatively healthy patients, results are less clear in the palliative care setting, and drug-drug interactions and side effects must be considered. Specific organ involvement should factor into drug use determination, as indicated in Chapters 6 and 13.

The primary disadvantage of all SSRI and SNRI treatments in the palliative care setting is the delayed efficacy. If the primary goal of care is improved quality of life in the short term, medications with delayed effects of four to six weeks may not produce the desired result. For that reason, medications whose side effects provide interim symptom relief may be preferable (see Table 18.4 in Chapter 18).

Psychostimulants

To bridge the gap between the start of an antidepressant and its peak efficacy, consulting psychiatrists should consider adding a psychostimulant (Rhondali et al., 2012). Fatigue and apathy may improve in as little as two days after the psychostimulant is started. In palliative care patients, low energy and motivation can easily be overlooked by patients as a normal and inevitable aspect of their experience of illness, along with frequent sleep disruption and daytime sleepiness. A patient's dismissal of these symptoms should not be compounded by physicians overlooking them as well, given that energy management is such a significant element of quality of life.

While randomized controlled trials are needed, amphetamine-based stimulants such as methylphenidate are more effective in our experience for both fatigue and concentration than pseudo-stimulants such as modafinil. Recent studies are encouraging regarding the safety and efficacy of psychostimulant use in adults. In 2007, the FDA issued warnings regarding the potential for adverse cardiac events in those with a history of cardiac abnormalities. Subsequent data regarding cardiac events are equivocal: a meta-analysis of studies of adults with ADHD found that cardiac events were rare (Franzen et al., 2012). It is common to start methylphenidate at 5 mg morning and midday, but it should be reduced to 2.5 mg morning and midday for the frail patient with low energy and motivation.

Anxiety and Post-Traumatic Stress Disorder

Symptoms commonly found in anxiety, such as poor concentration, rumination, difficulty falling asleep, increased energy, and agitation, often prove confusing in regard to etiology and the need for pharmacologic treatment. Much like the uncertainty in identifying depression in the palliative care setting, confusion about anxiety raises the risk of treating reasonable worry as anxiety, or conversely, mistaking disabling anxiety for a normal response to life-threatening illness. The consulting psychiatrist should reinforce with the medical team an understanding of this distinction, an awareness of the importance of the difference, and a willingness to work toward a common conceptualization of the symptoms and goals with the patient and other members of the team. As with stimulants for treatment of depressive symptoms such as low energy, benzodiazepines may be helpful in hastening symptom relief in patients with anxiety and panic. Caution should be exercised to use minimal dosing in order to avoid sedation, respiratory suppression, and delirium.

PTSD is no longer classified as an anxiety disorder in the fifth edition of the *Diagnostic and Statistical Manual of Mental Disorders* (*DSM-5*), but rather is part of trauma- and stressor-related disorders. Delirium associated with hospital admission, whether in the ICU or a lower-acuity setting, can be experienced as a traumatic event that may give rise to PTSD. In addition, recent studies have indicated that hospitalization for major medical illness and the threat to life presented therein can lead to PTSD (Mundy & Baum, 2004). In the past decade, studies regarding PTSD and hospitalization have shown that patients traumatized by their hospitalization avoid later medical care (Capuzzo et al., 2008). A short course of cognitive behavioral therapy may ameliorate PTSD symptoms during and after potentially traumatic hospitalizations and, moreover, may enable a patient to participate more fully in medical decision-making and care-seeking.

Progression of Delirium and Delirium Management in the Palliative Setting

Delirium is estimated to occur in up to two-thirds of hospitalized palliative patients (see Chapter 10 for details of presentation and management of delirium). It should be noted that it is very common for primary medical teams to mistake delirium (particularly hypoactive delirium) for depression, anxiety, or unwillingness to engage in treatment. Clarifying the diagnosis of delirium in these situations is therefore critical for appropriate patient care.

As in Chapters 10 (on delirium) and 18 (on psycho-oncology), first-line delirium management entails stabilization of the acute medical condition. Because eliminating the medical cause for delirium may not be possible in the palliative setting, the aim shifts to ameliorating the symptom and its impact. We can reduce or eliminate exacerbating influences on delirium by, for example, modulating opiate dosage, avoiding benzodiazepines, and limiting the utilization of other anticholinergic medications. Opiate modulation can prove to be particularly problematic, since pain is also a contributor to delirium. Behavioral interventions, such as surrounding the patient with objects that aid in orientation, decreasing the stimulation of the surrounding environment, and improving sensory deficits (glasses, hearing aids, etc.) are also common in palliative care.

While haloperidol remains the most studied and efficacious of the antipsychotics for managing delirium, more sedating antipsychotic agents may be useful in the palliative setting when a patient experiences concomitant agitation. In palliative care practice, a consultation-liaison (C-L) psychiatrist may be consulted on a patient who has already begun haloperidol but who, with worsening of the underlying medical illness, is now experiencing increasing agitation. In this instance, olanzapine can be substituted for haloperidol, providing a more calming effect. The next option is chlorpromazine, which is far more sedating but very effective for calming the symptoms of agitated delirium.

Increasingly, and especially in populations at high risk of recurrence, delirium management has shifted toward prevention. Comorbid symptoms such as cognitive dysfunction and nausea may lead a provider to select a medication that addresses both the current symptoms and the potential for future episodes of delirium. For example, haloperidol 0.5 mg twice a day for a hospitalized patient with infection, chronic nausea, and a previous episode of delirium could simultaneously treat the nausea and decrease the chance of future delirium.

Finally, as patients move from the needs of palliative care to hospice, some may experience what is known as terminal delirium, a steadily worsening state of delirium that will not improve prior to death. For these patients, terminal sedation using midazolam may be the only option.

Special Considerations for Capacity in the Palliative Care Setting

As indicated in Chapter 9, a patient's capacity can only be assessed regarding a specific decision at a specific point in time. For a patient to demonstrate capacity, the patient must be able to understand the information provided regarding treatment options, appreciate how the information applies to her situation, communicate her choice, and demonstrate reasoning that is consistent and free from acute cognitive and psychiatric symptoms. The degree to which the patient must demonstrate these elements is judged on a "sliding scale" determined by the relative risks and benefits of the patient's decision. For example, electing to begin dialysis when a patient is experiencing or is at risk for multi-systemic organ failure is a more complex decision than starting antibiotics for a bacterial infection (see Table 9.1 in Chapter 9); however, a decision to withdraw from dialysis, resulting in death, would require the highest level of capacity. Whatever a patient's capacity, we should remember that all of these decisions require consent, whether by the patient or her surrogate decision-maker.

All physicians are clinically and legally able to make capacity determinations. Psychiatrists are likely to be consulted for capacity determinations when a patient has a history of psychiatric illness, in part to determine whether psychiatric symptoms are influencing the patient's ability to process information. Capacity determinations are more often requested when patients reject courses of action recommended by treating physicians than when patients consent to physicians' recommended courses of action. In either case, capacity determinations should ultimately consider the relative risks and benefits: high-risk/low-benefit treatment options have higher standards for capacity than low-risk/high-benefit options, even when the patient, physician, or everyone involved prefers the former course of action.

Palliative care's specific capacity concerns arise from the complexity of the necessary decisions, the high risk of mortality for all options, and the importance of autonomy at the end of life. Making a decision that will hasten death may be completely reasonable under many circumstances, but may be complicated by differences in opinion between patients, their families, and their medical teams, as well as by patient histories. For example, capacity to refuse treatment in a patient with a history of suicidality is one of the great ethical debates of palliative care, but it is not just academic. Sometimes, prior lethality raises concerns for a patient's ability to weigh life and death decisions appropriately in the setting of a major illness. At other times, the concern is intrinsic to the situation: a patient's suicide attempt may result in the need for ongoing major medical intervention following resuscitation. Consulting psychiatrists must return to the definition of capacity and emphasize the moment at hand: we must evaluate the patient's ability to comprehend the complexity of the present situation, the current risks and benefits of a specific course of action, and whether or not psychiatric symptoms may be influencing the patient's present understanding or decision-making.

The consulting psychiatrist should also recognize that, given the complexity of medical decisions at the end of life, the patient—who is not a critical care specialist—will likely have limited comprehension of risks and benefits. We should seek to elicit a patient's desires for the end of life and identify a patient's values across time in order to determine whether current choices appear consistent with those values. A medical team may recommend an aggressive course of treatment with little chance of success, and the patient or family may want to refuse this (potentially inverting the typical risk/benefit consideration where death would always be the riskiest outcome). We can serve as interpreters, helping to bridge the divide between complicated medical considerations and expressed patient and family values, and recommending the course or courses of action that most adhere to those values.

Death and Dying

While hospice care itself is only a part of palliative care, complicated medical illness frequently brings death and the dying process to the forefront. One school of thought proposes that a person's anxiety about death is a governing force for much of life, and that perceived proximity to death affects how a person lives. Whether or not a person expresses thoughts about death has a lot to do with her own coping strategies, and the coping strategies of the people around her.

What might in another context appear to be a passive death wish may be a "normal" feature of a patient's adjustment to her own mortality. Indeed, a psychosomatic specialist is often consulted to assess lethality when a member of a treatment team has heard the expression of what he believes to be a death wish. Such scenarios should be expected for consulting psychiatrists working with seriously ill patients in any medical setting. Treatment teams should be reminded that, under some circumstances, a desire not to awaken from sleep may not represent active lethality so much as an expression of the desire for relief from the complexity of medical illness and its attendant suffering.

At the same time, the psychiatrist can help the patient to explore and address some of these stressors and work toward alleviating those that are mutable, while promoting acceptance of areas that cannot be changed. It can be helpful to consider the many losses that accompany worsening medical illness (e.g., loss of health, loss of function, loss of financial independence, loss of physical independence, and others) when considering the grieving process experienced by patients and their families. Death is not the only thing to be grieved, and grief-related therapies can be quite useful in easing suffering related to diminished quality of life.

Table 21.1 describes some of the therapeutic models that can be applied to patients who are experiencing grief or facing death. Some work well in the hospital setting (like normalization, supportive therapy, and brief cognitive behavioral interventions), while others are better suited to outpatient treatment (complicated grief therapy, meaning-making therapies, and brief psychodynamic therapy). A patient may benefit from one approach or from a combination of these approaches. Reaching out to other types of providers such as palliative psychologists, pastoral therapists, and alternative medicine practitioners can greatly enhance the patient's treatment.

Table 21.1 Philosophies of Death/Grief and Approaches to Treatment

Conceptual Framework	Approach to Death/Grief	Therapeutic Intervention
Existential	Anxiety derives from a lack of meaning	Meaning-making therapies - Lifebook and other narrative strategies
Cognitive	Anxiety derives from interpretation of the world through lens of loss	Cognitive behavioral therapy - Focus on changeable behaviors and intrusive thoughts
Attachment	Anxiety derives from disconnection to previously held attachments	Complicated grief therapy - Focus on loss and restoration of connection
Psychoanalytic	Anxiety derives from disconnect between ego and lost items	Brief psychodynamic therapy
Stage-based	Anxiety and depression must be experienced to successfully grieve	Normalization Supportive therapy
Spirituality	Multiple approaches to the meaning of death in the context of life; possibility of afterlife	Pastoral counseling
Other		Mindfulness/meditation Hypnosis

Conclusion

Forging an alliance between psychiatry and palliative care represents a natural outgrowth of both fields, given that each discipline focuses on quality of life interventions that attempt to address functional impairments and problematic symptoms, in addition to underlying etiology. In many ways, the role of psychiatry in the palliative care setting is akin to its practice in the general population. However, when applying psychiatric interventions and psychotropic medications in the palliative care population, it is especially important to consider both speed of response and the ability to address concurrent physical symptoms. It is also important to recognize the possible intensification of grief and death anxiety, and the role that these symptoms play in a patient's approach to coping, family, and life. With these unique considerations in mind, the consulting psychiatrist can collaborate with other providers to enhance or introduce valuable interventions for patients facing serious medical illness.

Key Points

- Palliative care and psychiatry are both fields that value the quality of a patient's life, and that focus on symptom relief and functional improvement. As such, their integration in the medical setting allows for broader and more nuanced patient care.
- Symptom-based care in the setting of major medical illness includes the treatment of depression, anxiety, delirium, pain, and nausea. Many of the treatments for these conditions overlap and can be thoughtfully combined.
- Delirium is frequently mistaken for many things, including depression, anxiety, and lack of participation in care. Recognizing and treating delirium effectively leads to quality of life improvement for patients, families, and medical staff.
- Determining patients' capacities to make life-or-death medical decisions, and advising effectively on those decisions, is one of the roles of a consultation-liaison psychiatrist.
- Major medical illnesses result in significant and varied losses. Psychiatrists can help patients to grieve those losses and cope with the proximity of death.

Disclosures

Dr. Patterson has no conflicts of interest.

Further Reading

American Psychiatric Association (2013). *Diagnostic and Statistical Manual of Mental Disorders*, 5th ed. Arlington, VA: American Psychiatric Publishing.

Cappuzo M, Bertacchini S, et al. (2008). Patients with PTSD after intensive care avoid hospital contact at two-year follow-up. *Acta Anaesth Scand.*, 15(2), 313–314.

Davydow D, Katon W, et al. (2009). Psychiatric morbidity and functional impairments in survivors of burns, traumatic injuries and ICU stays for other critical illnesses: A review of the literature. *Int Rev Psychiat.*, 21(6), 531–538.

Delgado-Guay M, Parsons H, et al. (2009). Symptom distress, interventions, and outcomes of intensive care unit cancer patients referred to a palliative care consult team. *Cancer*, 115(2), 437–445.

Franzen JD, Wetzel MW, et al. (2012). Psychostimulants for older adults: Certain agents improve apathy, ADHD, depression, and other conditions. *J Curr Psychiat.*, 11(1), 23–32.

Jubran A, Lawm G, et al. (2010). Post-traumatic stress disorder after weaning from prolonged mechanical ventilation. *Intens Care Med.*, 36(12), 2030–2037.

Mundy E, Baum A (2004). Medical disorders as a cause of psychological trauma and posttraumatic stress disorder. *Curr Opin Psychiat.*, 17(2), 123–127.

Ogawa A, Shimizu K, et al. (2010). Involvement of a psychiatric consultation service in a palliative care team at the Japanese Cancer Center Hospital. *Jpn J Clin Oncol.*, 40(12), 1139–1146.

Patterson K, Croom A, et al. (2014). Current state of psychiatric involvement on palliative care consult services: Results of a national survey. *J Pain Symptom Manag.*, 47(6), 1019–1027.

Rhondali W, Reich M, et al. (2012). A brief review on the use of antidepressants in palliative care. *Eur J Hosp Pharm.*, 19, 41–44.

Exercises

1. Which of the following conditions may be mistaken for delirium in the hospitalized palliative care patient?
   a. Depression
   b. Anxiety
   c. Personality pathology
   d. Lack of effort
   e. All of the above

2. A patient with a recent complicated and prolonged course requiring a lengthy ICU stay is found to be avoiding contact with his providers. While previously his values were consistent with being open and trusting toward his long-standing team, he now appears withdrawn and frequently misses his appointments. His wife is concerned about depression. Which of the following should *not* be carefully considered given his history?
   a. Delirium
   b. Schizophrenia
   c. PTSD
   d. Change in goals
   e. Panic

3. Which of the following is the best therapeutic modality to utilize for a patient who expresses a need to find a purpose in the face of a life-limiting illness?
   a. Cognitive behavioral therapy
   b. Interpersonal therapy
   c. Psychodynamic therapy
   d. Lifebook therapy
   e. Complicated grief therapy

Answers: (1) e (2) b (3) d

Future Directions in Psychosomatic Medicine

Christopher R. Dobbelstein, Ghennady V. Gushchin, Bradford Bobrin, and Kurt D. Ackerman

Introduction

As psychosomatic medicine (PM) specialists focus on caring for patients with comorbid psychiatric and general medical conditions, they holistically integrate the mental and physical aspects of their patients' health and help them to navigate both systems of healthcare. They do not differentiate between the care of the mind and body, since "the mind" is simply the function of the central nervous system (CNS) and "the body" is the organism as a whole.

Over the past few decades, specific molecular mechanisms have been identified that link the CNS with the rest of the body. We anticipate ongoing and startling advances in our understanding of neuroscience and physiology that will transform our understanding of disease processes and further blur the distinction between mind and body, and of psychiatry and other medical disciplines. The general medical community is increasingly adopting this holistic view of medicine, and divisions between behavioral and physical health systems are already becoming more permeable. PM specialists are at the forefront of these changes, bringing psychiatric expertise into every possible medical setting.

This chapter will highlight some examples of physiologic interrelationships between the CNS and the periphery that may affect PM practice over the coming decade. It will then describe innovative strategies that have been used to bring psychiatric expertise into general medical settings. Given the success of these models of care, we predict that they will eventually become commonplace, with PM specialists playing an integral role in their development and dissemination.

Physiologic Interrelationship of Mind and Body

Advancing from Cartesian Dualism to Psychoneuroimmunology

From ancient times, humans have understood that mental health and physical health are inextricably linked. In Western culture, this understanding was lost for centuries due to the prevailing Cartesian theory that mind and body are separate. Late nineteenth-century investigators, however, started to erode this dualism by demonstrating some of the physical mechanisms of the mind. These advances stimulated further studies of mental activity, the role of the CNS in maintaining homeostasis, and the physiological response of organisms to perceived threats (e.g., fight or flight reactions; Cannon, 1932).

Advances in immunology revolutionized medical science and our understanding of disease pathology. Although immune responses were found to be complex, genetically determined, and largely autonomous, reports that small hypothalamic lesions can alter immune reactions (Korneva & Khai, 1964) and that emotional factors can alter immune function, potentially contributing to disease (Solomon & Moon, 1964), suggested that neural, immune, and endocrine systems may be intricately linked. The interdisciplinary field of psychoneuroimmunology (PNI) thus developed to examine these interactions, which were found to be bidirectional. For example, "sickness behavior" (social withdrawal, decreased activity, somnolence, depressed mood, lack of appetite, and lack of motivation), which accompanies many infections, was found to be mediated by pro-inflammatory cytokines released by cells of the immune system. Current PNI research has expanded its scope to explore the clinical implications of neural-immune interactions in autoimmune disorders, allergy, aging, and cancer, as well homeostasis of the "microbiome." For example, peptic ulcer disease (PUD), once a classic "psychosomatic" illness of "neurogenic" nature, believed to be induced by stress, was later found to be associated with H. pylori infection. However, even though up to 70% of the general population are colonized with H. pylori, only a small number of these people become sick. This implies that neural-immune mechanisms may play a role in resisting the transition from H. pylori colonization to infection.

Figure 22.1, taken from a recent review and used with permission, provides an example of the complex mechanisms through which the immune system promotes learning, memory, neural plasticity, and neurogenesis, while stress and inflammation disrupt these processes (Yirmiya & Goshen, 2011). Note that interleukins, hormones, and neurotransmitters are active in both the CNS and the immune system, suggesting common modes of communication between mind and body.

Stress and Immunity

Stress alters immune function in complex ways, with studies suggesting that stress prolongs wound healing, decreases response to vaccination,

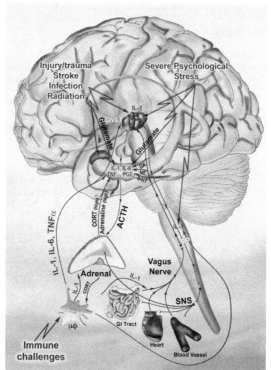

Figure 22.1 The immune and CNS systems impact health and disease via major bidirectional pathways and internal CNS circuits. Communication occurs between and within systems via molecules such as glutamate, norepinephrine (NE), dopamine (DA), and serotonin (5-HT). The CNS communicates with the immune system using both the sympathetic nervous system (SNS) and neuroendocrine systems (e.g., ACTH), with feedback to the CNS through glucocorticoids, the vagus nerve, and cytokines produced by macrophages (μφ) and other immune cells. Cytokines, including Interleukin-1 (IL-1), Interleukin-6 (IL-6), and Tumor Necrosis Factor (TNF-α), are produced locally in the brain and can impact the CNS from peripheral immune system activation at areas of decreased blood-brain-barrier such as the organum vasculosum of lamina terminalis (OVLT).

worsens autoimmune disease (e.g., rheumatoid arthritis, lupus, Graves, psoriasis, Crohn's, multiple sclerosis), increases susceptibility to viral infections (e.g., upper respiratory infections, Epstein-Barr virus, herpes simplex virus, cytomegalovirus), may affect HIV progression, and may decrease the ability to fight cancer.

Despite our incomplete understanding of how stress and the immune system interact, modifying stress and behavior has been shown to influence disease progression. For example, Fawzy (2003) demonstrated that a six-week group psychiatric intervention focused on coping skills and managing psychological distress in early stage melanoma patients (previously treated with standard medical care) resulted in longer survival versus non-intervention controls 10 years after the intervention. It is uncertain what mediated this increased survival, but intervention patients may have internalized coping skills, thereby decreasing stress and enhancing immune-mediated cancer surveillance.

Current PM specialists are building on these ideas as they pursue new opportunities for psychosocially focused interventions.

Conditioned Immune Modulation

Immune function can also be influenced via classical conditioning methods. For example, in a seminal PNI study, saccharin was paired with a single low dose of the chemotherapeutic drug cyclophosphamide. After continued exposure to saccharin (without cyclophosphamide), significant immunosuppression developed to the point where many of the exposed animals died of common infections. Similarly, if a visual cue is paired with antigen exposure to cause an allergic reaction, eventually this reaction can be provoked with the visual cue alone.

If conditioned stimuli can indeed suppress or induce an immune response independently of active agents, then perhaps this phenomenon can be harnessed to deliver optimal clinical efficacy but with fewer side effects. Recent studies have attempted to explore this prospect by substituting a placebo for immunologically active drugs. For example, Ader et al. (2010) used a placebo to decrease the cumulative steroid dose required to treat psoriasis. In this study, some participants received active drug at every administration, while others sometimes received active drug interspersed with placebo. The conditioned subjects achieved a similar response with lower doses of steroids, suggesting that the immune response of these subjects had been conditioned to be suppressed by the placebo.

Future investigators will need to explore how to separate the therapeutic aspects of conditioned immunosuppression from unwanted effects, an area of research that appears promising.

Looking Forward

As our understanding of brain circuitry, molecular biology, genetics, and psychoneuroimmunology grows, a new illness model will emerge that incorporates a holistic approach to the treatment of patients with comorbid conditions. This new approach will require a health delivery system without the current divisions between behavioral and physical health, and this system is already taking shape.

Innovations in the Dissemination of Psychiatric Expertise

The United States spends significantly more money on healthcare per capita than does any other country in the world, yet various measures of health in the United States reflect worse health outcomes than those of many other industrialized countries. In order to fix the systems that operate inefficiently, experts have proposed various strategies to align the goals of patients, providers, and payers to improve health while keeping costs low. The "triple aim" of healthcare reform is to (1) improve patients' experience of healthcare, (2) improve the health of populations, and (3) lower per capita costs. Decreased spending on healthcare would free up resources to be spent on other important social determinants of health such as education, housing, and the environment.

As noted earlier, it is increasingly evident that mental and physical health are inextricably linked. Any systematic effort to improve physical health must therefore improve mental health as well, and vice versa, since mental health problems significantly increase physical healthcare utilization and cost.

Unfortunately, many people with mental illness do not have access to adequate care. Innovative methods must therefore be developed to bring psychiatric expertise to those who need it. Three methods showing promise are computer-aided decision-making, telepsychiatry, and collaborative care. PM specialists possess the ideal skills to be leaders in these efforts.

Computer-Aided Decision-Making

Medical inpatients often have emergent psychiatric problems when psychiatric consultants are not available to evaluate and treat them. Similarly, patients with complex psychiatric problems frequently present to outpatient primary care practices in areas where access to psychiatric referral is limited. As robust electronic health record (EHR) systems become increasingly available, computer-directed order sets and clinical pathways will become important tools to guide medical staff as they provide psychiatric treatment.

Two examples show how these tools can help medical providers.

Example 1

A 26-year-old man presents to the emergency department (ED) with severe agitation, aggression, and paranoid delusions following bath salt ingestion. The ED staff may be unfamiliar with this toxidrome and may not know how to evaluate and treat him. He may not respond to typical doses of sedating agents and may thus present a danger to himself, staff, and other patients. Order sets for agitation and restraints can provide evidence-based psychiatric expertise to guide the medical staff as they provide urgent care for him.

Order sets are standardized groups of orders that may include comments to guide the physician and nursing staff regarding management of various clinical situations. They can include suggestions for diagnostic tests and procedures, medications, and precautions that follow best practice models. These are especially helpful during emergencies, when staff may not have time to consult the literature. Although medical teams might be familiar with many of these approaches, the availability of these orders as a group greatly increases the likelihood of safe and effective treatment.

- In this case, an order set for psychotic agitation might recommend vital signs frequency, nursing monitoring, labs for discerning the cause of delirium, EKG or telemetry, medication orders, and a link to an order set facilitating the appropriate use of restraints.

Other examples of psychiatric order sets that we find useful for inpatient medical settings include substance withdrawal protocols (severity scales, medications, vitamins), eating disorder dietary orders, clozapine management (with medication escalation and laboratory monitoring), behavioral health precautions, PO/IM combination and long-acting injectable orders, and order sets for delirium evaluation and prevention.

Example 2

A 48-year-old woman admitted with pneumonia does not disclose her alcohol use disorder when she initially presents to the ED. On hospital day three, the patient starts to show signs and symptoms of acute alcohol withdrawal. She becomes confused and confides significant substance use. As noted above, staff may use an alcohol withdrawal order set to guide their initial management of her withdrawal, but a computerized clinical pathway can provide additional guidance as the treatment course continues. This algorithm would be constructed based on an evidence-based clinical pathway designed by local experts.

Clinical pathways suggest the preferred sequence of interventions for a particular clinical situation. By decreasing unnecessary variation, they improve efficiency and quality of care. EHRs can use these pathways to guide management in a stepwise fashion, collecting inputs from available patient data.

- In this example, the patient's alcohol use history would be entered into the record. When staff type "alcohol," and select "alcohol withdrawal decision-support" in the orders matrix, the EHR initiates the pathway. It gathers information from the medical record related to the patient's risk of complicated withdrawal, including her amount of recent alcohol use, timing of her last drink, current Clinical Institute Withdrawal Assessment of Alcohol (CIWA-Ar) or Withdrawal Assessment Scale (WAS) score, history of seizures or delirium tremens, concurrent use of benzodiazepines or other drugs, current vital signs, and response to benzodiazepine treatment in the hospital (via past CIWA or WAS scores). Based on this input, the EHR generates a suggestion for initial withdrawal management (benzodiazepine front loading vs. benzodiazepine taper vs. PRN dosing of benzodiazepines based on ongoing CIWA or WAS scores). Reminders would also be provided for thiamine supplementation, labs, and ongoing vital sign monitoring.
- As staff enters subsequent CIWA or WAS scores into the EHR, it can generate alerts to prevent excessive sedation or under-treatment,

using graphs of CIWA or WAS scores and benzodiazepine administrations to illustrate the patient's status.
- If the patient's condition deteriorates, the decision-support module can recommend switching to a more intensive withdrawal treatment strategy, and can suggest consideration of ICU transfer if needed.

These computerized pathways require that the inputs be quantitative data (e.g., CIWA, pain scale, sedation/agitation scale, medication doses) and that the cause/effect relationships between inputs and suggestions be clearly established. Other examples of possible uses of computer-guided pathways for psychiatric treatment include management of agitation and pain control. We anticipate that additional pathways will be created in the future as evidence-based treatments are established.

In the outpatient setting, computer-generated pathways have guided PCPs to follow evidence-based guidelines for depression management using scores for depression severity, functional status, and side effects, with reminders to increase doses of FDA-approved medications at appropriate intervals. This kind of practice is still in development but may prove useful in a variety of settings.

Telepsychiatry

Telemedicine uses telephonic or video conferencing technology to link patients to medical specialists whose expertise is not otherwise available to the patient. Outpatient telepsychiatry has become an increasingly useful way to provide psychiatric expertise to patients in rural settings, skilled nursing facilities, emergency departments, and outpatient offices, including psychosomatic subspecialties such as transplant psychiatry. Given the paucity of psychosomatic psychiatrists in community hospitals, it can be expected that telepsychiatry will become an important tool to provide psychiatric consults to those who need them.

In outpatient telepsychiatry, the patient typically sits in a dedicated room equipped with a video camera, microphone, and monitor. An on-site assistant is helpful to provide patient support, collateral information, and assistance with technical issues. The telepsychiatric clinician (typically a psychiatrist or mid-level provider) has similar video communication equipment, as well as a second monitor that is used to review documentation, record notes, send prescriptions, or write orders. All information is exchanged via secure transmission lines.

In order to perform telepsychiatric consults in medical settings, a few modifications to the above system must be made:
- *Mobility*: It is often impossible to bring medically ill patients to a dedicated room, and so telemedicine equipment must be brought into hospital rooms. Some carts are too bulky to fit into some rooms, but smaller mobile devices will likely facilitate interactions in a variety of hospital settings.
- *Reimbursement*: Negotiating with insurance may be necessary, but some insurance companies have reimbursed for this service, particularly in rural areas.
- *Timing*: Stable patients can be scheduled for specific appointment times, but emergent situations may be less conducive to this kind of technology. In order for telepsychiatry to work in psychiatric

emergencies, both the on-site assistant and the psychiatric provider would need to be constantly available and have access to the appropriate equipment. In the future, consulting psychiatrists may carry secure tablet devices with them so that they can perform these consults at any time.

- *Practicing across state lines*: Licensing, malpractice, and prescribing regulations likely differ across states, complicating telemedicine practice.
- *Acceptance by the patient and requesting physicians*: Often it is the primary medical team and not the patient who requests the psychiatric consult. Adding the potential barrier of the lack of face-to-face contact may amplify the patient's unwillingness to be evaluated. Studies suggest, however, that telemedicine is well accepted in most situations. Given the increasing popularity of video conferencing among the general public, this barrier will likely decrease over time. Concerns have also been raised regarding whether telepsychiatric providers will accept this form of communication, especially since personal interactions is such an important part of psychiatric care. Preliminary studies from our institution suggest that psychiatrists adapt quickly to use of telemedicine and believe that patients able to receive equivalent care using this technique.

Telepsychiatry is already bringing outpatient psychiatric care to patients where services are scarce, and it is just a matter of time until it will be used in hospital settings as well.

Collaborative Care

Most mental healthcare is provided within primary care and not by psychiatry, but many mentally ill patients do not receive adequate treatment in this setting. This may be due to missed diagnoses, lack of timely medication adjustments, or difficulty referring patients to psychiatric experts.

In response to these shortcomings, investigators have tested various models of care in which psychiatrists are integrated into the primary care team. In the same way that liaison psychiatrists function as a part of sub-specialty teams (e.g., HIV, oncology, transplant), psychiatrists embedded in primary care clinics are increasingly involved in similar models of care, treating complicated patients face to face while providing guidance to the team about how to manage less difficult patients.

Hundreds of studies have been conducted in order to determine the optimal system of integrating psychiatric care into primary care. The shared principles of these collaborative care models include the following:

- Screening all patients in the practice for psychiatric disorders using validated instruments (e.g., PHQ-9 for depression, GAD-7 for anxiety, etc.);
- Frequent follow-up measurements to ensure psychiatric improvement;
- Use of a care manager embedded in the practice to proactively monitor patients for adherence and improvement using an electronic patient registry. Care managers can be specially trained nurses, social workers, or medical assistants, depending on local resources, and

they bear the responsibility of coordinating this graded increase in care and providing psychosocial interventions.

- Frequent meetings between the care manager and a psychiatrist to discuss patients who are not achieving remission so that the care manager can relay medication recommendations back to the PCP or perform psychosocial interventions;
- Face-to-face treatment by the psychiatrist for any patients who do not adequately respond to the care provided by the PCP and care manager. This can occur within the primary care clinic or offsite.

This so-called "stepped care" strategy of quickly optimizing treatment using increasing intensity of therapy and only using specialist care if needed has proven useful for both mental and physical health problems.

Collaborative care interventions for psychiatric illnesses improve the specific psychiatric symptoms that they target, and some have also produced improvements in patients' physical health as well. Models of collaborative care for both mental and physical problems (e.g., depression and diabetes), termed "blended interventions," capitalize on the theory that since these problems are often mutually reinforcing, optimal care requires treating both components. Indeed, studies of blended interventions that target both physical and mental facets of health have demonstrated multiplicative improvements in both outcomes.

A particularly promising feature of collaborative care is its effectiveness across a range of medical settings, demographic populations, diseases, and care modalities. To date, investigators have adapted collaborative care for use in academic medical centers, private practices, Veterans Administration facilities, home health, managed care organizations, safety net organizations, gynecology clinics, and Federally Qualified Health Centers. Populations studied have included urban and rural underserved communities, Hispanics, African Americans, and adolescents. In addition, collaborative care has been successfully applied in such illnesses as depression, anxiety, PTSD, bipolar disorder, ADHD, diabetes, cancer, HIV, pain, and heart disease. Care coordinators have been trained to perform telephone support, Internet-based support, group psycho-education, and face-to-face psychotherapy to suit diverse clinical and logistical parameters.

Collaborative care models are also cost-effective. While some interventions have saved money by reducing medical care utilization, others have cost more money than standard care. This increased spending, however, is on the order of a few cents to a few dollars per depression-free day, which is considered to be very cost-effective by current standards. Interestingly, some studies have required greater up-front cost but then have saved money over subsequent years due to decreased hospitalization rates and other healthcare expenditures. Cost savings may also occur outside the healthcare sector, such as through decreased homelessness or arrest rates. In order to promote collaborative care, many insurers now have ways for medical practices to charge for time spent by care managers and physicians on care coordination. Integrated payer/provider systems (e.g., Kaiser Permanente) are already using these models and have realized significant financial savings.

Many roles exist for psychiatrists in collaborative care, and PM principles and skills are useful for all of them. Besides supervising care managers, psychiatrists can also perform Internet-based consultations, participate in interdisciplinary team meetings, provide home visits, and round with the inpatient primary care teams in order to provide proactive psychiatric advice. Those who want further training in these skills can pursue sub-specialty primary care psychiatry fellowships during or after residency.

Conclusion

As patients and those who work in the healing arts have empirically known for many years, a person's mental status affects his or her physical health, and vice versa. Science has demonstrated this richly in recent years, especially in the field of PNI, and will likely continue to show that the CNS and periphery are inextricably linked. In the future, it is likely that healthcare providers will treat each person's mind and body as a whole, perhaps using stress reduction or conditioning strategies to augment health. Already psychiatry is being interwoven into the rest of healthcare, and this trend will only expand as technology and teamwork bring psychiatric expertise to those who need it. PM specialists will likely be on the vanguard of these changes, treating each person as an integrated whole.

Key Points

- "Mind" and "body" are inseparable aspects of whole human beings, and various fields, especially psychoneuroimmunology, will likely continue to elucidate the molecular mechanisms that link the CNS with the periphery.
- Stress has a complicated relationship with physical health, and stress reduction may improve physical health.
- Conditioning and the placebo effect may become important tools for decreasing the toxic side effects of medications.
- Optimal care of patients involves caring for their mental and physical needs in an integrated fashion, and PM specialists are working with their general medical colleagues to bring psychiatric care to those who need it.
- Computer-based order sets and decision support programs are one way in which non-psychiatric providers can access evidence-based psychiatric expertise at the moment when they need it.
- Telepsychiatry is already bringing psychiatric expertise to patients who live in areas with few psychiatrists. It is likely that telepsychiatry will be increasingly used in medical hospitals as well.
- Collaborative care involves proactively identifying patients with psychiatric disorders, monitoring them with validated instruments, optimizing treatment quickly, managing care using a mid-level provider, and overseeing the care manager with a psychiatrist. It involves teams of professionals working together to proactively care for patients.

Disclosures

Dr. Dobbelstein has no conflicts of interest to disclose.

Dr. Gushchin has no conflicts of interest to disclose.

Dr. Bobrin has no conflicts of interest to disclose.

Dr. Ackerman has no conflicts of interest to disclose.

Further Reading

Ader R, Cohen N (1975). Behaviorally conditioned immunosuppression. *Psychosom Med.*, *37*, 333–342.

Ader R, Mercurio MG, et al. (2010). Conditioned pharmacotherapeutic effects: A preliminary study. *Psychosom Med.*, *72*, 192–197.

Antoni MH (2013). Psychosocial intervention effects on adaptation, disease course and biobehavioral processes in cancer. *Brain Behav Immun.*, *30*, S88–S98.

Bergman LG, Fors UGH (2008). Decision support in psychiatry: A comparison between the diagnostic outcomes using a computerized decision support system versus manual diagnosis. *BMC Med Inform Decis Mak.*, *8*, 9.

Danzer R, Kelly KW (2007). Twenty years of research on cytokine-induced sickness behavior. *Brain Behav Immun.*, *21*, 153–160.

Fawzy FI, Canada AL, et al. (2003). Effects of a brief, structured psychiatric intervention on survival and recurrence at 10-year follow-up. *Arch Gen Psychiat.*, *60*, 100–103.

Green McDonald P, O'Connell M, et al. (2013). Psychoneuroimmunology and cancer: A decade of discovery, paradigm shifts, and methodological innovations. *Brain Behav Immun.*, *30*, S1–S9.

Glaser R, Kiecolt-Glaser JK (2005). Stress-induced immune dysfunction: Implication for health. *Nat Rev Immunol.*, *5*, 243–251.

Huffman JC, Niazi SK, et al. (2014). Essential articles on collaborative care models for the treatment of psychiatric disorders in medical settings: A publication by the Academy of Psychosomatic Medicine Research and Evidence-Based Practice Committee. *Psychosomatics*, *55*, 109–122.

IMPACT: Evidence-based depression care (June 6, 2012). Retrieved April 12, 2014, from http://impact-uw.org/.

Institute for Clinical Systems Improvement (2014). Retrieved April 12, 2014, from http://www.icsi.org/.

Katon W, Unützer J, et al. (2010). Collaborative depression care: History, evolution and ways to enhance dissemination and sustainability. *Gen Hosp Psychiat.*, *32*, 456–464.

Katon WJ (2013). Health reform and the Affordable Care Act: The importance of mental health treatment to achieving the triple aim. *J Psychosom Res.*, *74*, 533–537.

Korneva EA, Khai LM (1964). Effect of destruction of hypothalamic areas on immunogenesis. *Fed Proc.*, *23*, 88–92.

Solomon GF, Moos RH (1964). Emotions, immunity, and disease: A speculative theoretical integration. *Arch Gen Psychiat.*, *11*, 657–674.

Steptoe A, Hamer M, et al. (2007). The effects of acute psychological stress on circulating inflammatory factors in humans: A review and meta-analysis. *Brain Behav Immun.*, *21*, 901–912.

TEAMcare. (2014). Retrieved April 12, 2014, from http://www.teamcarehealth.org/.

Trivedi MH, Kern JK, et al. (2004). A computerized clinical decision support system as a means of implementing depression guidelines. *Psychiat Serv.*, *55*, 879–885.

Yirmiya R, Goshen I (2011). Immune modulation of learning, memory, neural plasticity and neurogenesis. *Brain Behav Immun.*, *25*, 181–213.

Exercises

1. Which of the following is true of telepsychiatry?
   a. Standard practice is to use video conferencing on your smart phone to do the consult.
   b. Telepsychiatry is performed through computer-based video conferencing from the home of the psychiatrist.
   c. Videoconferencing equipment is now the standard technology through which telepsychiatry is performed.
   d. None of the above

2. Severe stress can have which of these effects?
   a. Increased susceptibility to viral infections
   b. Decreased wound healing
   c. Decreased response to vaccination
   d. All of the above

3. Which of the following can be included in computer-based order sets?
   a. Communication to nursing to check for side effects
   b. Order testing for alcohol withdrawal
   c. Medications to treat agitation
   d. All of the above

4. Team-based care coordination for mental disorders has demonstrated which of the following results?
   a. Improved diagnosis
   b. Improved remission rates
   c. Decreased cost in the long run
   d. All of the above

5. A decision support program can be made to do all of the following except:
   a. Recommend antibiotics based on lab results
   b. Suggest off-label use of medications
   c. Warn about potential drug interactions
   d. Suggest an alternative strategy for treatment

Answers: (1) c (2) d (3) d (4) d (5) b

Glossary

5-HT	5-hydroxytrypatamine or serotonin
ACE	angiotensin-converting-enzyme
ACTH	adrenocorticotropic hormone
AD	Alzheimer's disease
ADH	antidiuretic hormone
ADHD	attention deficit hyperactivity disorder
AIDS	acquired immunodeficiency syndrome
AMA	against medical advice
ANA	anti-nuclear antibody
APA	American Psychiatric Association
APM	Academy of Psychosomatic Medicine
APP	Amyloid precursor protein
AUD	alcohol use disorder
AUDIT	Alcohol Use Disorders Identification Test
AV	atrioventricular
BAL	blood alcohol level
BDD	body dysmorphic disorder
BZD	benzodiazepine
bid	twice daily, from Latin, *bis in die*
BP	blood pressure
BUN	blood urea nitrogen
CABG	coronary artery bypass grafting
CAD	coronary artery disease
CADASIL	cerebral autosomol dominant arteriopathy with subcorticol infarction and leukoencephalopathy
CAM	confusion assessment method
CBC	complete blood count
CBT	cognitive behavioral therapy
CD	conversion disorder
CHF	congestive heart failure
CIWA-Ar	Clinical Institute Withdrawal Assessment of Alcohol Scale, Revised
C-L	consultation-liaison
CNS	central nervous system
COPD	chronic obstructive pulmonary disease
CPAP	continuous positive airway pressure
CPK	creatine phosphokinase

CrCl	creatinine clearance
CRH	corticotropin-releasing hormone
CSF	cerebrospinal fluid
CT	computed tomography
CVA	cerebrovascular accident (stroke)
CYP	cytochrome
DA	dopamine
DDAVP	1-deamino-8-D-arginine vasopressin (desmopressin)
DI	diabetes insipidis
DRS	Delirium Rating Scale
DSM	Diagnostic and Statistical Manual of Mental Disorders
DT	delirium tremens
EACLPP	European Association of Consultation-Liaison Psychiatry and Psychosomatics
EAPM	European Association of Psychosomatic Medicine
ECLW	European Consultation Liaison Workgroup
ECT	electroconvulsive therapy
ED	Emergency Department
EEG	electroencephalogram
EHR	electronic health record
EKG	electrocardiogram
EMG	electromyography
ENPM	European Network of Psychosomatic Medicine
EPS	extrapyramidal symptoms
ER	Emergency Room
ERP	exposure and response prevention
ESR	erythrocyte sedimentation rate
ESRD	end-stage renal disease
FD	factitious disorder
FDA	Food and Drug Administration
FDG	fluorodeoxyglucose
FTD	frontal-temporal dementia
FTLD	frontotemporal lobar degeneration
GABA	gamma-aminobutyric acid
GAD	generalized anxiety disorder
GFR	glomerular filtration rate
GH	growth hormone
GI	gastrointestinal
HAART	highly active antiretroviral therapy
HCV	hepatitis C virus

HD	hemodialysis
HE	hepatic encephalopathy
HG	hyperemesis gravidarum
HIV	human immunodeficiency virus
HPA	hypothalamic-pituitary-adrenal axis
HR	heart rate
HTN	hypertension
IAD	illness anxiety disorder
ICD	*International Classification of Diseases*
ICU	Intensive Care Unit
IFN-α	Interferon-alpha
IFN-γ	Interferon-gamma
IL	Interleukin
ILD	interstitial lung disease
IM	intramuscular
IQ	intelligence quotient
IV	intravenous
LBD	Lewy body disease
L-DOPA	L-3,4-dihydroxyphenylalanine
LFTs	Liver Function Tests
LP	lumbar puncture
LSD	lysergic acid diethylamide
MAO	monoamine oxidase
MAOI	monoamine oxidase inhibitor
MCI	mild cognitive impairment
MDD	major depressive disorder
MDMA	3,4-methylenedioxy-N-methyl amphetamine (Ecstasy, Molly)
MI	motivational interviewing
MI	myocardial infarction
MMSE	Mini-Mental Status Exam
MoCA	Montreal Cognitive Assessment
MRI	magnetic resonance imaging
MS	multiple sclerosis
MT	maintenance therapy
NAS	neonatal abstinence syndrome
NCD	neurocognitive disorder
NE	norepinephrine/noradrenaline
NIDA	National Institute on Drug Abuse
NIH	National Institute of Health

NM-ASSIST	NIDA Modified Alcohol, Smoking, and Substance Involvement Screening Test
NMDA	N-methyl-D-aspartate
NMS	neuroleptic malignant syndrome
NOS	not otherwise specified
NPH	normal pressure hydrocephalus
NSAID	non-steroidal anti-inflammatory drug
OCD	obsessive-compulsive disorder
OVLT	organum vasculosum of lamina terminalis
PAWSS	Prediction of Alcohol Withdrawal Severity Scale
PBA	pseudobulbar affect
PCA	patient-controlled analgesia
PCP	primary care provider
PCP	phencyclidine
PCR	polymerase chain reaction
pD	after dialysis
PD	panic disorder
PD	Parkinson's disease
PDR	Physician's Desk Reference
PET	positron emission tomography
PHQ	Patient Health Questionaire
PICC	peripherally inserted central catheter
PNI	psychoneuroimmunology
PO	per os, taken orally
PSEN	presenilin
PT/OT	physical therapy/occupational therapy
PTSD	post-traumatic stress disorder
PUD	peptic ulcer disease
QHS	every bedtime, from Latin, *quaque hora somni*
QTc	QT cardiac interval corrected for HR
RA	rheumatoid arthritis
REM	rapid eye movement
RPR	rapid plasma reagin (antibodies for syphilis organism)
SA	sinoatrial
SC	subcutaneous
SDH	subdural hematoma
SGA	second-generation antipsychotic
SIADH	syndrome of inappropriate antidiuretic hormone secretion
SL	sublingual
SLE	systemic lupus erythematosus

SNRI	serotonin and norepinephrine reuptake inhibitor
SNS	sympathetic nervous system
SPECT	single photon emission computed tomography
SSD	somatic symptom disorder
SSRI	selective serotonin reuptake inhibitor
SUD	substance use disorder
TBI	traumatic brain injury
TCA	tricyclic antidepressant
TD	Tardive dyskinesia
TdP	Torsade de Pointes
TIA	transient ischemic attack
tid	three times a day, from Latin, *ter in die*
TNF	tumor necrosis factor
TSH	thyroid stimulating hormone
UDS	Urine Drug Screen
VS	vital signs

Index

CPSIA information can be obtained
at www.ICGtesting.com
Printed in the USA
BVHW042333130319
542600BV00004B/9/P

9 780199 329311